VITAMINS AND HORMONES

VOLUME 41

VITAMINS AND HORMONES

ADVANCES IN RESEARCH AND APPLICATIONS

Editor-in-Chief

G. D. AURBACH

Metabolic Diseases Branch
National Institute of Arthritis,
Diabetes, and Digestive and Kidney Diseases
National Institutes of Health
Bethesda, Maryland

Editor

DONALD B. MCCORMICK

Department of Biochemistry
Emory University School of Medicine
Atlanta, Georgia

Volume 41
1984

ACADEMIC PRESS, INC. (Harcourt Brace Jovanovich, Publishers)

Orlando   San Diego   New York   London
Toronto   Montreal   Sydney   Tokyo

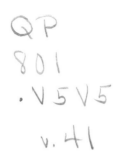

ACADEMIC PRESS, INC.
Orlando, Florida 32887

United Kingdom Edition published by
ACADEMIC PRESS, INC. (LONDON) LTD.
24/28 Oval Road, London NW1 7DX

LIBRARY OF CONGRESS CATALOG CARD NUMBER: 43-10535

ISBN 0-12-709841-0

PRINTED IN THE UNITED STATES OF AMERICA

84 85 86 87   9 8 7 6 5 4 3 2 1

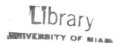

Former Editors

ROBERT S. HARRIS
Newton, Massachusetts

JOHN A. LORRAINE
University of Edinburgh
Edinburgh, Scotland

PAUL L. MUNSON
University of North Carolina
Chapel Hill, North Carolina

JOHN GLOVER
University of Liverpool
Liverpool, England

KENNETH V. THIMANN
University of California
Santa Cruz, California

IRA G. WOOL
University of Chicago
Chicago, Illinois

EGON DICZFALUSY
Karolinska Sjukhuset
Stockholm, Sweden

ROBERT OLSON
University of Pittsburgh School of Medicine
Pittsburgh, Pennsylvania

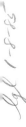

Contents

CONTRIBUTORS TO VOLUME 41 ix
PREFACE xi
ROBERT SAMUEL HARRIS, 1904–1983 xv

Brain Peptides

DOROTHY T. KRIEGER

I.	Introduction	1
II.	Methods for Delineation and Study of Brain Peptides	5
III.	Evolution and Brain Peptides	13
IV.	Ontogeny of Peptidergic Expression in Neural Tissues	16
V.	Biosynthesis of Neuropeptides..	17
VI.	Proteolytic Processing and Degradation of Peptides	24
VII.	Peptide Distribution..	27
VIII.	Functions of Brain Peptides..	30
IX.	Possible Therapeutic Implications of Brain Peptides	41
X.	Conclusion...	42
	References...	42
	Addendum...	275

Intracellular Mediators of Insulin Action

LEONARD JARETT AND FREDERICK L. KIECHLE

I.	Introduction	51
II.	Subcellular Systems...	52
III.	Whole Cell and Tissue Studies	60
IV.	Number of Mediators...	61
V.	Insulin-Sensitive Enzymes	64
VI.	Physical and Chemical Characteristics of the Mediator...............	68
VII.	Conclusion..	71
	References...	72

Relaxin

BRUCE E. KEMP AND HUGH D. NIALL

I.	Introduction	79
II.	Relaxin Genes	80
III.	Relaxin Covalent Structure	86

IV. Synthetic Relaxin 94
V. Mechanism of Action of Relaxin 97
VI. Relaxin Receptors 106
VII. Medical and Physiological Perspectives 107
References 109

Activation of Plasma Membrane Phosphatidylinositol Turnover by Hormones

JOHN N. FAIN

I. Introduction 117
II. Macrophages, Neutrophils, and Mast Cells 122
III. Brain Synaptosomes 125
IV. Hepatocytes 129
V. Adrenal Medulla 135
VI. Adrenal Glomerulosa Cells 137
VII. Adrenal Cortex 138
VIII. Platelets 139
IX. Blowfly Salivary Glands 144
X. Conclusion 150
References 152

The Chemistry and Physiology of Erythropoietin

JUDITH B. SHERWOOD

I. Introduction 161
II. Chemistry of Erythropoietin and Structure–Function Relationships 168
III. Purification of Erythropoietin 178
IV. Assays for Erythropoietin 186
V. Site of Erythropoietin Production 194
VI. Conclusions 202
References 203

Affinity Labeling of Receptors for Steroid and Thyroid Hormones

JOHN A. KATZENELLENBOGEN AND BENITA S. KATZENELLENBOGEN

I. Introduction 213
II. Strategies in Covalent Attachment 215
III. Affinity Labeling Studies on Receptor Properties
and Mechanism of Action 225
IV. Affinity Labeling Studies on Enzymes
and Extracellular Binding Proteins 253
V. Conclusion 266
References 267

INDEX 283

Contributors to Volume 41

Numbers in parentheses indicate the pages on which the authors' contributions begin.

JOHN N. FAIN, *Section of Biochemistry, Brown University, Providence, Rhode Island 02912* (117)

LEONARD JARETT, *Department of Pathology and Laboratory Medicine, University of Pennsylvania School of Medicine, Philadelphia, Pennsylvania 19104* (51)

BENITA S. KATZENELLENBOGEN, *Department of Physiology and Biophysics, University of Illinois and University of Illinois College of Medicine, Urbana, Illinois 61801* (213)

JOHN A. KATZENELLENBOGEN, *Department of Chemistry, University of Illinois, Urbana, Illinois 61801* (213)

BRUCE E. KEMP,[1] *Howard Florey Institute of Experimental Physiology and Medicine, University of Melbourne, Parkville, Victoria 3052, Australia* (79)

FREDERICK L. KIECHLE, *Department of Clinical Pathology, William Beaumont Hospital, Royal Oak, Michigan 48072* (51)

DOROTHY T. KRIEGER, *Division of Endocrinology, Mount Sinai Medical Center, New York, New York 10029* (1)

HUGH D. NIALL, *Howard Florey Institute of Experimental Physiology and Medicine, University of Melbourne, Parkville, Victoria 3052, Australia* (79)

JUDITH B. SHERWOOD, *Department of Medicine, Albert Einstein College of Medicine, Bronx, New York 10461* (161)

[1]Present address: Department of Medicine, University of Melbourne, Repatriation General Hospital, Heidelberg, Victoria 3081, Australia.

Preface

The subjects reviewed in this volume of *Vitamins and Hormones* reflect well the intent to present topics that are novel and current, and represent in broad scope the sciences that impinge on and embody endocrinology and nutrition. Several of the subjects represent "firsts" for this serial publication. Dr. Krieger has prepared a wide-ranging and thought-provoking discussion on brain peptides. The origins, biosynthesis, and CNS function of peptides newly discovered or newly found in the brain are of intense current interest. Similar interest has developed regarding the significance of phosphatidic acid and phosphoinositide metabolism in the mechanism of hormone action. Dr. Fain presents a valuable discourse on the hormone-induced activation of these processes with consequent increases in intracellular metabolism of triphosphoinositide with production of diacylglycerol and triphosphoinositol. The latter products may prove to be, like cyclic adenosine monophosphate, important intracellular messengers of hormone action. Less clear-cut is the mechanism of action of insulin. Drs. Jarett and Kiechle review the status of research on intracellular messengers for insulin action. A factor(s) enhancing the activities of intracellular enzymes involved in physiological responses to insulin is (are) released from cell membranes on the interaction of the hormone with its receptors. This substance(s) is acid and heat stable, of low molecular weight, and may represent the elusive intracellular messenger for insulin.

Drs. John and Benita Katzenellenbogen describe the utility and problems of affinity labeling of estrogen and thyroid hormone receptors. This approach has been used widely to identify, mark for purification, and study subunit structure of hormone receptors. Also reviewed for the first time in *Vitamins and Hormones* are the chemistry and physiology of erythropoietin. Dr. Sherwood discusses, in particular, the impact of radioimmunoassay on studies of this hormone and its implication for purification, determination of physiological control, and clinical research. Drs. Kemp and Niall discuss the chemistry, actions, and molecular biology of relaxin. They suggest that, ultimately, new clinical uses for relaxin may be found, particularly when the hormone can be produced in quantity, possibly through recombinant DNA-directed biosynthesis.

Science during the past year lost a beloved and admired colleague, Dr. Robert S. Harris. Dr. Harris was a man of many important accomplishments and served as one of the two original editors of *Vitamins and Hormones*. An outstanding summary, of interest to colleagues, friends, and readers of *Vitamins and Hormones*, of the life and works of Dr. Harris was prepared for this volume by Dr. Juan Navia. We are indebted to Dr. Navia who interrupted his busy schedule to write this tribute on very short notice. We also thank the staff of Academic Press for their excellent help in preparing this volume.

G. D. Aurbach
Donald B. McCormick

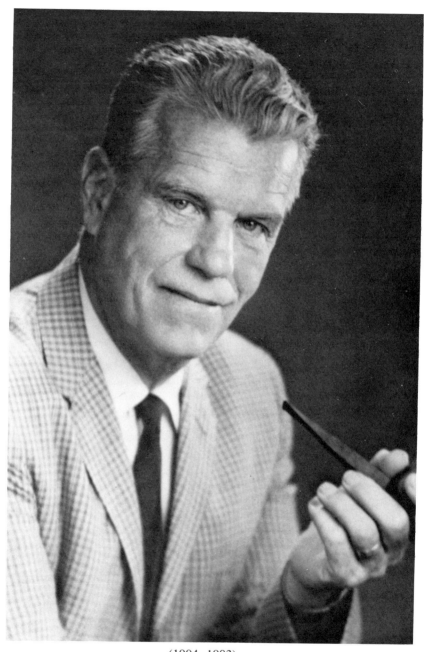

(1904–1983)

Robert Samuel Harris
(1904–1983)

By JUAN M. NAVIA

School of Public Health, Department of International Public Health Sciences, The John J. Sparkman Center for International Public Health Education, The University of Alabama in Birmingham, University Station, Birmingham, Alabama 35294

Few men have made a choice early in life, persevered with dedication and love in the pursuit of that goal, and completed successfully their self-appointed tasks within a lifetime. For Professor Robert S. Harris, a senior editor of *Vitamins and Hormones* during its first thirty-one years of existence, all of this was accomplished without neglect of family, friends, or personal love of music and sports. I would like to share with the readers a very personal recollection of this man who was my professor, friend, and colleague for more than thirty years. A review of his many contributions and the manner and style in which he accomplished them will inspire and teach us how one achieves a productive and fruitful life.

Bob Harris was born in Brookline, Massachusetts on May 10, 1904. At an early age he was attracted by the challenges and opportunities offered by a new scientific and technological academic institution in Cambridge, the Massachusetts Institute of Technology. MIT had been located in the Rogers building on Boylston Street since 1866. The move to Cambridge in June 1916 marked the end of one era and the beginning of another for the Massachusetts Institute of Technology. Prescott (1) describes Inauguration Day, which was attended by outstanding scientists and distinguished speakers such as Henry Cabot Lodge, who emphasized that "this great institution . . . will now enter upon a yet broader field of usefulness and contribute more generously even than in the past to the cause of learning and to the development of trained and educated men." Bob understood these academic ideals and was impressed by the tremendous technological achievements of the MIT faculty and alumni.

Many luminaries in science and technology attended the Golden Jubilee Banquet which was held in Symphony Hall on the evening of Inauguration Day. Charles A. Stone, president of the Alumni Association, addressed the participants:

> We are gathered here this evening to celebrate the fiftieth anniversary of the activity of the Massachusetts Institute of Technology. Pure science and technology have combined to make possible in 1916 many things which in 1866 the most courageous prophet would not have dared to predict.

> Perhaps the most marvelous of all achievements of science is the power to transmit the human voice 3000 miles or more. The courtesy of the American Telephone and Telegraph Company has made it possible for us to speak this evening, not only to alumni and guests in Boston, but also to the alumni gatherings in thirty-four cities in different parts of the States.

For the remainder of the evening communications were established always using the same formula: "Hello, New York." Walter Large replied "This is New York." "How many have you there Mr. Large?" "We have 130 members and guests." "Thank you." Then many other cities, even cities on the west coast, were contacted (1). To hear voices from these distant cities gave a sense of the intimacy of the entire MIT family and a thrilling realization of what science had accomplished in this special field.

The recording of these exciting events gives us a sense of the feelings, ideas, and events that instilled in Bob Harris the great desire to be part of this family of scientists and to dedicate his professional life with great love to the institution which at that time captured the mind of many aspiring scientists and engineers. In 1924, Bob Harris was accepted into MIT, and until his retirement this institution would be his academic home. He received a Bachelor of Science degree in 1928, and soon afterward he became a Research Assistant in the Department of Biology and Public Health. Three years later he became a Research Associate in the department, and began work on his Ph.D., which he completed in 1935. During his training, he specialized in nutritional biochemistry, and in 1937 he was named Assistant Professor of nutritional biochemistry in the Department of Biology and Public Health. Bob Harris started his career guided by his interest in the health and welfare of people and the need to apply his recently acquired scientific knowledge.

During the late 1930s and early 1940s, Secretary Henry Wallace and colleagues at the United States Department of Agriculture developed a national school lunch program in which "surplus" foods were used to supply lunches to many thousands of malnourished and undernourished school children. Dr. Harris was called on to participate in the discussion of the school lunch program to decide whether the real purpose of this program was to dispose of surplus foods or to feed children. Surplus foods alone seldom provide a balanced diet, so it was decided to supplement this supply with food concentrates obtained from other sources. Secretary Wallace proceeded to appoint Dr. Harris special Assistant to the Secretary of Agriculture, and a three-year research grant from the Rockefeller Foundation allowed the project to begin. Within one year an attractive food mixture resembling a cereal flake product was developed, which, together with a serving of fruit juice, served three times a day, would completely nourish a child. This inexpensive food mixture could feed a child at a cost of $16.00 per year. A year later, Dr. Harris and co-workers at MIT developed an inexpensive, palatable, nutritious soup mixture which contained skim milk, soy bean flour, precooked dried peas, spices, and selected vitamins and minerals. A teaspoonful of this soup powder, added to a cup of hot water, could supplement the nutritional intake of a child consuming a school lunch made up of surplus foods. The practical value of this soup was demonstrated by a study which compared one group of 343 children fed the regular lunch with another group of 426 children fed this lunch plus one cup of the special soup each day during the entire school term. This study (2) revealed the unsatisfactory nutritional status of the control group and the clear benefits of the soup supplement. Thousands of pounds of this powdered soup mixture would later be used during World War II to feed starving civilian populations in Europe!

It was at about this time that Dr. Harris met Dr. Kurt Jacoby, a man who would have great influence on his future editorial activities. The *Ergebnisse der Vitamin-und-Hormon Forschung* was first published by Akademische Verlagsgesellschaft in Germany in 1939. Because of World War II, only two volumes of this critical review were published. Mr. Walter Johnson and Dr. Jacoby, who had been associated with the German company, came to New York City and established Academic Press in 1942. Soon thereafter they invited Dr. Harris and Dr. Kenneth V. Thimann from Harvard University to edit a successor to the *Ergebnisse*. This new series would be an annual publication containing critical reviews of the rapidly expanding literature relating to vitamin and hormone research. They accepted the responsibility to become the first editors of *Vitamins and Hormones*. Professor Harris skillfully and critically edited thirty-one consecutive volumes (3) between 1943 and 1973 in collaboration with other scientists and academicians:

	Volumes published while serving	
Name and academic affiliation	As Editor	As Consulting Editor
Robert S. Harris, Massachusetts Institute of Technology	1–31	
Kenneth V. Thimann, Harvard University	1–17	18–31
G. F. Marrian, University of Edinburgh	10–17	18–25
Dwight J. Ingle, University of Chicago	18–19	—
Ira G. Wool, University of Chicago	18–27	28–31
John A. Lorraine, University of Edinburgh	21–27	28–31
Paul L. Munson, University of North Carolina	27–31	
Egon Diczfalusy, Karolinska Sjukhuset	28–31	
John Glover, University of Liverpool	29–31	

The fruitful relationship between Dr. Jacoby and Dr. Harris continued until Dr. Jacoby's death twenty-six years later. In the Preface to that year's volume, Bob called him "the golden thread in the fine fabric of Academic Press."

During the 1940s, Bob maintained his nutrition teaching and research activities at MIT, his editorial efforts with *Vitamins and Hormones,* and his travels as nutrition consultant to the Director of the Pan American Sanitary Bureau (PASB). He visited Dr. Francisco de P. Miranda, Director of the Nutrition Institute of Mexico, who knew about the work done by Professor Harris in developing the soup mixtures and who had an interest in using this approach to supplement the diet of Mexican school children. But implementation of such an approach required accurate data on the composition of Mexican foods and on the nutritional status of the Mexican people. Funds to support the necessary studies were provided by the W. K. Kellogg Foundation and distributed among the Nutrition Institute of Mexico, the PASB, and MIT. Training funds were also provided to allow young Mexican scientists to be trained in nutritional biochemistry, food science, and food analysis at MIT (4–9). Many foods of excellent nutritional quality were identified and a new approach to nutritional policy evolved based on the following principles: (a) the nutrition programs of a country should be based on the foods indigenous to the country, and (b) nutrition education in a country should be patterned around the food habits of the people and formulated on the known composition of native edible plants and animal products (10–12).

The experience in Mexico triggered the interest of Dr. W. Popenoe, then director of the Escuela Agrícola Panamericana in Honduras, who recognized the need to do similar studies in Central America. With the support of the United Fruit Company, samples of foods were collected by Dr. Louis Williams (Harvard University), stabilized by procedures that had been developed by Drs. S. Goldblith and Harris (13) at MIT, and analyzed for seventeen nutrients by a team under the leadership of Dr. Hazel Munsell, who later became a long-time collaborator of Dr. Harris. The results of the studies of 927 samples, representing over 200 varieties of edible plants, were published (14–16), and later provided the basis for the manuscript, "Plantas Comestibles de Centro América y Panamá" (17).

These critical studies demonstrated the importance of a food analysis program in which all edible plants and animals in a geographic area are analyzed for their content of critical nutrients. Some common foods were thereby defined as sources of nutrients in the local diet; still other foods were newly discovered by this survey, e.g., bledo (a pigweed), chaya, chipilin, frijol de arroz, hojas de ayote (squash leaves), puntas de camote, and pumitas de quicoy (growing tips of a sweet potato vine) (18). The program was very successful because it demonstrated that in just a few years it was possible to sample the flora and fauna of any region to determine their nutritional potential and to decide which of them should be developed agriculturally and added to the local diet.

These studies also led to the founding of the Institute of Nutrition of Central América and Panamá (INCAP). This outstanding research and training center located in Guatemala City continues to be a productive institution serving the needs and interests of the whole Central American region. Delegates from all six countries in the region convened in Guatemala City on February 18–20, 1946 and agreed to establish there the INCAP in cooperation with the PASB and the Kellogg Foundation. On September 18, 1946 a conference attended by representatives from MIT, PASB, and the Kellogg Foundation was held in Washington, D.C. Guatemala, El Salvador, and Honduras officially approved the plan, and the other countries soon took similar action.

The initial team consisted of one nutritional biochemist, one nutritional educator, one clinical nutritionist, and one agronomist. Their training program was administered by Professor Robert Harris, and classes were held at MIT and Harvard. By June 1948 the following teams had been chosen: Dr. Roberto Gandara (Guatemala) and Dr. Ernesto Borjas (Honduras) were assigned to the Harvard School of Public Health, and biochemist Dr. Guillermo Arroyave (Guatemala) and Dr. Salvador Pizzati (Honduras) were assigned to MIT with nutritionist Ms. Marina Flores (Guatemala).

While the young scientists were being trained at MIT and Harvard, plans were being made for the new building that would house INCAP. After completion of the building and the training of the staff, Dr. Nevin Scrimshaw assumed the Directorship of INCAP on July 1, 1949. Dr. Scrimshaw's strong and dynamic leadership completed the plans that Professor Harris had carefully formulated to make INCAP the most famous and successful of all nutrition institutes in the world.

These centers of excellence in nutrition conceived by Professor Harris in Central America led to the formation of a similar center in Cuba, where I had the privilege of working with him after my initial training at MIT. The program in Cuba was coordinated by the Fundación de Investigaciones Médicas (FIM) and the Finlay Institute. Dr. Tom Spies had been working on tropical sprue at the Calixto Garcia Hospital in Cuba, but little was known about the nutritional composition of foods. FIM, with the support of Dr. Robert Williams of the Williams–Waterman Fund, invited Professor Harris to develop a program similar to those that had been so successful in Mexico and Guatemala. Dr. Hady Lopez and I organized the food and nutrition laboratories and Dr. I. D. Clements (Harvard University) and Mr. Angel Valiente of the Harvard University Arboretum near Cienfuegos collected the samples. Within a few years the FIM Laboratories published data (19–21) which constituted the basis for the Tables of Nutrient Content of Cuban foods. Thus, the efforts of Professor Harris continued to expand and yield fruitful results in one country after another (see the Selected Bibliography).

Bob Harris had an untiring and enthusiastic love for his work which resulted in successful outcomes for most of his undertakings. Aside from his travels, his teaching, and his research on the nutritional role of vitamins, fats, and minerals, the results of which have appeared in over 294 scientific publications, he organized a number of conferences on vitamins and other topics, many of which were published in *Vitamins and Hormones*. He also worked with Dr. W. Sebrell (Columbia University) as coeditor of five volumes of *The Vitamins* (22), and still later edited the *Art and Science of Dental Caries Research* (23).

In the early 1960s Professor Harris developed still another program which would be as unique and important as any of the ones he had initiated earlier. For some time he had been interested in the relation of food and nutrition to oral diseases such as dental caries. Because he had done extensive research in mineral metabolism, he was extremely interested in the role of phosphates in dental caries (24, 25), and organized a conference with this theme at MIT in October 1962. After the proceedings of the conference were published (26), representatives from the National Institute of Dental Research (NIDR) in Bethesda suggested the establishment of an NIDR-supported training program at MIT. This would provide opportunities for dentists and scientists to expand their knowledge in the biomedical sciences and to receive sound research training in preparation for careers in dental education and dental research. The MIT Training Program in Oral Science was established in Fall 1963 and continued until Professor Harris retired in 1970. Via the program, Dr. Harris and co-workers organized conferences, symposia, and summer workshops which continue to serve as models for such academic activities in universities. Approximately twenty students were trained, and today most of them hold positions of leadership in academic institutions and industry. The trainees and research associates published many papers and abstracts during their fellowship tenure at MIT (see References). The productivity of the Oral Science program was firmly established by the time Bob left the program and went on to his post-retirement years.

Although he loved MIT dearly, after retirement he continued his work in science and academic endeavors outside that institution. In 1970, he became the William F. Lasby, Guest Professor in the Health Sciences at the University of Minnesota and Guest Professor in Oral Biology at the University of California School of Dentistry in Los Angeles. In 1974 he returned to his home in Waban, Massachusetts to spend his last days with his greatest loves: his wife Helen, his children, and his family, all of whom provided much love and support during his long battle with the cruel Alzheimer's disease he had developed.

Professor Harris's work was fully recognized not only by his peers in a number of professional societies such as the American Institute of Nutrition, the American Public Health Association, the Institute of Food Technologists, and the American Association for the Advancement of Science, but also by governments. He received from the President of Ecuador the rank of Official of the National Order "El Mérito"; from Cuba the rank of Commander of the Order of Carlos J. Finlay; and from Guatemala the rank of Commander of the Order of Rodolfo Robles.

Bob was exceptional not only by virtue of his many academic and professional achievements, but because despite his dedication to work he still found time to love his family, enjoy evenings at Symphony Hall, play an excellent game of golf or squash, and share with friends and family his house on Lake Winnipesaukee. Those of us who worked closely with him remember his arriving in the morning, lighting his pipe, and starting a day that could last for ten or more hours. He was able to read or write for long periods of time holding his red pen in the left hand to mark, cross, and rewrite. He used his scissors and tape to reconstruct disjointed, unclear protocols or reports into beautifully clear and organized manuscripts. At the end of the day, he would pack up his papers and journals in his old leather bag, and take them home to read and review later in the evening, if the urgency was great.

As well as being a distinguished scientist, Bob Harris was a kind and generous man. When I left Cuba in exile with my family, leaving behind everything we owned, he brought us into his home and gave us the strength and courage to face a new life. On our first Christmas away from home, he and Helen knocked on our door and brought us a Christmas tree with all the trimmings and presents for our children. We have kept these memories, but what we all remember most was his beautiful smile and the personal warmth he gave us that day, and every day.

Christmas was indeed his favorite time with its carols, holly, and happiness. Bob was a sensitive man who cared for his students, particularly foreign students whom he knew were especially homesick and lonesome for family and friends during that time of year. It was for this reason that he organized a Christmas party at his home every year for the international students in the MIT Department of Nutrition and Food Science. Once acquainted they began singing, and Bob's face would light up with happiness. He would sing and direct the first Christmas carols, and then we all would sing our own native Christmas songs in different languages to the delight of many and the blushing of others who had forgotten the lyrics! We loved him and he loved us.

Bob died on Christmas eve in 1983. On that day we said goodbye to a colleague who had worked hard on behalf of MIT, on behalf of the scientific community which he served with discipline and dedication, on behalf of the numerous students and trainees he taught and guided, and on behalf of the people in many regions of the world who have benefited from his untiring dedication to health and nutrition. Bob Harris has left a legacy that will always inspire others to continue to expand the work he carried out so fully and completely.

We echo Helen's words* when she said:

> Fortunate the man, most fortunate, who in his youth
> Makes his choice, the perfect choice
> And works throughout his years
> In happiness and dedication
> Never knowing how completely
> The endeavor enwraps, enfolds him
> Until he becomes the choice itself
> Accumulating vast knowledge, techniques, skills
> All to be shared. . . .
> Great the man who has long dreams, deep visions
> And time must now make us pause to sense
> That, more than most
> He has fullfilled them.

REFERENCES

1. Prescott, S. C. (1954). "When MIT was Boston Tech." The Technology Press, Cambridge, pp. 299–324.
2. Harris, R. S., Weeks, E, and Kinde, M. (1943). Effects of a supplementary food on the nutritional status of school children. *J. Am. Diet. Assoc.* **19**, 182–189.
3. Harris, R. S. *et al.* (Eds.) (1943–1973). *Vitamins and Hormones,* Volumes 1–31. Academic Press, New York.

*Excerpt from a tribute to Dr. Robert S. Harris by his wife Helen on his retirement from MIT in June 1969.

4. Cravioto, R. O., Lockhart, E. E., Anderson, R. K., Miranda, F.deP., and Harris, R. S. (1945). Composition of typical Mexican foods. *J. Nutr.* **29**, 317–329.

5. Harris, R. S. (1945). An approach to the nutrition problems of other nations. *Science* **102**, 42–44.

6. Cravioto, R. O., Anderson, R. K., Lockhart, E. E., and Harris, R. S. (1945). Nutritive value of the Mexican tortilla. *Science* **102**, 91–93.

7. Harris, R. S. (1946). The nutrition problem of Mexico. *J. Am. Diet. Assoc.* **22**, 974–976.

8. Anderson, R. K., Calvo, J., Serrano, G., and Payne, J. C. (1946). A study of the nutritional status and food habits of Otomi Indians in the Mezquital Valley of Mexico. *Am. J. Public Health* **36**, 883–903.

9. Lockhart, E. E., Miranda, F.deP., and Harris, R. S. (1946). The nutritional status of school children in Mexico city. *Fed. Proc., Fed. Am. Soc. Exp. Biol.* **5**, 235.

10. Harris, R. S. (1948). Food Composition and Nutrition Programs. *Nutr. Rev.* **6**, 33–35.

11. Harris, R. S. (1948). Progreso de la nutrición en Centro América. *Bol. Of. Sanit. Panam.* **27**, 902–911.

12. Harris, R. S. (1948). The foundation of nutrition in Central America. *Bol. Of. Sanit. Panam.* **27**, 97–101.

13. Goldblith, S. A., and Harris, R. S. (1948). Estimation of ascorbic acid in food preparations. *Anal. Chem.* **20**, 649–651.

14. Harris, R. S., and Munson, H. E. (1950). Edible plants of Central America. *J. Home Econ.* **42**, 629–631.

15. Munsell, H., Harris, R. S., *et al.* Composition of food plants of Central America and Panama. *Food Res.* **14**, 144–164, 1949; **15**, 16–33, 1950; **15**, 34–52, 1950; **15**, 263–296, 1950; **15**, 355–365, 1950; **15**, 379–404, 1950; **15**, 421–438, 1950; **15**, 439–453, 1950.

16. Harris, R. S. (1952). There is no indispensable food. *Congr. Rec.* **98**, 4289–4290.

17. INCAP–ICNND (1952). "Food Composition Table for Use in Latin America." INCAP, Guatemala City.

18. Harris, R. S. (1962). Influence of culture on man's diet. *Arch. Environ. Health* **5**, 144–152.

19. Navia, J. M., Lopez, H., Cimadevilla, M., Fernandez, E., Clement, I. D., Valiente, A., and Harris, R. S. (1955). Nutrient composition of Cuban foods. I. Foods of vegetable origin. *Food Res.* **20**, 97–113.

20. Navia, J. M., Lopez, H., Cimadevilla, M., Fernandez, E., Valiente, A., Clement, I. D., and Harris, R. S. (1957). Nutrient composition of Cuban foods. II. Foods of vegetable origin. *Food Res.* **22**, 131–144.

21. Lopez, H., Navia, J. M., Clement, I. D., and Harris, R. S. (1963). Nutrient composition of cuban foods. III. Foods of vegetable origin. *J. Food Sci.* **28**, 600–610.

22. Sebrell, W. H., and Harris, R. S. (Eds.) (1967–1972). "The Vitamins: Chemistry, Physiology, Pathology, Methods," Vols. I–V. Academic Press, New York.

23. Harris, R. S. (Ed.) (1968). "The Art and Science of Dental Caries Research." Academic Press, New York.

24. Nizel, A. E., and Harris, R. S. (1964). The effects of phosphates on experimental dental caries. A literature review. *J. Dent. Res.* **43**, 1123–1136.

25. Navia, J. M., and Harris, R. S. (1969). Longitudinal study of cariostatic effects of sodium trimetaphosphate and sodium fluoride when fed separately and together in diets of rats. *J. Dent. Res.* **48**, 183–191.

26. Harris, R. S. (1964). Proceedings of the Conference on Phosphates and Dental Caries. *J. Dent. Res. Suppl.* **43**, No. 6, Part 1, p. 995–1207.

SELECTED BIBLIOGRAPHY

Publications on Latin American foods published by Nutritional Biochemistry Laboratories, Massachusetts Institute of Technology, Cambridge, Massachusetts.

1. Cravioto, R. O., Lockhart, E. E., Anderson, R. K., de P. Miranda, F., and Harris, R. S. (1945). Composition of typical Mexican Foods. *J. Nutr.* **29**, 317–329.
2. Harris, R. S. (1945). An approach to the nutrition problems of other nations. *Science* **102**, 42–44.
3. Cravioto, R. O., Anderson, R. K., Lockhart, E. E., and Harris, R. S. (1945). Nutritive value of the Mexican tortilla. *Science* **102**, 91–93.
4. Cravioto, R. O., Lockhart, E. E., de P. Miranda, F., and Harris, R. S. (1945). Contanido nutritive de ciertos tipicos alimentos Mexicanos. *Bol. Of. Sanit. Panam.* **24**, 685–694.
5. Cravioto, R. O., Anderson, R. K., Lockhart, E. E., de P. Miranda, F., and Harris, R. S. (1945). Valor nutritive de la tortilla. *Bol. Of. Sanit. Panam.* **24**, 783–786.
6. Harris, R. S. (1946). The nutrition problem of Mexico. *J. Am. Diet. Assoc.* **22**, 974–976.
7. Anderson, R. K., Calvo, J., Serrano, G., and Payne, G. G. (1946). A study of the nutritional status and food habits of Otomi Indians in the Mesquital Valley of Mexico. *Am. J. Public Health* **36**, 883–903.
8. Harris, R. S. (1948). Food composition and nutrition programs. *Nutr. Rev.* **6**, 33–35.
9. Harris, R. S. (1948). Fundación de Nutrición de Centro América. *Bol. Of. Sanit. Panam.* **27**, 97–101.
10. Harris, R. S. (1948). Progreso de la nutrición en Centro América. *Bol. Of. Sanit. Panam.* **27**, 902–911.
11. Harris, R. S. (1949). Problemas de nutrición en otras naciones. *Pediatr. Amer.* **6**, 95–97.
12. Munsell, H. E., Williams, L. O., Guild, L. P., Troescher, C. G., Nightingale, G., and Harris, R. S. (1949). Composition of food plants of Central America. I. Honduras. *Food Res.* **14**, 144–164.
13. Munsell, H. E., Williams, L. O., Guild, L. P., Troescher, C. B., Nightingale, G., and Harris, R. S. (1949). Composición de la plantas alimenticias de las América Central. I. Honduras. *Bol. Of. Sanit. Panam.* **28**, 1253–1275.
14. Munsell, H. E., Williams, L. O., Guild, L. P., Troescher, C. B., Nightingale, G., and Harris, R. S. (1950). Composition of food plants of Central America. II. Guatemala. *Food Res.* **15**, 16–33.
15. Munsell, H. E., Williams, L. O., Guild, L. P., Troescher, C. B., Nightingale, G., and Harris, R. S. (1950). Composition of food plants of Central America. III. Guatemala. *Food Res.* **15**, 34–52.
16. Munsell, H. E., Williams, L. O., Guild, L. P., Troescher, C. B., Nightingale, G., Kelley, L. T., and Harris, R. S. (1950). Composition of food plants of Central America. IV. El Salvador. *Food Res.* **15**, 263–296.
17. Munsell, H. E., Williams, L. O., Guild, L. P., Throescher, C. B., and Harris, R. S. (1950). Composición de las plantas alimenticias de la America Central. II. Guatemala. *Bol. Of. Sanit. Panam.* **29**, 926–944.

18. Harris, R. S. (1950). Las plantas comestibles de Centro América y Panamá. *J. Home Econ.* **42**, 629–631.
19. Munsell, H. E., Williams, L. O., Guild, L. P., Throescher, C. B., and Harris, R. S. (1950). Composition of food plants of Central America. V. Nicaragua. *Food Res.* **15**, 355–368.
20. Munsell, H. E., Williams, L. O., Guild, L. P., Kelley, L. T., McNelly, A., and Harris, R. S. (1950). Composition of food plants of Central America. VI. Costa Rica. *Food Res.* **15**, 379–404.
21. Munsell, H. E., Williams, L. O., Guild, L. P., Kelley, L. T., and Harris, R. S. (1950). Composition of food plants of Central America. VII. Honduras. *Food Res.* **15**, 421–438.
22. Munsell, H. E., Williams, L. O., Guild, L. P., Kelley, L. T., and Harris, R. S. (1950). Composition of food plants of Central America. VIII. Guatemala. *Food Res.* **15**, 439–453.
23. Munsell, H. E., Williams, L. O., Guild, L. P., Troescher, C. B., Nightingale, G., and Harris, R. S. (1951). Composición de las plantas alimenticias de la América Central. III. Guatemala. *Bol. Of. Sanit. Panam.* **30**, 474–493.
24. Munsell, H. E., Williams, L. O., Guild, L. P., Troescher, C. B., Nightingale, G., Kelley, L. T., and Harris, R. S. (1952). Composición de las plantas alimenticias de la América Central. IV. El Salvador. *Bol. Of. Sanit. Panam.* **32**, 293–327.
25. Harris, R. S. (1952). The indigenous edible plants of Latin America. *Int. Z. Vitaminforsch.* **23**, 3.
26. Harris, R. S. (1952). There is No Indispensable Food. *Congr. Rec.* **98**, No. 115, 4289–4290 (June).
27. Munsell, H. E., Williams, L. O., Guild, L. P., Troescher, C. B., and Harris, R. S. (1953). Composición de las plantas alimenticias de la América Central. V. Nicaragua. *Bol. Of. Sanit. Panam.* **34**, 31–59.
28. Munsell, H. E., Williams, L. O., Guild, L. P., Kelley, L. T., McNally, A., and Harris, R. S. (1953). Composición de las plantas alimenticias de la América Central. VI. Costa Rica. *Bol. Of. Sanit. Panam.* **34**, 31–59.
29. Munsell, H. E., Williams, L. O., Guild, L. P., Kelley, L. T., McNally, A., and Harris, R. S. (1953). Composición de las plantas alimenticias de Centro América. VII. Honduras. *Bol. Of. Sanit. Panam.* **34**, No. 4, 352–371.
30. Munsell, H. E., Williams, L. O., Guild, L. P., Kelley, L. T., McNally, A., and Harris, R. S. (1953). Composición de las plantas alimenticias de Centro América. VIII. Guatemala. *Bol. Of. Sanit. Panam.* **34**, 492–507.
31. Harris, R. S. (1953). Importancia del análisis de los alimentos en la solución de problemas alimenticios. *Rev. Farm. Cuba* **31**, 59–60.
32. Munsell, H. E., Castillo, R., Zurita, C., and Portilla, J. M. (1953). Production, uses, and composition of foods of plant origin from Ecuador. *Food Res.* **18**, 319–342.
33. Navia, J. M., Lopez, H., Cimadevilla, M., Fernandez, E., Valiente, A., Clement, I. D., and Harris, R. S. (1955). Nutrient composition of Cuban foods. I. Foods of vegetable origin. *Food Res.* **20**, 97–113.

Publications related to oral science published by Oral Science Research Laboratories, Department of Nutrition and Food Science, Massachusetts Institute of Technology, Cambridge, Massachusetts.

1. Nizel, A. E., and Harris, R. S. (1950). Effect of foods grown in different areas on prevalence of dental caries in hamsters. *Arch. Biochem.* **26**, 155.

2. Nizel, A. E., and Harris, R. S. (1951). The caries-producing effect of similar foods grown in different soil areas. *N. Eng. J. Med.* **244**, 361.
3. Nizel, A. E., and Harris, R. S. (1953). Cariostatic effects of ashed foodstuffs fed in the diets of hamsters. *J. Dent. Res.* **32**, 672.
4. Nizel, A. E., and Harris, R. S. (1955). Effects of ashed foodstuffs on dental decay in hamsters. *J. Dent. Res.* **34**, 513.
5. Bulakul, N. (1956). Relation of lysine to dental caries. M.S. Thesis, MIT.
6. Gardner, D. S. (1956). Relation of food ash on the development of caries in hamsters. M.S. Thesis, MIT.
7. Harris, R. S., and Nizel, A. E. (1957). Effects of food ash and trace minerals upon dental caries in hamsters. *Proc. Int. Congr. Nutr. 4th,* 195.
8. Nizel, A. E., Keating, N., Sundstrom, C., and Harris, R. S. (1958). Effect of phosphate supplement to diet on development of hamster caries. *J. Dent. Res.* **37**, 35.
9. Nizel, A. E., and Harris, R. S. (1959). Effect of different levels of metaphosphoric acid on hamster caries. *J. Dent. Res.* **38**, 686.
10. Harris, R. S., and Nizel, A. E. (1959). Effects of food ash and trace minerals, especially phosphorus upon dental caries in hamsters. *J. Dent. Res.* **38**, 1142.
11. Nizel, A. E., and Harris, R. S. (1960). Effects of metaphosphoric acid in the diet of weanling hamsters upon dental caries development. *J. Am. Dent. Assoc.* **60**, 193.
12. Harris, R. S., and Nizel, A. E. (1960). Phosphorus and tooth decay. *Bull. Off. Nav. Res.* **14,**
13. Harris, R. S. (1960). Phosphorus and dental caries. *J. Dent. Res.* **39**, 1086.
14. Nizel, A. E., Harris, R. S., and Parker, J. M. (1960). Effects of metaphosphoric acid supplementation on morphology and caries incidence of hamster molars. *J. Dent. Res.* **39**, 725.
15. Harris, R. S., Nizel, A. E., and Parker, J. M. (1961). Residual cariostatic action of phosphates in hamster diets. *J. Dent. Res.* **40**, 698.
16. Nizel, A. E., Harris, R. S., and Parker, J. M. (1961). Inhibitory effect of disodium phosphate on dental caries in the rat. *J. Dent. Res.* **40**, 660.
17. Harris, R. S., Baker, N. J., and Nizel, A. E. (1962). Cariostatic effectiveness of fat-imbedded monopotassium phosphate in the diets of rats. *Proc. Int. Assoc. Dent. Res., abstr.* **125**, 40.
18. Nizel, A. E., Baker, N. J., and Harris, R. S. (1962). The effect of phosphate structure upon dental caries development in rats. *Proc. Int. Assoc. Dent. Res., abstr.* **236**, 63.
19. Harris, R. S. (1962). Influence of culture on man's diet. *Arch. Environ. Health* **5**, 155.
20. Harris, R. S., and Nizel, A. E. (1963). Effects of cation on the cariostatic activity of orthophosphate. *J. Am. Chem. Soc. Proc.* **34-C,** September.
21. Navia, J. M., Harris, R. S., Nizel, A. E., and Moor, J. R. (1963). Technique for removal of intact teeth from the jaws of experimental animals. *J. Dent. Res.* **42**, 1251.
22. Harris, R. S., and Navia, J. M. (1964). Foods, nutrition, trace metals and dental caries. *Proc. Am. Inst. Oral Biol.,* p. 32–50.
23. Harris, R. S., and Nizel, A. E. (1964). Metabolic significance of the Ca/P ratios of foods and diets. *J. Dent. Res.* **43**, 1090.
24. Nizel, A. E., and Harris, R. S. (1964). The effects of phosphates on experimental dental caries. A literature review. *J. Dent. Res.* **43**, 1123.
25. Nizel, A. E., Navia, J. M., Moor, J. R., and Harris, R. S. (1964). Quantitative technique for pulverizing rodent teeth. *J. Dent. Res.* **43**, 1257.
26. Nizel, A. E., Salazar, V. R., and Harris, R. S. (1964). Effects of particle size of

potassium phosphate on its cariogenic action when fed in the diets of rats. *J. Dent. Res.* **43**, 857.

27. Harris, R. S., and Nizel, A. E. (1965). Effects of cations on the cariostatic activity of orthophosphates. *J. Dent. Res.* **44**, 416–420.

28. Harris, R. S., Das, S. K., and Nizel, A. E. (1965). Cariostatic effects of three types of phosphates when fed singly or in combinations in the diets of rats. *J. Dent. Res.* **44**, 549–483.

29. Harris, R. S., Walsh, N. B., and Nizel, A. E. (1965). Cariostatic action of fat-imbedded potassium phosphate when fed in the diet of rats. *Arch. Oral Biol.* **10**, 477–483.

30. Salazar, V., Harris, R. S., and Nizel, A. E. (1965). Cariostatic action of organic phosphates when fed in the diet of rats. *Meet. IADR, 43rd Abstr.* **205.**

31. Harris, R. S., Francis, M. D., Konig, K., Nizel, A. E., Tanzer, F. S., Lopez, H., and Navia, J. M. (1965). Comparison of three methods for scoring cariostatic action of sodium trimetaphosphate and sodium fluoride when fed to rats. *Meet. IADR, 43rd, Abstr.* **207.**

32. Navia, J. M. (1965). Study of the cariostatic action of phosphates in rats. Ph.D. Thesis, MIT.

33. Harris, R. S. (1966). Dietary chemicals in relation to dental caries: Calcium and phosphorus. *Proc. Am. Chem. Soc.* **A23**, 1966.

34. Navia, J. M. (1966). Dietary chemicals in relation to dental caries: Trace minerals. *Proc. Am. Chem. Soc.* **A24**, 1966.

35. Das, S. K., and Harris, R. S. (1966). Fatty acids in fossil teeth. *Proc. Int. Assoc. Dent. Res.* **116**, 76.

36. Navia, J. M., Lopez, H., and Harris, R. S. (1966). Cariostatic effect of trimetaphosphate when fed to rats during different stages of tooth development. *Proc. Int. Assoc. Dent. Res.* **393**, 137.

37. Loesche, W. J., and Gibbons, R. J. (1966). Isolation of human cariogenic streptococci from urban and village Guatemalan children. *Proc. Int. Assoc. Dent. Res.,* **101.**

38. Das, S. K., and Harris, R. S. (1966). Lipids and fatty acids in teeth of different animal species. *Fed. Proc. Fed. Am. Soc. Exp. Biol.* **25**, 314.

39. Das, S. K., and Harris, R. S. (1967). Effects of food restriction on lipids and fatty acids of rat teeth. *Proc. Int. Congr. Nutr. 7th, 1966, 1967,* p. 66.

40. Lough, K. A., Navia, J. M., and Harris, R. S. (1966). Improved procedure for extracting food fatty acids. *J. Am. Oil Chem. Soc.* **43**, 627–631.

41. Harris, R. S., and Das, S. K. (1967). Effects of diet restriction on dental caries development in rats. *Meet. IADR 45th, Abstr.* **450.**

42. Harris, R. S., Nizel, A. E., Navia, J. M., and Das, S. K. (1967). Effects of dietary supplement of glycine on dental caries development in rats. *Proc. Int. Assoc. Dent. Res.* **451**, 151.

43. Navia, J. M., Lopez, H., and Harris, R. S. (1967). Evaluation of new diet for experimental caries research with rats. *Proc. Int. Assoc. Dent. Res.* **449**, 150.

44. Nizel, A. E., Salazar, V. R., and Harris, R. S. (1967). Effect of particle size on the cariostatic action of potassium acid phosphate. *Arch. Oral Biol.* **12**, 695–700.

45. Harris, R. S., Nizel, A. E., and Walsh, N. B. (1967). The effect of phosphate structure on dental caries development in rats. *J. Dent. Res.* **46**, 290–294.

46. Loesche, W. J., and Henry, C. A. (1967). Intracellular microbial polysaccharide production and dental caries in a Guatemalan Indian Village. *Arch. Oral Biol.* **12**, 189–194.

47. Henry, C. A., Walsh, N. B., Navia, J. M., and Harris, R. S. (1967). Effect of sodium

trimetaphosphate on oral flora of rats fed a caries producing diet. *Bacteriol. Proc.* **M36.**

48. Navia, J. M., Henry, C. A., Lopez, A., and Harris, R. S. (1967). Effects of magnesium chloride and sodium trimetaphosphate on caries development in rats. *Fed. Proc. Fed. Am. Soc. Exp. Biol.* **886,** 415.

49. Navia, J. M., Lopez, H., and Harris, R. S. (1968). Cariostatic effects of sodium trimetaphosphate when fed to rats during different stages of tooth development. *Arch. Oral Biol.* **13,** 779–768.

50. Cagnone, L. D., Harris, R. S., and Navia, J. M. (1968). Cariostatic effects of sodium orthophosphate and sodium trimetaphosphate: A comparison. *Proc. Int. Assoc. Dent. Res.* **364,** 128.

51. Navia, J. M., Cagnone, L. D., Lopez, H., and Harris, R. S. (1968). The effects of $MgCl_2$, $MnCl_2$, and Na trimetaphosphate on rat caries when fed alone or in combinations. *Proc. Int. Assoc. Dent. Res.* **361,** 128.

52. Harris, R. S., Navia, J. M., and Cagnone, L. D. (1968). Influence of caging on development of rat caries in studies involving minerals. *Proc. Int. Assoc. Dent. Res.* **362,** 128.

53. Henry, C. A., and Navia, J. M. (1968). Early development of rat caries and concurrent microbial changes. *Proc. Int. Assoc. Dent. Res.* **363,** 128.

54. Navia, J. M., Menaker, L., Seltzer, J., and Harris, R. S. (1968). Effects of $Na_2 SeO_3$ supplemented in the diet or the water on dental caries in rats. *Fed. Proc. Fed. Am. Soc. Exp. Biol.* **27,** 676.

55. Enwonwu, C. O., and Munro, H. N. (1968). Cytoplasmic action of hydrocortisone on liver RNA. *Fed. Proc. Fed. Am. Soc. Exp. Biol.* **27,** 416.

56. Harris, R. S., and Navia, J. M. (1968). Influences of vehicles and routes of administration on effectiveness of agents in the prevention of oral diseases in experimental animals. *Ann. N.Y. Acad. Sci.* **153,** 240–257.

57. Navia, J. M., Lopez, H., and Harris, R. S. (1969). Purified diet for dental caries research with rats. *J. Nutr.* **97,** 133–140.

58. Sutfin, L. V., Ogilvie, R. E., and Harris, R. S. (1969). Scanning electron microscope observations of the fracture surface of dental amalgam. *Proc. Int. Assoc. Dent. Res., Abstr.* **22,** 46.

59. DiOrio, L. P., and Navia, J. M. (1969). The influence of protein malnutrition on dental growth and development of infant rats. *Proc. Int. Assoc. Dent. Res., Abstr.* **92,** 63.

60. Navia, J. M., DiOrio, L. P., and Miller, S. A. (1969). Effects of low protein intake during gestation and lactation on growth and dentition of rat pups. *Proc. Int. Assoc. Dent. Res., Abstr.* **93,** 64.

61. Cagnone, L. D., Navia, J. M., and Harris, R. S. (1969). Longitudinal study of the cariostatic effects of sodium dihydrogen phosphate and sodium trimetaphospate. *Proc. Int. Assoc. Dent. Res., Abstr.* **93,** 64.

62. Nizel, A. E., King, G., Harris, R. S., and Navia, J. M. (1969). The effect of feeding fish protein concentrate (FPC) in different amounts on caries development in rats. *Proc. Int. Assoc. Dent. Res., Abstr.* **97,** 65.

63. Harris, R. S., and Navia, J. M. (1969). Effects of three phosphate compounds upon the caries activities of sugar and candies in rats. *Proc. Int. Assoc. Dent. Res., Abstr.* **10,** 66.

64. Kreitzman, S., and Navia, J. M. (1969). Alkaline phosphatase activity in a caries-promoting streptococcus. *Proc. Int. Assoc. Dent. Res., Abstr.* **123,** 71.

65. Saffir, A. J., Ogilvie, R. E., and Harris, R. S. (1969). Electron microprobe analysis of fluoride in teeth. *Proc. Int. Assoc. Dent. Res., Abstr.* **538**, 175.

66. Cagnone, L. D., Navia, J. M., and Harris, R. S. (1969). Cariostatic effects of NaH_2PO_4 and $Na_3(PO)_3$ when fed at different stages of tooth development. *Fed. Proc., Fed. Am. Soc. Exp. Biol.* **28, 374** (Abstr. 657).

67. Navia, J. M., and Harris, R. S. (1969). Longitudinal study of cariostatic effects of sodium trimetaphosphate and sodium fluoride when fed separately and together in the diets of rats. *J. Dent. Res.* **48**, 183–191.

68. Navia, J. M., DiOrio, L. P., and Miller, S. A. (1969). Effects of low protein intake during gestation and lactation on growth and dentition of rat pups. *Proc. Int. Assoc. Dent. Res. Abstr.* **93**, 64.

69. Grower, M. F., and Bransome, E. D., Jr. (1969). Selective effects of ACTH on synthesis of cytosol proteins in adrenal cortex: Similar *in vitro* and *in vitro* evidence. *Fed. Proc., Fed. Am. Soc. Exp. Biol.* **28**, 701 (Abstr. 2479).

70. Kreitzman, S. N., Irving, S., Navia, J. M., and Harris, R. S. (1969). Enzymatic release of phosphate from rat molar enamel by phosphoprotein phosphatase. *Nature (London)* **223**, 520–521.

71. Das, S. K., and Harris, R. S. (1970) Fatty acids in the tooth lipids of sixteen animal species. *J. Dent. Res.* **49**, 119–125.

72. Das, S. K., and Harris, R. S. (1969). Lipids and fatty acids in fossil teeth. *J. Dent. Res.* **49**, 126–130.

73. Navia, J. M., DiOrio, L. P., Menaker, L., and Miller, S. (1970). Effect of undernutrition during the perinatal period on caries development in the rat. *J. Dent. Res.* **49**, 1091–1098.

74. Morehart, R. E., Mata, L. J., Sinskey, A. J., and Harris, R. S. (1970). A microbiological and biochemical study of gingival crevice debris obtained from Guatemalan Mayan Indians. *J. Periodontol.* **41**, 644–649.

75. Harris, R. S. (1970). Fortification of foods and food products with anticaries agents. *J. Dent. Res.* **49**, 1340–1344.

76. Harris, R. S. (1970). Natural versus purified diets in research with non-human primates. *In* "Feeding and Nutrition of Nonhuman Primates," (R. S. Harris, ed.). Academic Press, New York.

77. Harris, R. S. (Ed.) (1970). "Feeding and Nutrition of Nonhuman Primates." Academic Press, New York.

78. Harris, R. S. (1970). Dietary chemicals in relation to dental caries. *Adv. Chem. Ser.* **94.**

79. Alam, S. Y., and Harris, R. S. (1972). Effects of nutrition on the composition of tooth lipids in rats. I. Effect of dietary carbohydrate on fatty acid composition of rat teeth. *J. Dent. Res.* **51**, 1474–1477.

80. Folke, L. E. A., Gawronski, T. H., Staat, R. H., and Harris, R. S. (1972). Effect of dietary sucrose on quantity and quality of plaque. *Scand. J. Res.* **80**, 529–533.

Brain Peptides

DOROTHY T. KRIEGER

Division of Endocrinology, Mount Sinai Medical Center,
New York, New York

I. Introduction 1
II. Methods for Delineation and Study of Brain Peptides 5
  A. Peptide Detection, Isolation, and Characterization 5
  B. Demonstration of Synthesis and Processing of Neuropeptides 8
  C. Electrophysiological Studies 9
  D. Detection of Peptide Receptors 10
  E. Neuroanatomical Techniques 10
  F. Summary 12
III. Evolution and Brain Peptides 13
IV. Ontogeny of Peptidergic Expression in Neural Tissues 16
V. Biosynthesis of Neuropeptides 17
  A. Introduction 17
  B. Sources of Polypeptide Diversity 18
  C. Examples of Neuropeptide Precursor Molecules and Their Synthesis .. 20
VI. Proteolytic Processing and Degradation of Peptides 24
VII. Peptide Distribution 27
VIII. Functions of Brain Peptides 30
  A. Effects on Major Homeostatic Systems 32
  B. Alterations of Brain Peptide Concentrations in CNS Disease 40
IX. Possible Therapeutic Implications of Brain Peptides 41
X. Conclusion 42
  References 42
  Addendum 275

I. INTRODUCTION

Cell-to-cell communication represents a major function of all living organisms, and is mediated primarily by chemical messengers. Such communication is achieved through several mechanisms: paracrine (diffusion of the messenger between individual or groups of cells), endocrine (secretion of messenger from its site of production in glandular cells into the circulation to act on distant targets), or synaptic. (See Addendum 1, p. 275.) The mediators of paracrine communication are "local tissue factors," of endocrine communication, "hormones," and of synaptic communication, "neurotransmitters." "Neurohormone" describes messengers secreted into the circulation by neurons rather than by glandular cells.

1

Until recently, it was thought that synaptic communication was solely mediated by monoamines (norepinephrine, epinephrine, dopamine, and serotonin), a number of excitatory and inhibitory amino acids, and acetylcholine. Prior to the last decade the only peptide described within the brain was substance P, found also in the gastrointestinal tract.

Over forty years ago, Scharrer and Scharrer (1940) promulgated the concept that nerves could secrete hormones. This, however, referred to secretion of peptide products into the bloodstream. Such neurosecretory cells were initially described in the vertebrate hypothalamus. Palay

YEAR	TRANSMITTER		% OF BRAIN SYNAPSES
1920	ACETYLCHOLINE		5 - 10
	EPINEPHRINE		
1930			
1940			
1950	NOREPINEPHRINE		0.5
	AMINO ACIDS	GABA GLUTAMIC ACID ASPARTIC ACID	25 - 40
1960	DOPAMINE		0.5
1970	SUBSTANCE P SEROTONIN		0.5
1			
2			
3			
4	"HYPOTHALAMIC RELEASING HORMONES"	TRH LHRH SRIF	
5	ENKEPHALIN		
6	VIP, CCK		
7	ACTH		
8	OTHER PITUITARY HORMONES INSULIN VASOPRESSIN, OXYTOCIN ANGIOTENSIN		
9	GLUCAGON		
1980			
1	CORTICOTROPIN-RELEASING HORMONE		
2	GROWTH HORMONE-RELEASING HORMONE		
3			

FIG. 1. Chronology for the description of neurotransmitters and neuropeptides in the central nervous system. The left-hand column represents percentages of synapses affected as estimated by Snyder (1980). Reproduced from Krieger (1983b), with permission.

(1945) and Bargman (1960) showed that vertebrate hypothalamic neurons projected to the posterior pituitary lobe. It was inferred that the hypothalamic neurons were the source of vasopressin and oxytocin, classically found in this lobe, which were then secreted into the circulation from storage sites in nerve terminals. Only recently has it been recognized that projections from these same hypothalamic neurons exist elsewhere in the central nervous system, where vasopressin and oxytocin may act via local neural actions, i.e., as neurotransmitters.

A large number of peptides recently have been found in the vertebrate nervous system (Fig. 1). It has been estimated (Snyder, 1980) that nonpeptide neurotransmitters may account for 40–50% of the synapses in the central nervous system; elucidation of roles for neuropeptides already discovered and for those yet to be discovered should provide major new insights into the understanding of neural function. There have been suggestions that such neuropeptides function as neurotransmitters and/or neuromodulators (see Section VIII). Peptides are released from nerve terminals by mechanisms resembling the calcium-dependent stimulus–secretion coupling phenomena described for conventional neurotransmitters (Iversen *et al.*, 1980). Electrophysiological data indicate that neuropeptides act in part by generating rapid effects on neural membranes. Other studies indicate that they may affect the turnover of other neurotransmitters, and by such means or others modulate the postsynaptic effects of the latter.

The major categories of brain peptides described to date are listed in Table I. This classification is somewhat arbitrary and based on previous attributions for given peptide locations. For example, it is now appreciated that the "hypothalamic releasing hormones"—which were isolated in confirmation of the suggestion of hypothalamic control of anterior pituitary function—show, in the main, wide extrahypothalamic distribution. The extrahypothalamic distribution of so-called posterior pituitary hormones (and their associated neurophysins) was already cited. Furthermore it is apparent that a number of peptides found originally in secretory elements of the gastrointestinal tract exist in the brain as well as in gastrointestinal neurons. For the most part, studies to date have indicated that the gut–brain peptides from the two tissues have identical amino acid sequences. There is less information with regard to the presence of CNS receptors for these peptides and some evidence that the nature of such receptors may differ from those for the given peptide in non-CNS tissues. Moreover, peptides considered previously to be produced solely within the anterior pituitary are synthesized also within the central nervous system. Whether there is concurrent regulation and interaction of all of the

TABLE I

CATEGORIES OF MAMMALIAN BRAIN PEPTIDES[a]

Hypothalamic-releasing hormones	Gastrointestinal peptides
Thyrotropin-releasing hormone	Vasoactive intestinal polypeptide
Gonadotropin-releasing hormone	Cholecystokinin
Somatostatin	Gastrin
Corticotropin-releasing hormone	Substance P
Growth hormone-releasing hormone	Neurotensin
	Met-enkephalin
Neurohypophyseal hormones	Leu-enkephalin
Vasopressin	Insulin
Oxytocin	Glucagon
Neurophysin(s)	Bombesin
	Secretin
Pituitary peptides	Somatostatin
Adrenocorticotropic hormone	TRH
β-Endorphin	Motilin
α-Melanocyte-stimulating hormone	Pancreatic polypeptide
Prolactin	
Luteinizing hormone	Growth factors
Growth hormone	IGF_2
Thyrotropin	EGF
	FGF
Opioid peptides	Endothelial cell growth factor
Dynorphin	
β-Endorphin	Others
Met-enkephalin	Angiotensin II
Leu-enkephalin	Bombesin
	Bradykinin
Invertebrate peptides	Carnosine
FMRF amide	Sleep peptide(s)
Hydra head activator	CGRP (calcitonin gene-related peptide)
	Neuropeptide Yy

[a]Reproduced from Krieger (1983b), with permission.

cells that synthesize and release a given peptide remains to be seen. Lastly, peptides originally thought to exist only in invertebrates have now been found within the vertebrate central nervous system; the converse also is true.

Concentrations of brain peptides as well as "pituitary" peptides in brain are several orders of magnitude less than those of previously defined neurotransmitters (acetylcholine, monoamines, and amino acids). Of those peptides initially described in the gastrointestinal tract, only CCK appears to show concentrations in the CNS greater than its concentration in gastrointestinal tract. But the relatively low concentrations of peptides in the CNS by no means minimize their importance therein. Glandular content of peptide hormones is high in order to allow for great dilution in the circulation. In the central nervous system, these peptides act over short distances with much less dilution. It should also be realized that the concentration of a peptide really gives no information as to turnover rate. Finally specific regional concentrations of peptides (many yet to be determined) may be greater than found in gross areas of the central nervous system.

The multitude of brain peptides identified presents us with numerous candidates in search of physiological functions. Moreover, identification of precursor polypeptide molecules and their genes, discovery of alternate processing pathways for a given peptide precursor in different tissues (Krieger, 1983a), delineation of primary RNA transcripts that are processed differently in neural vs nonneural tissues (Amara *et al.*, 1982), and elucidation of gene families giving rise to products expressing coordinate behavior (Scheller *et al.*, 1983) add exciting new dimensions to studies on peptide evolution and gene expression, within and without the central nervous system.

II. Methods for Delineation and Study of Brain Peptides

New techniques and recognition of pitfalls in older ones have greatly facilitated progress. A major emphasis has been detection and verification of a given peptide location in nervous tissue and proof of whether existence therein represents transport from without or local synthesis. Only peptides synthesized within the brain are clearly candidates for, neurotransmitters although peptides arising from other sources could also be important in physiology. Biosynthesis, it is now recognized, may produce different peptides from one region to another by virtue of differential processing of precursor molecules. The following sections deal with the types of studies used to detect brain peptides, their synthesis, processing, and regulation.

A. Peptide Detection, Isolation, and Characterization

1. *Radioimmunoassay and Physicochemical Characterization*

Radioimmunoassay and immunohistochemistry have been the major techniques applied to detect peptides recognized originally in other tissues or phyla in vertebrate brain. The advent of monoclonal antibodies has, in many instances, circumvented the earlier problem of antisera heterogeneity and has allowed for more specific identification of immunologic determinants for a given antiserum. The validity of radioimmunoassay for peptide detection ultimately can be established only through structural identity between the "unknown" assay material and the peptide of interest. Lacking this, one can use certain cross-checks such as analysis with multiple antibodies with specificities for different portions of the molecule in question, as well as with independent assays (such as radioreceptor assay or bioassay). The latter assays, however, are also limited in interpretation since a peptide in brain may be only structurally related (with shared antigenic determinants), not identical, to that in another tissue.

Physicochemical characterization (utilizing many chromatographic and electrophoretic methods to compare unknown and standard) of immunoreactive material detected is a valuable procedure to establish identity of at least some portion of the detected substance. Many of the peptides in question exist in picomolar or femtomolar concentrations; regional assays and assays of microdissected areas (see Section VII) can be valuable in detecting major differences in concentration between given areas. The introduction and availability of high-performance liquid chromatography, of high resolution and efficiency for submicrogram amounts of peptide, have greatly facilitated analysis of tissues. New sensitive methods of amino acid analysis can be performed with as little as 5–10 pmol of pure peptide. The molecular weight of a peptide can be determined from 10 pmol of sample by fast atom bombardment mass spectroscopy, and subnanomole amounts of peptide can be sequenced with modern high-sensitivity methods.

2. Detection of "New" Peptides

We discussed above the characterization of known peptides. (See Addendum 2, p. 275.) A new strategy to seek new peptides has been described by Viktor Mutt and co-workers and is based on the hypothesis that peptides bearing C-terminal amides are biologically important. Using a novel chemical method to detect such terminal amides (Tatemoto and Mutt, 1978), hitherto uncharacterized peptides were isolated from intestine and brain (Tatemoto et al., 1982). One of the peptides so isolated exists in brain in relatively high concentration, as high as found for other peptides already described therein. Further searches based on knowledge of the cell biology of the nervous system (i.e., bioassay) should lead to detection and ultimate chemical characterization of substances important in growth and differentiation.

Further peptides will be found through analysis of precursor mRNAs or genes that encode them. Determination of the cDNA structures of POMC and of pro-enkephalin A and B revealed therein hitherto unknown peptides, i.e., γ-MSH in the former and multiple forms of enkephalin peptides in the latter. A new brain peptide, the calcitonin gene-related product, has been recognized through sequencing the gene for calcitonin.

3. *Immunohistochemistry*

Immunohistochemistry provides a valuable dimension in visualizing neuropeptides or their component parts (by light microscopy) in specific nerve cells or in subcellular organelles (by electron microscopy). Application of neuroanatomy combined with immunohistochemistry can establish the source, transport, and terminal fields of neuronal peptides (see Palkovits, 1983, for review) (see Section II,E). It should be appreciated that recognized cross-reactivity of a given antiserum under radioimmunoassay conditions cannot be directly translated to immunohistochemistry because (1) higher concentrations of antisera are employed in immunohistochemistry, exposing the tissue to different antibody populations of varying affinity (antibodies of low affinity are insignificant at the high dilutions of heterogeneous antisera employed in immunoassay), (2) the specificity of purified antigen tracer is lost in immunohistochemistry, and (3) the antigen may be altered by tissue fixation methods. Further, it is now also recognized that specificity in immunohistochemistry is not guaranteed by adsorption controls. These are necessary but further controls are facilitated by use of "purified" antibodies obtained by either immunoaffinity or hybridoma techniques (if antibodies are of appropriate affinity for immunohistochemical studies). A control for fixation technique has been introduced recently by assessing staining of a given molecular species on a solid-phase chemically analogous model of fixed tissue (Elde, 1983; Schneider *et al.,* 1979; Schippe and Tilders, 1983). The problem of such fixation is especially acute in studies at the electron microscopic level. In many instances, the procedures required for maintaining the peptide *in situ* and preserving ultrastructural morphology may compromise the antigenicity of the neuropeptide. Until recently, this has necessitated a compromise approach, that of "preembedding" staining; the tissue is embedded subsequent to staining for electron microscopy. This method for examining ultrastructural features of peptidergic neurons was subject to diffusion of the antigen or of the reaction product, thereby limiting conclusions about storage and release compartments for the peptide. New fixation techniques, as well as the use of the rapid ultra-low temperature freezing and freeze-drying method prior to embedding, may ameliorate these problems.

An exciting finding has been the identification, using sequential immunostaining methods, of the simultaneous localization of two or more antigens in the same tissue section [i.e., within a heterogeneous cell group in a given brain nuclear area and, indeed, within the same cell or nerve fiber (see Hokfelt *et al.*, 1980)]. Immunohistochemistry may also be combined with autoradiography to colocalize radioactively labeled ligands and antibodies to neuropeptides; this can be employed at either the light or electron microscopic level. Autoradiography is also a powerful method to localize neurotransmitter receptors.

A new technique, conceptually similar to immunocytochemistry, is that of *in situ* hybridization cytochemistry. A radioactive cDNA probe is used to reveal mRNA. With use of the two methods combined it will be possible to find both expressed message and peptide product within the same cell, and to study the switching on or off of genes during the course of development.

There has been only limited use of neuroanatomical techniques combined with immunohistochemistry. In some instances, the low concentrations of peptides in axons can be enhanced by transection; pile-up of peptide proximal to the site of section can then be demonstrated immunohistochemically. The projection fields of a given neuron(s) can be identified by retrograde injection of horseradish peroxidase or immunofluorescent dyes; this combined with immunostaining allows characterization of the identified neuronal cell body by establishing the nature of the transmitter.

B. DEMONSTRATION OF SYNTHESIS AND PROCESSING OF NEUROPEPTIDES

Two major definitive approaches to demonstrate synthesis are currently available. One involves tissue incubation with labeled amino acids and demonstration of their incorporation into the peptide precursor or product of interest. Recombinant DNA methodology has been a powerful tool. cDNA probes can be used to identify specific mRNA within the nervous system and to establish thereby that local neural peptide synthesis likely exists. It has also been possible to obtain mRNAs from neural tissue known to encode particular peptides, and, by sequencing the analagous cDNA clone, to deduce structures of precursor molecules. Structural analysis of these precursor molecules, and identification of likely specific enzyme cleavage sites (see Section VI), can imply the nature of processing and of potential peptide products. Such processing can be investigated through *in vitro* or *in vivo* (or both) pulse-labeling experiments, and physicochemical characterization of the synthesized forms (i.e., by size, charge, and products derived from tryptic digestion). The characterization of the processing enzymes involved and the validation of their specificity remain major challenges.

C. ELECTROPHYSIOLOGICAL STUDIES

The methods as applied to brain peptides are the same as those previously used in studying other neurotransmitters. Much information has been obtained from intracellular recordings. Studies in the CNS are limited because precise local delivery of pharmacological agents is difficult (due to the blood–brain barrier) and one cannot control the extracellular environment. Some of these problems have been circumvented by the use of brain slices maintained in suitable artificial medium. This approach allows recording and drug application under visual control and provides a stable and long-lasting system. The chemical composition of the media can be manipulated and, unlike recording in the intact nervous system, drug delivery electrodes can be separated from recording electrodes. The major problem with this approach is that afferent inputs from regions outside the slice cannot be evaluated. Interpretation also may be questioned because peptides maintained at a defined concentration may cause desensitization, unlike studies wherein delivery is accomplished in brief pulses by pressure or by current administration.

The use of cultured neurons offers the advantage of direct visual control and obviates the problem of diffusion barriers. The question of heterogeneity of neurons within a given population, however, still remains. The addition of the "patch clamp" technique to studies of cultured neurons allows the detection of currents flowing through individual channels within a small patch of membrane. One can study thereby the intracellular or extracellular surface of the membrane, or even gain access to the cell interior. The effect of ionic composition on current as well as the conductance of a single channel can be studied during the period that a single channel remains open, and kinetic parameters involved in processes of desensitization can be measured.

Since peptides are found in the peripheral nervous system, a simpler model can be developed utilizing preparations of autonomic ganglia. It is much easier therein to test whether a given peptide fulfills the criteria for a neurotransmitter (see Section VIII). Such a substance must exist in presynaptic cells, must be released therefrom upon stimulation, and must produce physiological changes in postsynaptic cells identical to those produced by stimulation of the presynaptic cell. The nerve-evoked response should be blocked by specific antagonists. Such observations are necessary before one can ascribe a particular function to a peptide and also provide significant information as to which of multiple neurotransmitters coexisting in a given neuron mediate a specific response.

Studies of brain tissue show that as with conventional neurotransmitters the greatest concentrations of neuropeptides are found in nerve terminals or synaptosomal fractions. *In vitro* incubation studies of synaptosomes indicate that neuropeptides are released with neuronal depolarization induced either by high potassium or electrical stimulation. Such release is dependent on cellular uptake of calcium. Release can be stimulated or inhibited by application of the "conventional" neurotransmitters (norepinephrine, acetylcholine, and dopamine), indicating some type of interaction between the neurotransmitters and the peptides.

D. Detection of Peptide Receptors

Several techniques allow identification of receptors. Ligands labeled with either ^3H or ^{125}I to high specific radioactivity have been utilized in incubations with peptidase inhibitors to reduce degradation of tracer peptides. High specific activity antagonists, as well as agonists, employed in competition with structural analogs of the transmitter of interest, have helped define the existence of multiple types of tissue receptors for a given transmitter. Such receptors can also be characterized *in vitro* by autoradiography using high specific activity ligand. Recent successful solubilization of receptors may lead to isolation and purification, and resolution of the question of whether, as has been suggested, there are multiple types of receptor for a given ligand or whether the multiple forms detected represent different configurations of the same receptor. Fluorescent ligands have also been used to visualize physical characteristics of receptor binding, with the demonstration that receptor cross-linking and aggregation appear to be essential for triggering biological responses for some receptor–ligand systems. Such labeled ligands can also be used to study the patterns and mobility of receptors on cells and, in many instances, to monitor subsequent internalization.

E. Neuroanatomical Techniques

A number of such techniques have been devised (see Palkovits, 1983, for review) which can be combined with and supplement those of immunocytochemistry (as already cited in Section II,A,3) and neurophysiology.

1. Demonstration of Neural Pathways

There are several different approaches to the delineation of neural pathways within the nervous system. Neuropeptide-containing pathways are implied by detection of peptides in microdissected (see below) brain areas after lesioning distant regions or transection of neuronal afferents to areas under study. These approaches may show small changes in peptide concentrations not detectable histochemically. Tracts can also be traced by stimulating with microelectrodes stereotactically implanted leading to excitation of the terminal fields and localizing thereby neuropeptide-containing cell bodies. The nerve degeneration technique (transection of an axon originating in the cell body causes degeneration of the axon distally) can be used to localize the innervation fields of neurons and neuronal pathways. Degenerating fibers are identified by selective silver impregnation and examination at the light microscopic level. Tracing can also be achieved after retrograde or anterograde injection of tracers. In the former, horseradish peroxidase, fluorescent dye, or radiolabeled material can be injected stereotaxically into the presumed projection field of the cell or cell group, and accumulation of tracer substance in the cell body characterized by immunostaining or autoradiography. In anterograde tracing the same materials or labeled amino acids can be injected intracellularly by iontophoresis or pressure microinjection, making it possible to visualize axons and projection fields. (Such intracellular marking techniques are also used to identify recorded neurons in brain.) We previously discussed visualization of cell bodies, projecting fields, and afferents of the cells in the same section, by a combination of immunostaining of cell bodies, retrograde tracing, and techniques for recognition of afferent terminals of cell bodies. Functional pathways also may be delineated using 2-deoxy-D-[^{14}C]glucose whereby local cerebral glucose utilization in the brain can be traced by autoradiography. Such studies can be performed after selective lesioning, pathway transection, drug treatment, or specific stimulation of brain regions and pathways.

2. Microdissection

Microdissection allows analysis of discrete brain areas on a greatly defined basis. This is performed on 300-μm-thick sections; as little as 10 μg of brain tissue can be removed with a single punch. Tissue so obtained can be analyzed for neuropeptide or transmitter content, for biosynthesis of neuropeptides after injection of precursor into the brain, or for receptor studies.

3. Stereotaxic Techniques

Other neuroanatomical techniques utilize stereotaxic maneuvers (1) for direct application by pressure microinjection or microiontophoresis of substances with physiological or pharmacological function; (2) for injection of labeled material to demonstrate local synthesis; (3) for implantation of a push–pull perfusion system (the given brain region of a conscious, freely moving animal is superfused with a trace amount of the labeled substance and the newly synthesized and *in situ* released product is collected in serial samples); (4) for chronic studies in which implanted electrodes are placed for chronic stimulation; and (5) for production of mechanical, electrolytic, or toxin-induced lesions. The latter utilize neurotoxins that are relative selective for neurons containing a given transmitter or for perikarya rather than fibers in a given area. Another surgical technique, that of deafferentation of portions of the nervous system, can allow differentiation between intrinsic deafferentated areas and those regulated by incoming inputs.

4. *Quantitation of Cell Number and Density*

Major new efforts have been applied to quantitate cell numbers and density within the central nervous system under basal conditions and after experimental manipulation. Several automatic or computer-aided devices available are utilized to characterize cell packing density (cell number/unit volume), total number of neuropeptide-containing neurons in a particular brain nucleus, and total number of neuropeptide-containing neurons as percentage of total cell number in a brain nucleus (in certain brain nuclei this percentage is greater than 100%, indicating, as has already been noted, the coexistence of neuropeptides or of neuropeptides and neurotransmitters in the same cell). Such computerized image analysis also has been developed to enumerate silver grains in autoradiographic studies. Such techniques are being considered for determination of nerve terminal density, synapse density, or the number of neuronal afferents existing on neuropeptide-containing neurons.

F. Summary

We have discussed several methods, including recent technical advances, for studying brain peptides. It is now possible to seek answers to questions that previously could only be formulated. It is anticipated that the scope of such investigations will advance still further. The plethora of new transmitter candidates requires a conceptual re-evaluation of neuronal function. Results with simple organisms may give insight into functional interrelations in more complex ones. Studies at the cellular level must now be related to those on the whole organism. The ability to characterize, localize, and assess interrelationships and functional roles of known peptides and peptides still to be identified should provide better understanding of neuronal specialization, communication, and physiological function in the normal subject. Such knowledge may lead to elucidation of disease abnormalities related to distribution and nature of CNS peptides.

III. EVOLUTION AND BRAIN PEPTIDES

There is now great interest in the origin and evolution of brain peptides and of polypeptide hormones per se. The voluminous literature on these subjects can only be considered briefly here. Two major questions arise: one, the significance of finding in vertebrate nervous tissue peptides classically recognized as glandular in origin; two, the finding of peptides classically recognized as vertebrate now in invertebrate neurons (in species which lack an endocrine system).

A further challenge has been identification of peptides similar to invertebrate peptides (i.e., ACTH, β-endorphin, insulin, vasopressin, and relaxin) in unicellular organisms, and reports that such unicellular organisms possess peptide receptors. It has been proposed (LeRoith et al., 1983) that these peptides serve as primitive elements of intracellular communication in these unicellular organisms (see Fig. 2). With the phyletic appearance of a neuronal system (in multicellular invertebrates probably arriving at the coelenterate stage), some of

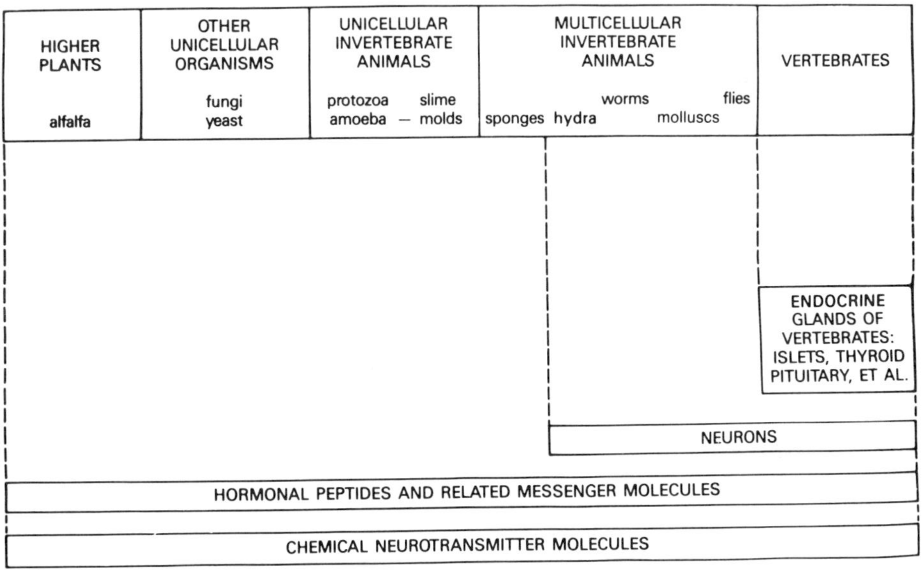

HIGHER PLANTS	OTHER UNICELLULAR ORGANISMS	UNICELLULAR INVERTEBRATE ANIMALS	MULTICELLULAR INVERTEBRATE ANIMALS		VERTEBRATES
alfalfa	fungi yeast	protozoa slime amoeba — molds	sponges hydra	worms flies molluscs	

ENDOCRINE GLANDS OF VERTEBRATES: ISLETS, THYROID PITUITARY, ET AL.

NEURONS

HORMONAL PEPTIDES AND RELATED MESSENGER MOLECULES

CHEMICAL NEUROTRANSMITTER MOLECULES

FIG. 2. Evolution of biochemical elements of the endocrine system and the nervous system. Reproduced from LeRoith et al. (1982), with permission.

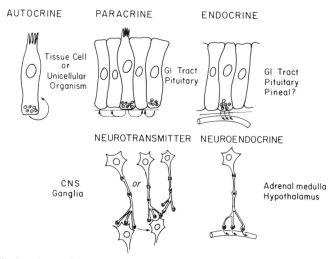

FIG. 3. Modes of peptide secretion. In autocrine secretion, the products act locally on the cell of origin. In paracrine secretion the product reaches neighboring cells, by extracellular fluid transport systems or via intracellular gap junctions. In endocrine secretion, the product reaches distant target tissue through the circulation. In neuronal cells (lower portion of figure), cell-to-cell communication is effected via axodendritic or presynaptic axoaxonic synapses; this is a subtype of paracrine communication (neurotransmitter). In neurohumoral secretion (neuroendocrine) a neuronal product reaches other tissues through the bloodstream. Representative tissues utilizing such forms of communication are cited. Reproduced from Krieger (1983a), with permission.

these messenger molecules become functionally organized as neurotransmitters, and in some instances as neurohormones. With the later advent of the endocrine system (in vertebrates), some of these same peptides have become localized in glandular structures and are secreted as hormones; others remain within neurons and acquire endocrine regulatory functions (Dockray *et al.*, 1981). TRH exists in the brain of species lacking a pituitary gland (Jackson and Reichlin, 1974); neurohormonal function via secretion into the pituitary portal plexus is acquired later in evolution than the presumed neurotransmitter function in brain. This is illustrated in Fig. 2, indicating the evolutionary time scale for such organization and in Fig. 3, indicating the types of cellular communication mediated by a given hormone, whether dispersed from different tissues of different species or from different tissues of the same species (see below). For example, peptides derived from proopiomelanocortin in invertebrate neurons (and in *Tetrahymena*) may act via neurotransmitter and autocrine mechanisms, respectively, while in invertebrates they may subsume neurotransmitter (in brain), paracrine (in reproductive and gastrointestinal tract), hormonal (in pituitary), or possibly neurohormonal roles (e.g., existence in pituitary portal blood). In some instances, evolution has changed the morphological configuration of a peptide-secreting cell. The pinealocyte [whose peptide product(s) is still incompletely defined] in lower vertebrates is a photoreceptor with afferent nerve connections, but in mammals is devoid of either of these attributes and takes on the characteristics of a typical glandular cell secreting hormone.

It is of interest that invertebrate peptides (localized to neurons in these species) may be found in some instances in vertebrate tissues within both glandular and neuronal elements, and in others solely within neuronal elements. Peptides found in vertebrates solely in endocrine tissue are found only in neuronal tissues in invertebrates. These observations are in keeping with the evidence (Fig. 2) that the anatomical elements of an epithelial endocrine system are a vertebrate phenomenon, while neuronal organization appears with the early multicellular invertebrates. It should be stressed, however, that neurosecretory elements in invertebrates subsume some "endocrine" type functions.

The processing of a given peptide (see below) also appears to undergo evolutionary changes. As one example, caerulein is a decapeptide isolated from frog skin. This peptide is identical, save for one amino acid substitution and N-terminal modification, to the octapeptide terminal portion of cholecystokinin, which is a 39-amino acid peptide. In vertebrate species, cholecystokinin is processed to CCK-8, CCK-33, or CCK-39 in the gastrointestinal tract, while it is processed to CCK-8 in brain, similar to the processing in frog skin. Additionally, gastrin and CCK share the same pentapeptide C-terminal sequence.

The target cell for a given peptide may undergo evolutionary change. For example, prolactin in teleosts is concerned with regulation of fluid balance, whereas in mammals it is concerned with the regulation of secretory epithelium of the mammary gland and has lost, for the most part, its effects on fluid homeostasis. (See Addendum 3, p. 275.)

Studies of peptide structure across multiple species show that portions of a peptide sequence are maintained throughout evolution and the sequences so conserved are those functionally active. Common sequences shared by different peptides within a species (i.e., cholecystokinin, gastrin, glucagon, secretin, and VIP), and peptide sequences serving similar functions in different species (i.e., secretin and VIP stimulate pancreatic function in mammals and birds, respectively, but VIP is ineffective in mammals, as is secretin in birds), may evolve by the phenomena of gene duplication or of point mutation with amino acid substitution. [Among such peptide families the peptide identified as of neuronal tissue (i.e., VIP in the "secretin" family) is presumed to be the ancestral molecule (Barrington, 1982).]

Although the molecular mechanisms of gene duplication are not yet fully understood, they involve unequal crossover events in sister chromatids, or the insertion of transposable elements containing intact genes or DNA regions that initiate or terminate transcription. One can estimate elapsed evolutionary time from the point of divergence of two proteins by comparing amino acid structures of related proteins, or nucleotide sequences of their mRNAs, and by inferring the length of time required for mutations to cause a given percentage change in amino acids in sequence. Sometimes results of such analyses do not agree with those of the fossil record, or studies on evolution of two different peptides may produce divergent data on time and course of speciation. Other concepts, such as that of unequal crossover, may be invoked to explain such discrepancies.

IV. ONTOGENY OF PEPTIDERGIC EXPRESSION IN NEURAL TISSUES

Recent studies show that neurotransmitter expression in autonomic and sensory neurons is influenced by embryonic microenvironment encountered by neural crest cells (the progenitors of such neurons) during migration as well as at the subsequent definitive site of localization (Le Douarin, 1980). Grafts of neural crest areas destined to become catecholaminergic neurons to areas destined to become cholinergic cells give rise to cholinergic populations; the converse is also true. Normally cholinergic regions grafted to sites committed to catecholaminergic function subserve the latter. On the other hand, it is possible that some noradrenergic traits are expressed by cultured crest neuroblasts even lacking a normal embryonic environment. There is also evidence of mutability of neuronal phenotype in the neonatal period. Some embryonic gut cells may transiently express catecholaminergic characteristics during development (Teitelman, 1981); the subsequent fate of such cells has been unclear.

There is very little information about factors involved in expression of peptidergic neurons. Preliminary evidence suggests that some of the embryonic gut cells, i.e., those present in embryonal pancreas, which transiently express a dopaminergic phenotype, also express insulin or glucagon, thus indicating derivation of peptidergic cells from a catecholamine precursor-type cell (Teitelman et al., 1982). Such studies may be complementary to those in rats showing that catecholaminergic expression is detected at an earlier embryonic age in brain and peripheral nerve (i.e., E 10.5) (Cochard *et al.*, 1978) than is peptidergic expression (i.e., E 16 for Substance P and somatostatin) (Black, 1978). These findings, however, are based only on immunohistochemical and radioimmunoassay techniques, and do not militate against the existence of nonimmunoreactive precursor molecules for such peptides earlier in gestation. [Reversal of transmitter expression had previously been shown for sympathetic neurons when they were cultured in the presence of certain types of nonneuronal cells (Patterson and Chun, 1977).] It is reported that embryonic chick dorsal root ganglia containing Substance P and somatostatin cultured with ganglionic nonneuronal cells show increases in neuronal content of somatostatin without any change in content of Substance P (Mudge, 1981). (See Addendum 4, p. 275.)

V. BIOSYNTHESIS OF NEUROPEPTIDES

A. INTRODUCTION

The importance of proving biosynthesis within the CNS of brain peptides was discussed in Sections I and II,B. Synthesis appears to be governed by the same general mechanisms as have been described for all polypeptide hormones and proceeds through posttranslational proteolytic cleavage of larger precursor molecules. The precursor, representing the initial translation product, is termed the "pre-protein," and contains a signal sequence at the N-terminus of the polypeptide. Signal sequences serve to translocate the translated product into the RER cisterna; subsequent cleavage by a "signal peptidase" yields the "pro-protein," which serves as the precursor molecule for component peptides. It appears that most of the pro-proteins express little, if any, inherent biological activity.

Neuropeptide synthesis, like that for all polypeptides, takes place on ribosomes within the perikaryon at a considerable distance from the secretory site at the axon terminal. This contrasts with the circumstances of local synthesis, uptake, and recycling mechanisms at the axon terminal of enzymatically synthesized neurotransmitters such as acetylcholine and the biogenic amines. (Genomic control of these latter neurotransmitters is exerted by perikaryal synthesis of the enzymes involved in the synthesis of the neurotransmitters.) A major question remains unanswered with regard to coordinate regulation of the disparate modes of synthesis of these different types of neuroactive substances released from axon terminals, since both types of molecule coexist within the same neuron, and possibly within the same secretory vesicles (Pelletier *et al.*, 1981) (see below).

The concept that peptides and other exported proteins are derived from posttranslational proteolytic cleavages of larger precursor molecules was based on pulse–chase studies utilizing radioactive amino acids. Results showed that a larger labeled form of the peptide was synthesized initially and radioactivity in that fraction decreased as the amount of the final product increased. Precursors and products were characterized on the basis of size and charge and by use of specific immunological probes. Precursor and product contained similar immunoreactivities, or a given precursor could contain two different immunoreactive regions one detected with one antiserum and one with another (e.g., endorphin and ACTH, products of the ACTH precursor molecule, proopiomelanocortin). This approach requires that significant synthesis takes place to incorporate labeled amino acids at detectable levels. Further progress made use of *in vitro* translation experiments with purified mRNA in heterologous cell-free translation systems. Selective immunoprecipitation by specific antibodies to the newly synthesized proteins then allows identification of the products formed. This method requires finding sufficient mRNA within the tissue of interest to yield sufficient product to be detected by immunoprecipitation. For several peptides within the central nervous system, concentrations are too low for this purpose. Recombinant DNA technology with amplification of nucleotide by cloning can be applied to even small amounts of mRNA template. Sequencing the cDNA clone allows elucidation of the entire amino acid sequence of precursor molecules, yielding knowledge of prohormones and products not contemplated heretofore.

The organization of genes coding for polypeptide hormones thus is of importance. Although it is not possible to detail here all the major recent advances in this field, studies with other polypeptides and proteins yield principles of significance for research on brain peptides as well.

B. Sources of Polypeptide Diversity

Diversity of polypeptide hormones can arise from multiple mechanisms: existence of multigene families, variation in splicing of a primary transcript, and alterations in posttranslational processing (see Section VI).

1. *Multigene Families*

Multigene families represent units which overlap in function, are homologous in structure, and are often tandemly arranged (Hood *et al.,* 1975). Whereas single genes encode for single chemically homogeneous products, multigene families can encode for a series of products with virtually identical sequences required as multiple copies (histone genes are an example) or for very similar products with functions slightly modified by evolution, e.g., the gene family comprising growth hormone, prolactin, and chorionic somatotropin (placental lactogen). Other classes of multigene families can code for heterogenous arrays of closely related molecules, allowing for a wide range of specificities, e.g., the antibody V-region genes, with further amplification through somatic rearrangements of the other DNA segments (i.e., the V, D, and J segments) (Robertson, 1982).

Of great interest is the possibility that similar types of gene families will be found within the central nervous system. A recently discovered multigene family may represent a model for how behavior can vary in response to diverse stimuli. This gene family encodes for peptides controlling egg laying in the organism *Aplysia,* and was identified through the use of cDNA probes to mRNA isolated from a specific neuron in the *Aplysia* abdominal ganglion. The A and B peptides are found in a glandular structure, the atrial gland. These peptides stimulate the bag cells (collections of neural cells) that release, in addition to other peptides, egg-laying hormone (ELH). Bag cell products act on contiguous neurons and are also secreted into the hemolymph. The coordinate action of A and B peptides and ELH controls behavior typically associated with egg deposition. This behavior consists of—in addition to egg deposition—head waving, respiratory pumping, walking, and eating. It has been determined that the gene encoding ELH and the genes for A and B peptides show approximately 90% sequence homology in their mRNA transcripts. Each of these three gene products contains sequences coding for A and B peptides, as well for ELH. In peptides A and B, single base changes produce added cleavage sites or frame shifts, causing premature termination. For each of these genes, there is the potential, via posttranslational cleavage, to give rise to a number of active peptide products beyond the recognized A-, B-, and ELH-like peptides. Thus, although genes for these three peptides share significant homology, they have so diverged that different member genes express functionally related but only partially overlapping sets of peptides (arising via posttranslational processing; see below). This greatly expands the informational potential of the genome.

This family of genes may thus represent a unit coding for multiple peptides to express information controlling a pattern of actions (Scheller *et al.*, 1982) involved in egg laying. It is also possible that each gene product may be separately regulated to respond to a given stimulus requiring only one portion of egg-laying behaviour (i.e., respiratory pumping or walking). Of further interest is that the precursor protein contains a sequence for another 12-amino acid peptide (flanked by pairs of basic amino acids) that corresponds precisely to the partial sequence of a peptide isolated from *Aplysia* abdominal ganglion, which has excitatory actions on a network of abdominal ganglion neurons and their target cells (Aswad, 1978). It remains to be seen if the multiple peptides described as being involved in a given vertebrate behavioral system (see Section VIII) are similarly interrelated and regulated.

2. *Splicing Choices within a Primary Transcript*

Splicing choices within given primary transcripts are known for the major adenovirus transcription unit and the heavy chains of immunoglobulin (Darnell, 1982). Recently, a similar process has been described for the calcitonin gene (Amara *et al.*, 1982). This gene contains four coding exons within the primary transcript (referred to sequentially as C, D, calcitonin/CCP, and CGRP). It is postulated that there are two poly(A) sites, one between calcitonin/CCP and CGRP, and the other downstream from CGRP. Alternative processing of this transcript involves termination at the first-described poly(A) site in the thyroid, yielding calcitonin, while in hypothalamus, processing appears to involve an alternative splicing event, in which exons C and D are joined to CGRP, with splicing out of the exon coding for calcitonin, eventually yielding CGRP, a previously unknown peptide now found in widespread distribution throughout the central nervous system. The mechanism responsible for such alternative splicing in the two tissues is still unknown.

C. EXAMPLES OF NEUROPEPTIDE PRECURSOR MOLECULES AND THEIR SYNTHESIS

Precursor molecules are known for ACTH and related peptides (i.e., POMC), the enkephalins (the pre-pro-enkephalins A and B), somatostatin, vasopressin, oxytocin, substance P, and calcitonin. Elucidation of the structure of bovine POMC from the cloned cDNA sequence (Noda *et al.*, 1982) showed that it contained sequences not only for ACTH and β-lipotropin, previously described (Mains *et al.*, 1977), but

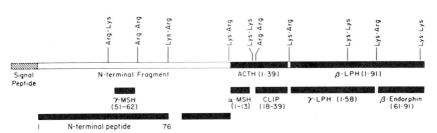

FIG. 4. Schematic representation of the bovine proopiomelanocortin precursor molecule (Nakanishi *et al.*, 1979). Dibasic amino acids represent potential cleavage sites by trypsin-like enzymes. The peptides potentially generated by such trypsin-like cleavages are indicated below the intact proopiomelanocortin structure. Reproduced from Krieger (1983a), with permission.

also for an N-terminal fragment (see Fig. 4) containing within it an MSH-like sequence. Also accounted for are the α-MSH and β-MSH sequences known to occur within ACTH and β-LPH, respectively. A high-molecular-weight precursor is also found in brain, although its genomic structure has not yet been detailed. mRNA hybridizing [Northern blot analysis (Civielli *et al.*, 1982) or *in situ* hybridization technique (Gee *et al.*, 1983)] to a pituitary-derived cDNA probe has been found. Our laboratory further has found *in vivo* (Liotta *et al.*, 1983) and *in vitro* (Liotta *et al.*, 1980) in hypothalamic cells incorporation of labeled amino acids into high-molecular-weight material containing both ACTH and β-endorphin antigenic determinants. α-MSH-like and β-endorphin-like material also appeared to be major products. Characterization by SDS gel electrophoresis, gel filtration, peptide mapping, and isoelectric focusing indicated that the precursor material in brain was similar to that synthesized in pituitary in size and charge. Thus synthesis of precursor material in hypothalamus is similar to that in pituitary.

Elucidation of the cDNA structure of mammalian pre-pro-enkephalin A (from adrenal medulla) (Comb *et al.*, 1982; Gubler *et al.*, 1982; Noda *et al.*, 1982) and pre-pro-enkephalin B (from hypothalamus) (Kadidani *et al.*, 1982) has clarified the origin of all of the multiple Met- and Leu-enkephalin-containing forms reported for the central nervous system as well as for the adrenal medulla. The structures of these precursors are indicated in Fig. 5. Pairs of dibasic amino acids represent sites of potential proteolytic cleavage allowing generation of numerous enkephalin-containing forms. The general organization of these genes and the POMC gene is similar. Structural analysis has unequivocally established the existence of separate precursors for the endorphin-, enkephalin-, and dynorphin-related opioids.

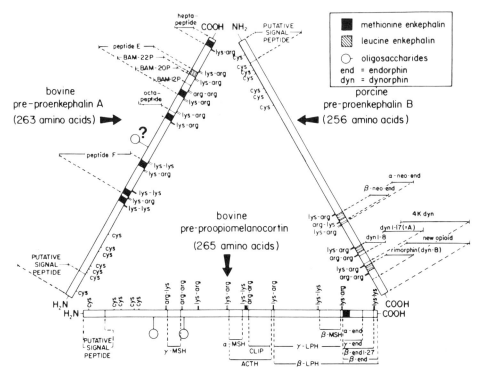

FIG. 5. Schematic representation of bovine pre-proopiomelanocortin, bovine pre-pro-enkephalin A, and porcine pre-pro-enkephalin B. The heptapeptide is Met-enkephalin-Arg[6]-Phe[7]; the octapeptide is Met-enkephalin-Arg[6]-Gly[7]-Leu[8]; BAM-P, bovine adrenal medulla peptides. Reproduced from Hollt (1983), with permission.

Somatostatin was one of the first neuropeptides isolated; it was initially described as a tetradecapeptide. It next became evident that this tetradecapeptide forms part of an NH_2-terminally expanded molecule consisting of 28 amino acids, potentially giving rise to the tetradecapeptide SS-14 (occupying the C-terminal portion of the extended peptide), as well as a dodecapeptide occupying the N-terminal portion of the SS-28 molecule (1–12). All three of these forms (Benoit et al., 1982; Morrison et al., 1983), as well as four other forms (4.4–5.5K) representing N-terminal extensions of SS-28 or SS-28 (1–12) are known (Benoit et al., 1982) in brain. Studies with antibodies specific for the first three forms indicate that they are differentially distributed; SS-28 occurs preferentially in cell bodies and SS-28 (1–12) in terminals. The density of the latter two far exceeds that of SS-14 (Morrison et al., 1983), the peptide form putatively found in brain and therein initially characterized physiologically. These findings are compatible with reports indicating that SS-28 is more potent than SS-14 as an inhibitor of growth hormone release (Meyers *et al.*, 1980), and in other central actions (Brown *et al.*, 1981a). Thus far, based on recombinant DNA techniques, there appear to be at least five different genes coding for somatostatin, one in mammals (determined from a rat thyroid carcinoma producing somatostatin), two or three in anglerfish pancreatic islets, and two in catfish islets. The mammalian form comprises a leader sequences of 24 amino acids at the amino terminus, a pro-region of 64 amino acids, and the SS-28 sequence at the carboxyl terminus. An antibody to determinants in the segment before SS-28 revealed a CNS distribution identical to that of immunoreactive somatostatin-14 (Lechan *et al.*, 1983). It appears that the phenotype of somatostatin-14 is well conserved, and so is SS-28 in part; there is less conservation of segments 5' to the SS-28 sequence.

Incubation of hypothalamic cells with [^{3}H]phenylalanine revealed a 15K molecule in addition to the SS-14 and SS-28 somatostatin segments. Pulse–chase experiments indicate a transfer of label from the 15K material to material corresponding to the SS-28 forms (Zingg and Patel, 1982). Recent evidence (Robbins *et al.*, 1983) suggests that SS-28 may not be an obligatory intermediate in the synthesis of SS-14.

A precursor for TRH has been identified in frog skin (Richter *et al.*, 1984). The deduced polypeptide of 123 amino acids for the tripeptide TRH (pGlu-His-Pro-NH$_2$) contains three copies of the sequences Lys-Arg-Gln-His-Pro-$^{Lys}_{Arg}$-Arg and a fourth incomplete copy at the carboxyl end. Therefore, the TRH precursor joins the list of polyproteins that can be processed to yield more than one molecule of end product.

The existence of precursor molecules for vasopressin and oxytocin, containing their respective neurophysins, had been suggested as early as 1964 (Sachs and Takabatake, 1964). More recent studies utilizing the pulse–chase method revealed precursor molecules with molecular weights of approximately 20K that are processed during axonal transport, to 10K fragments encompassing the peptides and their respective neurophysins (Brownstein *et al.*, 1980). A structure for the precursor was proposed, based on results with cyanogen bromide cleavage, showing a vasopressin–neurophysin–glycopeptide order (Russel *et al.*, 1981). This arrangement has been confirmed with the elucidation of the primary structures of the pre-prohormones obtained through sequencing the cDNAs encoding for the hypothalamic mRNAs (Land *et al.*, 1982). The rat gene for the arginine vasopressin–neurophysin precursor has most recently been cloned. It contains three exons, each of which codes for one of the three conserved functional domains of the precursor, namely, arginine vasopressin, neurophysin, and the glyco-protein (Schmale *et al.*, 1983).

VI. PROTEOLYTIC PROCESSING AND DEGRADATION OF PEPTIDES

"Processing," the liberation of active peptide substances from pre-cursors by proteolytic enzymes (proteases), takes place, at least in the context of this article, intracellularly. This is one mechanism that can account for the large diversity of known peptide products. Degrada-tion, on the other hand, represents loss of defined biological activity, the product exhibiting no new defined biological activity (degradation is synonymous with termination of action). It is generally held that in processing endopeptidases are involved, whereas in peptide degrada-tion, both endopeptidases and exopeptidases are involved. Endogenous protease inhibitors also are found in tissues (Pontremoli *et al.*, 1983). It is possible that a number of factors separately involved in activation of either proteases or their inhibitors may regulate expression of peptides in different tissues, and in normal and abnormal physiology. (See Ad-dendum 5, p. 275.)

It is thought that most precursor molecules are cleaved to their component peptides at the stage of secretory processing within the Golgi apparatus and the developing secretory granules; in some cases the RER appears to be involved. (It is not clear whether enzymes in-volved in processing exist in the soluble phase of the granule contain-ing the precursor, are in separate granules that fuse with the precur-sor-containing granule, or are membrane-bound.) Cleavage usually takes place at points in the peptide backbone where there are pairs of basic amino acids. (Arg rather than Lys may be preferred at the car-boxyl site of the pair.) A POMC-converting enzyme has been partially purified from bovine intermediate lobe secretory vesicles, which is in-hibited by a thiol blocker (Loh and Parish, 1984). A similar activity has been found in neural lobe secretory vesicles.

Other types of posttranslational enzymatic modifications will be mentioned but not discussed further in this section. These include amidation, cyclization of glutamic acid to form pyroglutamate, acetyla-tion, sulfation, glycosylation, methylation, and phosphorylation. Some of these modifications, such as acetylation, greatly modify the func-tional activity of a given peptide product. Deacetylation of α-MSH greatly decreases the melanophore-stimulating activity (Hofmann, 1974); α-N-acetylation of β-endorphin reduces its affinity for opiate receptors by a factor of 10^{-3} (Akil *et al.*, 1981). Other such modifications may introduce conformational changes that could alter accessibility to processing enzymes. Acetylation, amidation, and glycosylation may also prolong half-lives of peptides by making them more resistant to proteolytic degradation.

It is generally held that several different types of enzymes are involved in processing. Some contain serine at active sites (trypsin, kallikrein, plasmin), others thiols (cathepsin-B-like), and still others metalloproteases. The enzymes are characterized by substrate specificity and type of inhibitor. Although some information exists on enzymes involved in extra-CNS sites (see Chertow, 1981, for review) (i.e., proopiomelanocortin in pituitary, insulin in pancreas, somatostatin in pancreas) and much less in CNS sites, no specific enzyme has been isolated, biochemically characterized, or appropriately localized. Recently, a high-molecular-weight neutral endopeptidase complex was found in pituitary, which on polyacrylamide gel electrophoresis under dissociating conditions revealed five components, with molecular weights of 24–28K and which exhibited three distinct activities: chymotrypsin-like, trypsin-like, and a peptidyl glutamylpeptide bond hydrolyzing. It is suggested that separate catalytic units are responsible for the observed activities, but that the integrity of the complex is important for the expression of all activities. A similar complex has been characterized in brain (Orlowski and Wilk, 1981). It is apparent that definitive characterization of enzymes in tissues of interest and development of specific inhibitors thereto are needed in order to develop physiological and therapeutic insight.

Posttranslational processing is perhaps best illustrated by the proopiomelanocortin molecule (see Fig. 4). In the anterior pituitary, the major demonstrable products are the N-terminal glycopeptide, ACTH, and β-lipotropin. In the intermediate lobe found in certain species, ACTH is cleaved further to α-MSH and the corticotropin-like intermediate lobe peptide (CLIP); β-LPH is cleaved to γ-LPH and β-endorphin. Virtually all of these cleavages occur at pairs of basic amino acid residues flanking biologically active peptides. Such cleavage may represent action of a trypsin-like enzyme but, since the active peptides do not terminate in arginine or lysine, it is proposed that other carboxypeptidase B-like enzymes hydrolyze basic residues from the C-termini exposed by action of the trypsin-like enzyme. There is no explanation yet for the differences in processing of proopiomelanocortin between the anterior lobe on the one hand and the intermediate lobe on the other. Genomic regulation of enzyme expression and content may well be involved in controlling such posttranslational processing.

Further posttranslational modification is represented in acetylation of β-endorphin and α-MSH. Acetylated α-MSH, the form most prevalent in the intermediate lobe, is a much more potent melanotropic hormone (Hofmann, 1974) than deacetyl α-MSH; acetylated β-endorphin, the major β-endorphin form in the intermediate lobe, shows, as discussed above, only 1/1000 of the affinity of the unacetylated form for its receptor. Processing of POMC within the hypothalamus appears to be initially similar to that found in the intermediate lobe, since α-MSH and β-endorphin are the major forms found. On the other hand in the hypothalamus they exist predominantly as unacetylated forms (Evans *et al.,* 1982; Weber *et al.,* 1981). Differing modes of posttranslational processing provide a mechanism whereby in different tissues the same precursor molecule can give rise to different products thereby serving different functions.

The degradative systems are especially important for CNS peptides and their postulated neurotransmitter functions. Unlike the "classical" neurotransmitters, for which there are reuptake mechanisms and enzymatic degradation mechanisms to terminate actions, we know of no reuptake mechanisms for CNS peptides. Termination of action for peptide hormones of the general endocrine system appears to proceed not by degradation of peptide at receptor sites but rather by internalization of hormone receptor complexes which then interact with intracellular organelles in the target cell. Although this mechanism may exist in the CNS extracellular peptidase action may be the more important mechanism for termination of action. Enzymes involved might reside near pre- or postsynaptic peptide receptors in membrane-bound form. Most of our knowledge of peptidases in neural tissue has been gained with enkephalinases. Both enkephalin pentapeptides (Met-enkephalin, H-Tyr-Gly-Gly-Phe-Met-OH, and Leu-enkephalin, H-Tyr-Gly-Gly-Phe-Leu-OH) are inactivated at Tyr-Gly by an enkephalin aminopeptidase, "enkephalinase-B," and at Gly-Phe (by enkephalinase-A). The latter accounts for less than 25% of enkephalin metabolism, but receives most attention since it is membrane bound, is uneven in distribution among regions of the brain, and appears to be closely associated with opioid receptors (Schwartz *et al.,* 1981). There are no data, however, showing a quantitative relationship between change in excitability in enkephalin-sensitive preparations and kinetics of enkephalinase activity. Although enkephalinase inhibitors enhance enkephalin activity and concentration, specificity and selectivity of the enzyme are yet to be established. Studies on anatomical distribution, and substrate specificity, might help establish "functional specificity."

There is evidence that Tyr-Gly cleavage in LHRH is catalyzed by a metalloendopeptidase, and that the activity of this enzyme can be regulated by different hormonal feedback paradigms (Advis *et al.*, 1983). Although other peptidases have been isolated from neural tissues— proline endopeptidase, Substance P endopeptidase, in addition to other peptidases noted above—there is no compelling evidence (and none for enkephalinases) that such enzymes exist exclusively in neural tissue or are specific for any given peptide.

VII. PEPTIDE DISTRIBUTION

We cannot present here detailed descriptions on distribution of the many neuropeptides found within the central nervous system, but will offer several generalizations. The hypothalamus contains the highest concentrations of peptides, termed "hypothalamic releasing hormones," and this is the tissue wherein they were first sought, based on the hypothesis that CNS control of anterior pituitary function was mediated by substances elaborated therefrom. We now realize that "hypothalamic" releasing hormones are widespread in distribution throughout the central nervous system, wherein they presumably subserve functions (see Section VIII) beyond those recognized as classical within the hypothalmus. Indeed, TRH has been found within the nervous system of species prior to the appearance of a pituitary gland (Jackson and Reichlin, 1974). Moreover it is now apparent that cell bodies of the hypothalamic magnocellular nuclei containing vasopressin and oxytocin emanate projections not only to the posterior lobe (the classical receptor tissue for these hormones) but also diffusely to regions throughout the central nervous system and into the spinal cord. Again there is the suggestion that such extrahypothalamic projections subserve functions other than those specified by the posterior pituitary projections. Highest CNS concentrations of proopiomelanocortin-related peptides, of bombesin, and of neurotensin are also found within the hypothalamus (see Fig. 6). Other peptides, such as cholecystokinin and vasoactive intestinal polypeptide (VIP), show highest concentrations within the cerebral cortex. Certain peptides are found in moderate to high concentrations within the limbic system, whereas significant concentrations for only somatostatin, enkephalin, Substance P, and cholecystokinin have been found within the medulla and pons. These data have been obtained primarily in animal studies. There are indications that significant concentrations can be found within human brain (measured with radioimmunoassays) obtained a short time postmortem; such concentrations seem similar to those determined in laboratory animals (Edwardson and McDermott, 1982).

Immunocytochemical studies (note there are species differences)

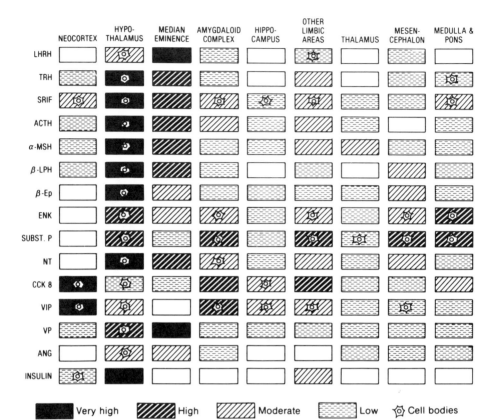

FIG. 6. Relative concentrations of neuropeptides in selected central nervous system areas. The amygdaloid complex and hippocampus are considered part of the limbic system. The median eminence refers to a specialized area of the hypothalamus located in the inferior portion of the third ventricle, containing endings of the hypophysiotropic and other neurons in the capillaries of the hypophyseal portal circulation. Also depicted are those areas in which cell bodies containing the designated peptides have been demonstrated immunocytochemically. SRIF, Somatostatin; β-Ep, β-endorphin; Enk, enkephalin; NT, neurotensin; VIP, vasoactive intestinal polypeptide; VP, vasopressin; ANG, angiotensin; ACTH, adrenocorticotropic hormone; α-MSH, α-melanocyte-stimulating hormone. For the neurotransmitters, releasing hormones, Substance P, and enkephalin, chemical identity has been established. ACTH precursor molecule and other "pituitary" hormones contained therein have been established by immunocytochemical, immunoassay, biosynthetic, and cDNA hybridization techniques. Other peptides cited have thus far been characterized by immunoassay or immunocytochemistry. The data cited for vasopressin and oxytocin, long known to exist in the magnocellular nuclei and the tuberohypophyseal tract, represent more widespread CNS distribution. Reproduced from Krieger (1983b), with permission.

show, in the main, that the cell bodies containing certain neuropeptides, (i.e., vasopressin and oxytocin and their respective neurophysins, the family of peptides derived from proopiomelanocortin, and gonadotropin-releasing hormone) are confined to the hypothalamus but give rise to long projections throughout the CNS accounting for the concentrations of these peptides reported in these other CNS areas. In contrast, other peptides (i.e., Substance P, VIP, enkephalin, CCK, and neurotensin), as well as some of the "hypothalamic" releasing hormones (i.e., somatostatin and thyrotropin-releasing hormone), are found in cell bodies distributed widely throughout the brain and spinal cord showing short projection systems.

Hokfelt *et al.* (1980) have made a major contribution toward peptide localization proving the coexistence of neuropeptides and neurotransmitters within the same cell and, indeed, within given peripheral nerves. (Coexistence of peptides and biogenic amines had previously been found within endocrine cells of the gastrointestinal tract.) Serotonin has been found, together with Substance P and TRH, in neurons of the medulla oblongata, CCK and dopamine in cells of the mesencephalon, somatostatin or enkephalin with norepinephrine in sympathetic ganglia, and VIP and acetylcholine within autonomic ganglia. Very recently, CRF was found in some cells of the magnocellular nuclei together with vasopressin. In studies on subcellular distribution it was found that neuropeptide concentrations are greatest in nerve terminal or synaptosome fractions. In such terminals, there are large and small synaptic vesicles (100–150 and 30–50 nm, respectively). It has been questioned whether the neuropeptide and neurotransmitter exist within the same secretory granule or in separate populations of granules. Recently, Pelletier *et al.* (1981) have provided evidence for the coexistence of serotonin and Substance P within the same dense-core secretory granule. This raises fundamental questions concerning mechanisms of storage. Although it is known that there is an active reuptake process from the synaptic cleft for neurotransmitters, especially monoamines, with repackaging within secretory granules, and that synthesis of neurotransmitters occurs within terminals, no such process has been described for neuropeptides. The latter are characteristically synthesized in the cell body, and subsequently transported to the Golgi for packaging in secretory granules.

The functional significance of neuropeptide–neurotransmitter coexistence remains to be explored. Release of each concurrently regulated would allow for interaction between neuropeptides and neurotransmitters. A model of such interaction is represented by vasoactive intestinal polypeptide and acetylcholine. VIP in physiologically relevant concentrations produces a 10,000-fold increase in the affinity of acetyl-choline for muscarinic receptors in the cat submandibular gland (Lundberg *et al.,* 1982). Moreover, long-term treatment with atropine (producing muscarinic receptor blockade) increases the numbers of both VIP and muscarinic receptors in the salivary gland (Hedlund *et al.,* 1983) and causes peptidergic as well as muscarinic supersensitivity. Another possible coordination is found between secretory and vasodilatory (cat submandibular glands and nasal mucosa) functions of acetylcholine and VIP (Lundberg, 1981). Antiserum against VIP partially blocks the atropine-resistant vasodilation produced by parasympathetic activity (Lundberg, 1981).

VIII. FUNCTIONS OF BRAIN PEPTIDES

One major question concerns the physiological significance of the many peptides now recognized within the central nervous system. To date it has not been possible to characterize CNS receptors for all of the described neuropeptides. Imbedded within this question are the problems of how one defines neurotransmitters and how they act? Neurotransmitters are classically considered to be substances liberated at presynaptic terminals, which diffuse across the narrow synaptic gap and act on the postsynaptic membrane (Iversen *et al.,* 1980). Their actions are localized to the synaptic regions and their effects are milliseconds in duration. Termination of action is accomplished by removal of the transmitter, by enzymatic degradation, or through reuptake into the presynaptic terminal. Transmitters may, however, be capable of a wider range of action. The duration of action for many putative neurotransmitters, including amines and most peptides, may extend to seconds, minutes, or longer (considerably outlasting the period of application), and the distance between release sites and target cells may be several micrometers (Kuffler, 1980). A broader classification, as noted in Section II,C, would connote a substance in the presynaptic cell, released therefrom by stimulation and depolarization, causing physiological changes in postsynaptic cells identical to those produced by stimulating presynaptic cells. Specific antagonists should block the nerve-evoked response. The term "neuromodulator" has been applied to substances without traditional transmitter action. There is, however, no uniform definition for such and it may be taken to imply diverse properties. Peptides considered neuromodulators (1) modify known actions of "classical" conventional fast neurotransmitters (peptides coexisting with "classical" neurotransmitters modulate receptors for conventional neurotransmitters); (2) may block the release of transmitters via presynaptic endings on terminals releasing such transmitters; or (3) may alter the turnover of other neurotransmitters (Deyo et al., 1979; Kadar et al., 1981; Moroni et al., 1977; Van Loon and De Souza, 1978). Moreover, neuropeptides located in terminals of the median eminence of the hypothalamus and in the tuberohypophyseal tract can affect pituitary hormone secretion (McCann, 1980) and potentially produce secondary effects on the nervous system mediated by target cell hormones.

The best evidence that peptides are conventional neurotransmitters has been obtained with LHRH found in sympathetic ganglia. An LHRH-like peptide is released from ganglia by nerve stimulation via a calcium-dependent process and acts directly on sympathetic neurons to produce a depolarizing response lasting for minutes. This peptide probably functions as a transmitter for the long-lasting, late, slow excitatory postsynaptic potential (EPSP) observed after nerve stimulation. The responses to LHRH and the late slow EPSP are associated with similar conductance changes in membranes and alterations in excitability of the neuron. Both responses are blocked by LHRH analogs (Jan and Jan, 1981) that inhibit LHRH-induced release of LH from gonadotrophs.

The possible functional significance of brain peptides can be deduced also from the observation (see Fig. 1) (Snyder, 1980) that norepinephrine and dopamine act as neurotransmitters at only 1% of brain synapses, serotonin at a similarly low fraction, and acetylcholine at no more than 5–10% of synapses. The bulk of the CNS transmitters known are amino acid congenes, acting at 25–40% of synapses, depending on brain region. Thus peptide neurotransmitters may prove to account for the majority of neurophysiologic functions mediated through synaptic sites still to be classified, and may act via effects on these "classical" neurotransmitters. Much is to be learned through elucidating the functions of such brain peptides.

Two types of studies have been performed to assess the function of brain peptides. In one a peptide is given, usually intraventricularly or intracerebrally, and its effects are observed on a behavior. Do these represent pharmacological or physiological effects? In some instances, antagonists or antiserum to a particular peptide are given to assess endogenous function of peptides. These studies may be hampered by lack of specific antagonists. Another approach is to determine concentrations of peptides in diseases of the central nervous system; postmortem samples of cerebral tissue or cerebrospinal fluid are analyzed. There are problems with this approach also. The first is that a given peptide may not be stable through the lapse of time to autopsy. For many peptides this fortunately does not appear to be a major consideration. Cerebrospinal fluid, more readily accessible, may be more suitable for analysis. Most of such studies, however, are performed on lumbar fluid, and in view of the distribution of peptides throughout the neuraxis, measurements at this level may reflect peptides from the spinal cord rather than the brain. Further, there may be alterations in a localized disease area not reflected in assays on cerebrospinal fluid. There may also be dynamic changes in peptide secretion into CSF as well as active or passive transport of a given peptide to blood and CSF. (See Addendum 6, p. 275.)

A. EFFECTS ON MAJOR HOMEOSTATIC SYSTEMS

Although brain peptides may affect diverse homeostatic systems, only selective aspects can be considered here. Each system is affected by multiple peptides and by conventional neurotransmitters. The interactions among these factors and how they regulate a given system are challenging topics for research.

1. *Pain*

Information perceived as pain reaches the central nervous system via peripheral nerves terminating in the dorsal horn of the spinal cord. Dorsal horn cells send processes to the substantia gelatinosa of the central nervous system. Dorsal horn cells also receive input from other neurons originating within the dorsal horn, as well as descending inputs from brainstem centers, specifically from the nucleus Raphe magnus and the nucleus reticularis paragigantocellularis. Diverse peptides have been found at each level of this chain (Jessel, 1983). For example, Substance P, somatostatin, VIP, CCK-8, and angiotensin have been detected in primary sensory neurons. Dorsal horn neurons contain enkephalin, Substance P, CCK-8, somatostatin, neurotensin, bombesin, and pancreatic polypeptide. Binding sites for calcitonin are present in CNS areas anatomically involved in the transmission of nociceptive information (Pecile *et al.*, 1984). Finally, in the supraspinal pathway which descends to the dorsal horn, Substance P, TRH, enkephalins, oxytocin, vasopressin, and angiotensin have been found. Interrelations of these peptides in pain perception are extremely complex. There is good evidence that Substance P is a sensory transmitter released by certain classes of afferent neurons. Enkephalin and related opioid peptides, as noted above, act to inhibit dorsal horn neurons, and this may explain the analgesic actions of these compounds. Little is known of the functions of the many other peptides in the dorsal horn.

2. Memory, Learning, and Adaptive Behavior

Even before it was known that peptides are synthesized in the CNS there were many reports that systemic or intraventricular administration of ACTH, α-MSH, or vasopressin could correct the impairment caused by hypophysectomy of conditioned avoidance behavior (i.e., facilitate learning). Similar behavioral effects (i.e., facilitation of learning) were also produced by these peptides in normal animals. Such effects could be induced by fragments or analogs devoid of any endocrine effects. ACTH fragments 4-7 and 4-10, sequences common to ACTH, α-MSH, the β-MSH-like part of β-lipotropin, and γ-MSH, were effective (Bohus, 1979). The presence of phenylalanine in position 7 plays a key role in the behavioral effects of such fragments. These fragments seemed involved in short-term memory processes, while similar effects of vasopressin implied function in long-term memory (de Kloet and de Wied, 1980).

Similar studies have now been performed with endogenous opioids prompted by reports that morphine (an opiate alkaloid) affected behavior and the likelihood that ACTH fragments and endorphin, both derived from the common precursor molecule, proopiomelanocortin, coexist in the brain. The latter area of study has yielded some confusing results. The initial description indicated that opiate alkaloids disrupted learning behavior, but naloxone facilitated such behavior (Messing et al., 1981). Facilitation of learning has been reported for α- and β-endorphin and for minute doses of Met- and Leu-enkephalin, given subcutaneously. The effects of the enkephalins and of α-endorphin were not reversed by naloxone. γ-Endorphin (also believed to be derived from β-endorphin) generally produced opposite effects (de Wied et al., 1978b; Koob and Bloom, 1983; Koob et al., 1981). Some of the observed discrepancies may be related to the test conditions: aversive motivation or positive reward. In the latter, there appear to be differences, at least for γ-endorphin, in effects on food-motivated vs thirst-motivated learning. The prolonged effects of peptides given subcutaneously is surprising in view of the rapid disappearance of these peptides from blood. The discrepant effects of opiate alkaloids vs endorphin on behavior are also puzzling. Perhaps different receptor subtypes are affected by each of the compounds (see de Wied, 1982). One report indicated that des-tyrosine γ-endorphin, devoid of opiate receptor interaction, can facilitate extinction (de Wied et al., 1978a); this has not been confirmed. The sometimes opposite effects of ACTH(4-7)-like peptides and of β-endorphin-like peptides are mirrored by reports that these classes of compound affect concentrations of brain neurotransmitters, cAMP, and neuronal firing rates in opposing directions. These findings, and the opposite effects of α- and γ-endorphin, raise the question as to whether processing of POMC-derived peptides differs according to terminal area, receptor distribution, or in local feedback modulatory control.

One group (de Wied, 1976) has observed that subcutaneous or intracerebroventricular administration of vasopressin delays extinction in active or passive avoidance testing, that the reverse effects are produced by vasopressin antiserum, that Brattleboro rats (genetically deficient in vasopressin) are defective in passive avoidance behavior, and that an analog, desglycinamide lysine vasopressin, devoid of endocrine effect, produces behavioral effects similar to those of vasopressin (Van Wimersma Greidanus *et al.,* 1975a,b). It has been suggested that vasopressin acts centrally by modulating neurotransmission in catecholamine systems distributed throughout the dorsal adrenergic bundle. The role of oxytocin in some of these experimental paradigms requires further study, since it produces behavioral effects opposite to those of vasopressin (Bohus *et al.,* 1978). In contrast to these studies, Bloom *et al.* (1976) have reported that arginine vasopressin given systemically affects not only learning, but also overt behavior such as locomotion, blood pressure, and food reward. They suggest that central effects of vasopressin on learning are mediated via responses to afferent stimuli, not direct effects on neural elements (Koob and Bloom, 1983). A pressor antagonist analog of arginine vasopressin abolishes the behavioral effects of AVP given subcutaneously (Koob *et al.,* 1981). The latter group also suggested that central catecholaminergic effects of intracerebroventricularly administered vasopressin may be secondary to actions on blood pressure regulation.

Results with other peptides are also controversial. That the effects of ACTH fragments appear is apparent with the use of the reproducible dextro-7-isomer of ACTH(4-7). It produces effects similar to those of the levo-isomer in avoidance acquisition, but opposite effects on extinction. Perhaps different receptor types are involved here too. There are also reports indicating that ACTH and its fragments interact with opiate receptors (Terenius, 1975).

Although these peptides apparently act in cognitive function, specificity of response, peripheral vs central effects, and biochemical and physiological mechanisms require extended investigation. Applicability to human learning and memory also must be assessed. Some reports propose and others deny that systemic administration of ACTH(4-10) increases attention and visual discrimination (Bohus, 1979; Sandman *et al.,* 1976). Most studies have been performed in young, healthy volunteers. Others in elderly persons whose cognitive functions are disturbed may provide more significant information. Administration of lysine vasopressin (Legros *et al.*, 1978) or a synthetic analog, 1-de-amino-D-Arg^8 vasopressin (Weingartner *et al.*, 1981), led to improved performance in tests measuring long-term memory and in memory of patients suffering retrograde amnesia (Oliveros *et al.*, 1978). Still unexplained is the long-lived effect of a single dose of vasopressin on behavior.

The recently discovered corticotropin-releasing factor may also affect central behavioral activation. It remains to be determined whether these effects are mediated by changes in concentrations of POMC-related peptides, in vasopressin, or by stimulatory effects of CRF on adrenal medullary secretion of catecholamines.

3. *Psychiatric Disease*

Early theories about central monoamines as etiological factors in psychiatric conditions prompted similar considerations that brain peptides might be involved. Some suggested that TRH was effective in depression but these reports have not been substantiated (Prange *et al.*, 1978). The discoveries that endogenous opioids exist, that opiate receptors are abundant in certain brain areas, e.g., limbic system (putatively influences emotion), that interactions between opioid and monoamine systems are possible, and that opiates affect behavior have engendered considerable interest. Bloom *et al.* (1976) initially suggested that postural rigidity in rats given intracisternal injections of β-endorphin was similar to the catatonia of schizophrenia. It was inferred that schizophrenia might be associated with excessive brain endorphin activity. Jacquet and Marks (1976), however, interpreted such rigidity as analagous to catalepsy induced by neuroleptic properties of endorphin, and suggested that schizophrenia might reflect a deficiency of endorphin. There is little information to suggest that these peptides influence affect in normal human subjects. Schizophrenia will be the only affective disorder considered in this section. There is even less information concerning opioids in other psychiatric conditions, such as mania or depression. The role of endogenous opioids in learning behavior has been briefly reviewed in the preceding section.

Studies in schizophrenic subjects have suggested either increased or decreased opioid activity. Terenius *et al.* (1976) found increased opioid-like activity in cerebrospinal fluid obtained from untreated schizophrenic subjects. The opioid-like activities were in fractions distinct from those containing β-endorphin and enkephalins. Concentrations decreased in two patients who improved with therapy. In another report, increased concentrations were found only in acute, not chronic, schizophrenia (Domschke *et al.*, 1979). Other investigators find no change in CSF opioid content in this group. In many studies, however, neither characterization of the opioid nor definition of diagnosis was adequate. Treatment with naloxone has been tried in schizophrenia with reductions in hallucinations in response to high-doses of the drug (Berger *et al.*, 1981; Davis *et al.*, 1979). Naloxone acts predominantly on (μ) opiate receptors. If, as suggested, the (δ) receptor mediates behavioral effects, one would not expect naloxone to be effective in this condition; specific antagonists of (δ) receptors should offer greater potential for this purpose.

In still other studies the hypothesis was tested that there might be an opioid deficiency in schizophrenia. Intravenous administration of β-endorphin has given inconclusive results (Berger *et al.*, 1980; Gerner *et al.*, 1980; Pickar *et al.*, 1981). Administration of β-endorphin on a short-term basis to patients with chronic disease may not be the best method to assess therapeutic efficacy, since the peptide is rapidly degraded. De Wied *et al.* (1978a) proposed that schizophrenics cannot convert β-endorphin to des-tyrosine γ-endorphin, which they postulate normally functions as a neuroleptic agent. Although they reported encouraging clinical responses utilizing des-tyrosine γ-endorphin for treatment of schizophrenia, results of others do not agree (Tamminga *et al.*, 1981). Des-tyrosine γ-endorphin does not bind to classic opiate receptors, but does bind to dopamine receptors, which may be in keeping with the proposal that dopaminergic activity is disturbed in this disease.)

4. *Feeding*

Early studies on appetite implicated a medial hypothalamic "satiety center," receiving stimulatory serotonergic inputs and inhibitory adrenergic inputs, and a lateral hypothalamic "feeding center," receiving prominent dopaminergic inputs. There appear to be reciprocal interactions between these two areas, characterized by mutual inhibition. Activation of one area causes inhibition of the other; suppression of one causes activation of the other.

More recently, it has been proposed that several peptides, within and without the CNS, regulate feeding behavior. The C-terminal octapeptide of cholecystokinin (CCK-8), the predominant form of cholecystokinin within the brain (found also with intact cholecystokinin-39 in the intestinal tract), has been the most intensively studied. Both peripheral and central CCK-8 appear to be involved in feeding behavior. Parenteral administration of CCK-8 suppresses sham feeding in animals (Debas *et al.*, 1975; Gibbs *et al.*, 1973) and this effect is blocked by vagotomy in some species (Smith *et al.*, 1981). It has been postulated that the effects of CCK are mediated by information reaching the brain via vagal afferent fibers, perhaps in response to the decrease in gastric emptying occasioned by cholecystokinin (Moran and McHugh, 1982).

There is also evidence that brain CCK is involved in feeding behavior; in sheep, but not in rats, injection of antibody to CCK into the lateral ventricles inhibits normal postprandial satiety and stimulates food intake (Della-Fera *et al.*, 1981). There is no conclusive evidence, however, that the brain content of CCK changes in parallel with altered nutritional or feeding states or in experimental models of obesity (Schneider *et al.*, 1979). CCK receptors increase in the hypothalamus of fasted mice (Saito *et al.*, 1981), but not rats (Hays and Paul, 1981). Receptor content is increased in the cortex but not the hypothalamus in forms of genetically induced obesity in rodents (Hays and Paul, 1981; Saito *et al.*, 1981).

CCK may also bind to opiate receptors (Schiller *et al.*, 1978) and opioids have been implicated as major regulators in central stimulation of food intake. Administration of opioid peptides into discrete regions of the central nervous system stimulates feeding (Grandison and Guidotti, 1977). Moreover, high concentrations of endorphins have been found in Zucker fatty rats (Gibson *et al.*, 1981), and fasting leads to decreased hypothalamic content of β-endorphin. There are no reports yet that obesity or nutritional state affect opiate receptor number or affinity. Since β-endorphin can affect turnover of central monoamines and since the latter may regulate feeding behavior, further studies on control of these systems by β-endorphin are needed.

There are also many peptides potentially involved in controlling satiety. Insulin (when administered centrally), bombesin, calcitonin, CRF, or TRH can decrease feeding. The site of action of these peptides has been presumed to be within the CNS, but it is controversial whether these effects are mediated directly on the satiety center, by interaction with catecholaminergic systems, or by inhibition of endogenous substance(s) (i.e., opioids) that stimulate feeding. (See Addendum 7, p. 275.) Finally, some of these peptides may affect glucoregulation. Hypoglycemia is a potent stimulus to feeding behavior, and hyperglycemia may effect satiety. The only clinical correlate for these studies has been the effect of CCK-8, which, given peripherally, decreases food intake in obese men (Pi-Sunyer *et al.*, 1982).

5. Temperature Regulation

Elevation, reduction, or maintenance of normal body temperature requires coordination of mechanisms for heat production and heat loss. Such mechanisms represent a complex interplay between peripheral and central receptors. Information received via peripheral afferent receptor systems presumably is integrated and compared against a central nervous system thermoregulatory set-point; appropriate changes in heat production or heat loss are then brought about by neural effector mechanisms. These responses may be regulated by changing the central set-point at which heat loss or conservation is elicited, or by activation of efferent thermoregulatory pathways. Heat production is enhanced by increased cellular metabolism; heat loss is effected by increased blood flow to areas of heat transfer with coordinate processes of piloerection and sweating modulating heat exchange. There are also behavioral mechanisms for increasing or decreasing heat transfer involving choice of thermal environment.

The controlling areas of the CNS appear to be mainly the anterior hypothalamus, especially the preoptic area, the septum, and the brainstem reticular formation. Earlier studies emphasized the importance of serotonergic and noradrenergic involvement, respectively, in the increase or decrease of body temperature. Many substances believed to affect body temperature may act through a common mechanism. A decrease in hypothalamic calcium concentration or an increase in sodium concentration elevates core temperature (Myers and Tytell, 1972), whereas the converse takes place with increased hypothalamic calcium concentration (Hanegan and Williams, 1973). Prostaglandins, reported to be thermogenic, facilitate mitochondrial calcium uptake, causing a decrease in local concentrations of calcium.

Brain peptides may also be involved in regulation of body temperature (see Clark and Lipton, 1983, for review), although there is no information on specific locus or mode of action. Effects of a given peptide can vary, depending on ambient temperature at the time of administration; there is also variation of effect and potency between species. The following represents a brief summary of those peptides which have been most extensively studied.

Intracranial injection of TRH causes hyperthermia (Brown et al., 1977) and in some studies, but not others, reverses the hypothermic effect of bombesin, neurotensin (Brown et al., 1981b), or β-endorphin (Holaday et al., 1977). These effects of TRH were also found in hypothysectomized animals, implying central rather than a peripheral effects secondary to increased thyroid hormone release. Endogenous prostaglandins may be involved since TRH-induced hyperthermia is prevented by indomethacin (Cohn et al., 1980). Administration of anti-TRH serum into the lateral ventricle causes a decrease of core body temperature (Prasad et al., 1980), implying that TRH acts physiologically; administration of a neurotensin antibody produces an increase in core body temperature (Wallace et al., 1981).

The hypothermic effect of β-endorphin and other opioids has already been noted. These effects are dose dependent, high doses producing hypothermia and low doses causing hyperthermia (Bloom and Tseng, 1981; Holaday et al., 1978a; Huidibro-Toro and Way, 1979). Tolerance may develop to the effect of a given opioid and cross-tolerance between opioids (Huidibro-Toro and Way, 1979). Naloxone reverses some thermoregulatory effects of β-endorphin, but not the effects of enkephalins on body temperature. Naloxone also produces disordered thermoregulation in animals exposed to cold or hot environments; thus endogenous opioids may be involved in temperature adaptation (Holaday *et al.*, 1978b).

Recently interest has developed in endogenous vasopressin as an antipyretic agent. Intracranial (septal region) administration of arginine vasopressin prevents pyrogen-induced fever in sheep (Cooper *et al.*, 1979) and this effect is enhanced by perfusion of the same area with antivasopressin serum. Release of vasopressin into the septal area has been detected after induction of fever in studies utilizing the push–pull cannula perfusion techniques (Veale *et al.*, 1981). In the rabbit, however, injection of AVP causes hyperthermia, not antipyresis (Bernardini *et al.*, 1983).

Central administration of α-MSH and ACTH also induces hypothermia in normal or adrenalectomized animals. Like the findings with vasopressin, the concentration of α-MSH within the septum rises during fever (Samson *et al.*, 1981), and microinjection of the peptide into this region reduces fever (Glyn-Ballinger *et al.*, 1983). Surprisingly peripheral or intragastric administration also is effective (Murphy and Lipton, 1982).

6. *Blood Pressure*

A multitude of factors may be involved in maintenance of blood pressure and in derangements leading to hypertension. In addition to renal, adrenal, and dietary factors, the CNS is important in blood pressure control. Previous studies on control implicate carotid and aortic baroreceptors and their linkage in a centrally mediated reflex arc involving the nucleus of the solitary tract. Glutamic acid was proposed as the neurotransmitter of the primary baroreceptor afferents. Peripheral and central catecholamines are involved in the regulation of vascular reactivity, as well as in the control of renin secretion, and the peripheral angiotensin system also may effect central regulation of blood pressure and fluid volume.

Several newly described brain peptides also may be involved. Central administration of angiotensin increases blood pressure, and this is blocked by the inhibitor saralasin. Intraventricular saralasin, as well as Captopril (the angiotensin-converting enzyme inhibitor), decreases blood pressure in the spontaneously hypertensive rat of a stroke-prone strain (Ganten *et al.*, 1981). There are no data as to possible interactions between the peripheral and central renin-angiotensin systems.

Opioids have also been implicated in the control of blood pressure. We will discuss here only central effects, although actions of peripheral opioids (especially adrenal medullary enkephalins) have also been described. Much of the evidence comes from studies using the opioid antagonist naloxone to reverse manifestations of diverse forms of hypotensive shock (endotoxic shock, hemorrhagic shock, spinal shock) (Holaday, 1983). These experiments do not, however, identify the specific opioids involved. TRH (Holaday *et al.*, 1981), to an even greater degree than naloxone, also reverses the hypotension of shock. Clonidine, an α-adrenergic agonist which increases central β-endorphin levels (Kunos *et al.*, 1981), can reduce blood pressure of spontaneously hypertensive rats (Farsang *et al.*, 1980). The above findings may have some clinical applicability in view of a recent report in which continuous naloxone infusion reversed hypotension in a ventilator-dependent patient (Higgins *et al.*, 1983). (See Addendum 8, p. 275.)

7. *Summary*

From the foregoing, it is apparent that behavior patterns are governed by diverse peptides. The hierarchy of involvement and interrelationships between the several components affecting a given behavior remain to be determined. The possibility exists that some groups among the several peptides involved in expression of a particular behavioral pattern may represent products of a single gene family. This may become apparent with the rapid application of recombinant DNA technology to neurobiological questions. For many of the peptides described physiological function is yet to be established; for others, yet to be proposed. As further knowledge is gained about the active forms of these peptides (which may differ from their forms in other tissues) in the CNS, about details of topographical distribution, physiological regulation, and studies with specific antagonists, new understanding should be forthcoming.

B. Alterations of Brain Peptide Concentrations in CNS Disease

Changes in concentration of peptides in brain are being studied for use as possible markers in neurological diseases, in view of their ubiquity, effect on other transmitters, and reported behavioral effects. As in other neurochemical studies, it should be apparent that measurement of tissue concentrations does not reflect changes in turnover. Although still in its infancy, this field has contributed data on two major neurological diseases of unknown etiology: Alzheimer's disease (representing a degenerative disorder of the nervous system) and Huntington's disease (an autosomal dominant hereditary disorder). In Alzheimer's disease, there appears to be a decrease in concentration of somatostatin within the cerebral cortex in areas affected by the neuritic plaques and neurofibrillary tangles characteristic of this disease, as well as in mid-temporal gyrus and hippocampus. Prior to these studies, the most consistent abnormality associated with this disease was a cholinergic deficit secondary to a loss of cholineacetyl transferase (CHAT). Correlations have been found (Davies and Terry, 1981) between loss of CHAT and somatostatin in four of eight brain regions examined. The content of two other peptides with prominent cortical distribution (CCK-8 and VIP) appears to be normal (Davies and Terry, 1981; Perry *et al.*, 1981). Huntington's disease, characterized by marked neuronal loss in the basal ganglia, shows in the same region decreases in CCK-8, Substance P, and enkephalin and increased concentrations of somatostatin (Aronin *et al.*, 1983; Emson *et al.*, 1980a,b). The reduced peptide concentrations thus do not appear to represent merely neuronal loss. CCK receptor binding also is reduced in both the basal ganglia and cortex of patients with Huntington's disease, whereas it is normal in patients with Alzheimer's disease (Hays and Paul, 1982). A TRH analog has been reported to be effective in the treatment of degenerative myoconus epilepsy (Inanaga and Inoue, 1981; Matsuishi *et al.*, 1983) and in one clinical variant of congenital muscular dystrophy (Fukuyama *et al.*, 1981; Korinthenberg and Palm, 1983). There are no data on CNS-TRH content in these conditions. These findings may be compatible with the reported effect of TRH on depressing excitability of cerebral neurons (Renaud *et al.*, 1979).

Low TRH levels in CSH have been reported in patients with amyotrophic lateral sclerosis (King-Engel *et al.*, 1983), and clinical improvement (over the period of infusion) in this condition has been reported after the administration of very high intravenous doses of TRH. No data on CFS TRH levels or serum thyroid hormones during or following infusion were given.

Though not an example of CNS disease, increased plasma growth hormone concentrations have been reported in diabetic retinopathy (Hansen *et al.*, 1974), with excellent correlation between CSF and plasma concentrations, while there is a reported neural Substance P deficiency in diabetic retinopathy (Clements *et al.*, 1984). Despite the caveats re significance of CSF peptide levels (see p. 31), alterations of CSF and peripheral peptides have been reported in several neurological syndromes (see Post *et al.*, 1982 for review), no correlations of such levels with those in CNS have been reported.

Direct effects of brain peptides on CNS structures are discussed in Addendum 9 (p. 275).

IX. POSSIBLE THERAPEUTIC IMPLICATIONS OF BRAIN PEPTIDES

Given the effects of brain peptides diverse homeostatic systems affected by disease, one might expect that there are potentials for therapy with peptides in conditions characterized by malfunctioning of these systems (e.g., hypertension, obesity, anorexia, hyperpyrexia, pain, psychiatric and learning disabilities). Realization of such potential will require surmounting problems of the multiplicity of neuroactive substances involved in regulating a given system, and the multiplicity of behavioral effects of a given peptide. Analogs specific for a given effect and lasting in duration of effect must be developed (note the short half-lives of naturally occurring substances). The latter may be accomplished by designing compounds with reduced rates of peripheral degradation or with greater receptor affinity, and by use of inhibitors of degrading enzymes. Specific antagonists may be valuable in conditions caused by excessive production of peptide. The blood–brain barrier to peptide access may be circumvented by chemical modification or administration of increased amounts of peptide. Finally, since neurotransmitters and peptides may be coordinately released, and a given behavior may require coordinate expression, interactions between substances that are coreleased need be considered.

X. CONCLUSION

A number of peptides are now recognized that arise within the brain; some have been described previously in other species or outside the CNS. Mechanism(s) of action as well as the functional role within the CNS are yet to be characterized. Peptides affecting centrally on homeostatic systems appear to act in concert with other previously described neurotransmitters, as well as with other more recently characterized neuropeptides. An understanding of such interactions will add to our knowledge of the intricacy of central nervous system function. Further physiological and pharmacological studies are needed to determine the role of these peptides in health and disease, and to provide new therapeutic approaches to CNS disorders.

REFERENCES

Advis, J. P., Krause, J. W., and McKelvy, J. R. (1983). Evidence that endopeptidase-catalyzed luteinizing hormone-releasing hormone cleavage contributes to the regulation of median eminence LHRH levels during positive steroid feedback. *Endocrinology* **112**, 1147–1149.

Akil, H., Young, W., and Watson, S. J. (1981). Opiate binding properties of naturally occuring N- and C-terminus modified beta-endorphins. *Peptides* **2**, 289–292.

Amara, S. G., Jonas, V., Rosenfeld, M. G., Ong, E. S., and Evans, R. M. (1982). Alternative RNA processing in calcitonin gene expression generates mRNAs encoding different polypeptide products. *Nature (London)* **298**, 240–244.

Aronin, N., Cooper, P. E., Lorenz, L. J., Bird, E. D., Sagar, S. M., Leeman, S. E., and Martin, J. B. (1983). Somatostatin is increased in the basal ganglia in Huntington disease. *Ann. Neurol.* **13**, 519–526.

Aswad, D. W. (1978). Biosynthesis and processing of presumed neurosecretory proteins in single identified neurons of *Aplysia californica*. *J. Neurobiol.* **9**, 267–284.

Bargman, W. (1960). The neurosecretory system of the diencephalon. *Endeavor* **19**, 125–133.

Barrington, E. J. W. (1982). Evolutionary and comparative aspects of gut and brain peptides. *Br. Med. Bull.* **38**, 227–232.

Benoit, R., Ling, N., Alford, B., and Guillemin, R. (1982). Seven peptides derived from pro-somatostatin in rat brain. *Biochem. Biophys. Res. Commun.* **107**, 944–950.

Berger, P. A., Watson, S. J., Akil, H., Elliott, G. R., Rubin, R., Pfefferbaum, A., Davis, K. L., Barchas, J. D., and Li, C. J. (1980). Beta-endorphin and schizophrenia. *Arch. Gen. Psychiatry* **37**, 635–640.

Berger, P. A., Watson, S. J., Akil, H., and Barchas, J. D. (1981). The effects of naloxone in chronic schizophrenia. *Am. J. Psychiatry* **138**, 913–918.

Bernardini, G. L., Lipton, J. M., and Clark, W. G. (1983). Intracerebroventricular and septal injections of arginine vasopressin are not antipyretic in the rabbit. *Peptides* (in press).

Black, I. B. (1978). Regulation of autonomic development. *Annu. Rev. Neurosci.* **1**, 183–214.

Bloom, A. S., and Tseng, L. (1981). Effects of beta-endorphin on body temperature in mice at different ambient temperatures. *Peptides* **2**, 293–297.

Bloom, F., Segal, D., Ling, N., and Guillemin, R. (1976). Endorphins: Profound behavioral effects in rats suggest new etiological factors in mental illness. *Science* **194**, 630–632.

Bohus, B. (1979). Effects of ACTH-like neuropeptides on animal behavior and man. *Pharmacology* **18**, 113–122.

Bohus, B., Urban, I., Van Wimersma Greidanus, Tj.B., and De Wied, D. (1978). Opposite effects of oxytocin and vasopressin on avoidance behavior and hippocampal theta rhythm in the rat. *Neuropharmacology* **17**, 239–247.

Brown, M., Rivier, J., and Vale, W. (1977). Actions of bombesin, thyrotropin releasing factor, prostaglandin E_2 and naloxone on thermoregulation in the rat. *Life Sci.* **20**, 1681–1687.

Brown, M., Rivier, J., and Vale, W. (1981a). Somatostatin-28: Selective action on the pancreatic beta-cell and brain. *Endocrinology* **108**, 2391–2396.

Brown, M. R., Tache, Y., Rivier, J., and Pittman, Q. (1981b). Peptides and regulation of body temperature. *In* "Neurosecretion and Brain Peptides: Implications for Brain Functions and Neurological Disease" (J. B. Martin, S. Reichlin, and K. L. Bick, eds.), pp. 397–408. Raven, New York.

Brownstein, M. J., Russell, J. T., and Gainer, H. (1980). Synthesis, transport and release of posterior pituitary hormones. *Science* **207**, 373–378.

Chertow, B. (1981). The role of lysosomes and proteases in hormone secretion and degradation. *Endocr. Rev.* **2**, 137–173.

Civielli, O., Bernberg, N., and Herbert, E. (1982). Detection and quantitation of pro-opiomelanocortin mRNA in pituitary and brain tissues from different species. *J. Biol. Chem.* **297**, 6783–6787.

Clark, W. G., and Lipton, J. M. (1983). Brain and pituitary peptides in thermoregulation. *Pharmacol. Ther.* **22**, 249–297.

Clements, R., Leeman, S., and Aronin, N. (1984). Neural substance P (SP) deficiency in diabetic neuropathy. *In* "7th International Congress of Endocrinology Abstracts," p. 624. Elsevier, Amsterdam.

Cochard, P., Goldstein, M., and Black, I. B. (1978). Ontogenetic appearance of tyrosine hydroxylase and catecholamines in the rat embryo. *Proc. Natl. Acad. Sci. U.S.A.* **75**, 2986–2990.

Cohn, M. L., Cohn, M., and Taube, D. (1980). Thyrotropin releasing hormone induced hyperthermia in the rat inhibited by lysine acetylsalicylate and indomethacin. In "Thermoregulatory Mechanisms and Their Therapeutic Implications" (B. Cox, P. Lomax, A. S. Milton, and E. Schonbaum, eds.), pp. 198–201. Karger, Basel.

Comb, M., Seeburg, P. H., Adelman, J., Eiden, L., and Herbert, E. (1982). Primary structure of the human Met- and Leu-enkephalin precursor and its mRNA. Nature (London) 295, 663–666.

Cooper, K. E., Kasting, N. W., Lederis, K., and Veale, W. L. (1979). Evidence supporting a role for endogenous vasopressin in natural suppression of fever in the sheep. J. Physiol. (London) 295, 33–45.

Darnell, J. E., Jr. (1982). Variety in the level of gene control in eukaryotic cells. Nature (London) 297, 365–371.

Davies, P., and Terry, R. D. (1981). Cortical somatostatin-like immunoreactivity in cases of Alzheimer's disease and senile dementia of the Alzheimer type. Neurobiol. Aging 2, 9–14.

Davis, G. C., Bunney, W. E., Jr., Buchsbaum, M. S., De Fraites, E. G., Duncan, W., Gillin, J. C., van Kammen, D. P., Kleinman, J., Murphy, D. L., Post, R. M., Reus, V., and Wyatt, R. J. (1979). Use of narcotic antagonists to study the role of endorphins in normals and psychiatric patients. In "Endorphins in Mental Health Research" (E. Usdin, W. E. Bunnery, Jr., and N. S. Kline, eds.), pp. 393–406. Macmillan, New York.

Debas, H. T., Farrooq, O., and Grossman, M. I. (1975). Inhibition of gastric emptying is a physiological action of cholecystokinin. Gastroenterology 68, 1211–1217.

de Kloet, R., and de Wied, D. (1980). The brain as target tissue for hormones of pituitary origin: Behavioral and biochemical studies. In "Frontiers in Neuroendocrinology" (L. Martini and W. F. Ganong, eds.), Vol. 6, pp. 157–201. Raven, New York.

Della-Fera, M. A., Baile, C., Schneider, B. S., and Grinker, J. A. (1981). Cholecystokinin antibody injected in cerebral ventricles stimulates feeding in sheep. Science 212, 687–689.

de Wied, D. (1976). Impaired development of tolerance to morphine analgesia in rats with hereditary diabetes insipidus. Psychopharmacologica 46, 27–29.

de Wied, D. (1982). Neuropeptides and psychopathology. Eur. J. Clin. Invest. 12, 281–284.

de Wied, D., Bohus, B., van Ree, J. M., Kovacs, G. L., and Greven, H. M. (1978a). Neuroleptic-like activity of [Des-Tyr]-γ-endorphin in rats. Lancet 1, 1046 (letter).

de Wied, D., Kovacs, G. L., Van Ree, J. M., and Greven, H. M. (1978b). Neuroleptic activity of the neuropeptide beta-LPH62-77 ([Des-Tyr¹] gamma-endorphin; DT gamma E). Eur. J. Pharmacol. 49, 427–436.

Deyo, S. N., Swift, R. M., and Miller, R. J. (1979). Morphine and endorphin modulate dopamine turnover in rat median eminence. Proc. Natl. Acad. Sci. U.S.A. 76, 3006–3009.

Dockray, G. J., Vaillant, C., and Williams, R. G. (1981). New vertebrate braingut peptide related to a molluscan neuropeptide and an opioid peptide. Nature (London) 293, 656–657.

Domschke, W., Dickschas, A., and Mitznegg, P. (1979). CSF beta-endorphin in schizophrenia. Lancet 1, 1024 (letter).

Edwardson, J. A., and McDermott, J. R. (1982). Neurochemical pathology of brain peptides. Br. Med. Bull. 38, 259–264.

Elde, R. (1983). Immunocytochemistry. In "Brain Peptides" (D. T. Krieger, J. B. Martin, and M. J. Brownstein, eds.), pp. 485–494. Wiley, New York.

Emson, P. C., Arregui, A., Clement-Jones, V., Sandberg, B. E. B., and Rossor, M. (1980a).

Regional distribution of methionine-enkephalin and substances P-like immunoreactivity in normal brain and in Huntington's disease. *Brain Res.* **199,** 147–160.

Emson, P. C., Rehfeld, J. F., Langevin, H., and Rossor, M. (1980b). Reduction in cholecystokinin-like immunoreactivity in the basal ganglia in Huntington's disease. *Brain Res.* **198,** 497–500.

Evans, C. J., Lorenz, R., Weber, E., and Barchas, J. D. (1982). Variants of alpha-melanocyte stimulating hormone in rat brain and pituitary: Evidence that acetylated α-MSH exists only in the intermediate lobe of pituitary. *Biochem. Biophys. Res. Commun.* **106,** 910–919.

Farsang, Cs., Ramirez-Gonzalez, M. D., Mucci, L., and Kunos, G. (1980). Possible role of an endogenous opiate in the cardiovascular effects of central *alpha* adrenoceptor stimulation in spontaneously hypertensive rats. *J. Pharmacol. Exp. Ther.* **214,** 203–208.

Fukuyama, Y., Osawa, B., and Suzuki, H. (1981). Congenital progressive muscular dystrophy of the Fukuyama-type—Clinical, genetic and pathological considerations. *Brain Dev.* **3,** 1–29.

Gambert, S. R., Garthwaite, T. L., Pontzer, C. H., and Hagen, T. C. (1980). Fasting associated with decrease in hypothalamic β-endorphin. *Science* **210,** 1271–1272.

Ganten, D., Speck, G., Mann, J. F. E., and Unger, G. R. (1981). Role of the renin-angiotensin system in central mechanisms of blood pressure control. *In* "Frontiers in Hypertension Research" (J. H. Laragh, F. R. Beuler, and D. W. Seldin, eds.), pp. 268–273. Springer-Verlag, Berlin and New York.

Gee, C. E., Chen, C.-L.C., Roberts, J. L., Thompson, R., and Watson, S. J. (1983). Identification of POMC neurons in the rat hypothalmus by *in situ* hybridization. *Nature (London)* **306,** 374–376.

Gerner, R. H., Catlin, D. H., Gorelick, D. A., Hui, K. K., and Li, C. H. (1980). Beta-endorphin. Intravenous infusion causes behavioral change in psychiatric patients. *Arch. Gen. Psychiatry* **37,** 642–647.

Gibbs, J., Young, R. C., and Smith, G. P. (1973). Cholecystokinin elicits satiety in rats with open gastric fistulas. *Nature (London)* **245,** 323–325.

Gibson, M. J., Liotta, A. S., and Krieger, D. T. (1981). The Zucker fa/fa rat: Absent circadian corticosterone periodicity and elevated β-endorphin concentrations in brain and intermediate lobe. *Neuropeptides* **1,** 349–362.

Glyn-Ballinger, J. R., Bernardini, G. L., and Lipton, J. M. (1983). α-MSH injected into the septal region reduces fever in rabbits. *Peptides* (in press).

Grandison, L., and Guidotti, A. (1977). Stimulation of food intake by muscimol and beta endorphin. *Neuropharmacology* **161,** 533–536.

Gubler, U., Seeburg, P., Hoffman, B. J., Gage, L. P., and Udenfriend, S. (1982). Molecular cloning established proenkephalin as precursor of enkephalin-containing peptides. *Nature (London)* **295,** 306–308.

Hanegan, J. L., and Williams, B. A., (1973). Brain calcium: Role in temperature regulation. *Science* **181,** 663–664.

Hansen, A. P., Soenksen, P. H., and Knopf, R. F. (1974). *In* "Hormone de Croissance (5e Symposium de Megeve, 8–10 mars) (Synthese du 83 Congres de la Federation Internationale due Diabete, Bruxelles, juillet 1973)," (J. M. Brogard, ed.), pp. 153–155. International Diabetes Federations, Geneva.

Hayes, S. E., and Paul, S. M. (1981). Cholecystokinin receptors are increased in cerebral cortex of genetically obese rodents. *Eur. J. Pharmacol.* **70,** 591–592.

Hayes, S. E., and Paul, S. M. (1982). CCK receptors and human neurological disease. *Life Sci.* **31,** 319–322.

Hedlund, B., Abens, J., and Bartfai, T. (1983). Vasoactive intestinal polypeptide and muscarinic receptors: Supersensitivity induced by long-term atropine treatment. *Science* **220**, 519–521.

Higgins, T. L., Sivak, E. D., O'Neil, D. M., Graves, J. W., and Foutch, D. G. (1983). Reversal of hypotension by continuous naloxone infusion in a ventilator-dependent patient. *Ann. Intern. Med.* **98**, 47–48.

Hofmann, K. (1974). Relations between chemical structure and function of adrenocorticotropin and melanocyte-stimulating hormones. *Handb. Physiol. Sect. 7: Endocrinol.* **4**, 28–58.

Hokfelt, T., Johansson, O., Ljungdahl, A., Lundberg, J. M., and Schultzberg, M. (1980). Peptidergic neurones. *Nature (London)* **284**, 515–521.

Holaday, J. W. (1983). Cardiovascular consequences of endogenous opiate antagonism. *Biochem. Pharmacol.* **32**, 575–585.

Holaday, J. W., Tseng, L.-F., Loh, H. H., and Li, C. H. (1977). Thyrotropin releasing hormone antagonizes β-endorphin hypothermia and catalepsy. *Life Sci.* **22**, 1537–1543.

Holaday, J. W., Loh, H., and Li, C. H. (1978a). Unique behavioral effects of beta endorphin and their relationship to thermoregulation and hypothalamic function. *Life Sci.* **22**, 1525–1536.

Holaday, J. W., Wei, E., Loh, H., and Li, C. H. (1978b). Endorphins may function in heat adaptation. *Proc. Natl. Acad. Sci. U.S.A.* **75**, 2923–2927.

Holaday, J. W., D'Amato, R. J., and Faden, A. I. (1981). Thyrotropin-releasing hormone improves cardiovascular function in experimental endotoxic and hemorrhagic shock. *Science* **213**, 216–218.

Hollt, V. (1983). Multiple endogenous opioid peptides. *Trends Neurosci.* **6**, 24–26.

Hood, L., Campbell, J. H., and Elgin, S. C. R. (1975). The organization and expression in evolution of antibody genes and other multigene families. *Annu. Rev. Genet.* **9**, 305–353.

Huidobro-Toro, J. P., and Way, E. L. (1979). Studies on the hyperthermic response of beta-endorphin in mice. *J. Pharmacol. Exp. Ther.* **211**, 50–58.

Iversen, L. L., Lee, C. M., Gilbert, R. F., Hunt, S., and Emson, P. C. (1980). Regulation of neuropeptide release. *Proc. R. Soc. London Ser. B* **210**, 91–111.

Jackson, I., and Reichlin, S. (1974). Thyrotropin-releasing hormone (TRH): Distribution in hypothalamic and extrahypothalamic brain tissues of mammalian and submammalian chordata. *Endocrinology* **95**, 854–862.

Jacquet, Y. F., and Marks, N. (1976). The C-fragment of β-lipotropin: An endogenous neuroleptic or antipsychotogen. *Science* **194**, 632–634.

Jan, L. Y., and Jan, Y. N. (1981). Role of an LHRH-like peptide as a neurotransmitter in sympathetic ganglia of the frog. *Fed. Proc., Fed. Am. Soc. Exp. Biol.* **40**, 2560–2564.

Jessel, T. M. (1983). Neuropeptide function in neurons that transmit and regulate nociceptive information. *In* "Brain Peptides" (D. T. Krieger, J. D. Martin, and M. J. Brownstein, eds.), pp. 315–332. Wiley, New York.

Kadar, T., Feketa, M., Balazs, M., and Telegdy, G. (1981). Influence of intracerebroventricular administration of TRH and TRH antiserum on dopamine, norepinephrine and serotonin contents of different brain structures in rats. *In* "Advances in Physiological Science, Vol. 14. Endocrinology Neuroendocrinology, Neuropeptides-II" (E. Stark, G. B. Makara, B. Halasz, and G. Rappay, eds.), pp. 259–263. Pergamon, Oxford.

Kakidani, H., Furutani, Y., Takahashi, H., Noda, M., Morimoto, Y., Hirose, T. Asaia, M., Inayama, S., Nakanishi, S., and Numa, S. (1982). Cloning and sequence analysis of cDNA for porcine β-neo-endirphin/dynorphin precursor. *Nature (London)* **298**, 245–249.

King-Engel, W., Siddique, T., and Nicoloff, J. T. (1983). Effect on weakness and spasticity in amyotrophic lateral sclerosis of thyrotropin-releasing hormone. *Lancet* II, 73–75.

Koob, G., and Bloom, F. E. (1983). Memory, learning, and adaptive behaviors. *In* "Brain Peptides" (D. T. Krieger, J. B. Martin, and M. J. Brownstein, eds.), pp. 369–388. Wiley, New York.

Koob, G. F., LeMoal, M., and Bloom, R. D. (1981). Enkephalin and endorphin influences on appetite and adversive conditioning. *In* "Endogenous Peptides and Learning and Memory Processes" (J. L. Martinez, R. A. Jensen, R. B. Messing, H. Ricter, and J. L. McGaugh, eds.), pp. 249–267. Academic Press, New York.

Korinthenberg, R., and Palm, D. (1983). Congenital muscular dystrophy. *Brain Dev.* 5, 429 (letter).

Krieger, D. T. (1983a). The multiple faces of pro-opiomelanocortin, a prototype precursor molecule. *Clin. Res.* 31, 342–353.

Krieger, D. T. (1983b). Brain peptides: What, where, and why? *Science* 222, 975–985.

Kuffler, S. W. (1980). Slow synaptic responses in autonomic ganglia and the pursuit of a peptidergic transmitter. *J. Exp. Biol.* 89, 257–276.

Kunos, G., Fasang, Cs., and Ramirez-Gonzalez, M. D. (1981). β-endorphin: Possible involvement in the antihypertensive effects of central α-receptor activation. *Science* 211, 82–84.

Land, H., Schutz, G., Schmale, H., and Richter, D. (1982). Nucleotide sequence of cloned cDNA encoding bovine arginine vasopressin-neurophysin II precursor. *Nature (London)* 295, 299–303.

Lechan, R. M., Goodman, R. H., Rosenblatt, M., Reichlin, S., and Habener, J. F. (1983). Prosomatostatin-specific antigen in rat brain: Localization by immunocytochemical staining with an antiserum to a synthetic sequence of preprosomatostatin. *Proc. Natl. Acad. Sci. U.S.A.* 80, 2780–2784.

Le Douarin, N. M. (1980). The ontogeny of the neural crest in avian embryo chimaeras. *Nature (London)* 286, 663–669.

Legros, J. J., Gilot, P., Seron, X., Claessens, J., Adam, A., Moeglen, J. M., Audibert, A., and Berchier, B. (1978). Influence of vasopressin on learning and memory. *Lancet* 1, 41–42.

LeRoith, D., Shiloach, J., and Roth, J. (1982). Is there an earlier phylogenetic precursor that is common to both the nervous and endocrine systems? *Peptides* 3, 211–215.

LeRoith, D., Shiloach, J., Berlowitz, M., Frohman, L. A., Liotta, A. S., Krieger, D. T., and Roth, J. (1983). Are messenger molecules in microbes the ancestors of the vertebrate hormones and tissue factors? *Fed. Proc., Fed. Am. Soc. Exp. Biol.* 42, 2602–2607.

Liotta, A. S., Loudes, C., McKelvy, J. F., and Krieger, D. T. (1980). Biosynthesis of precursor corticotropin/endorphin, corticotropin, α-melanotropin, β-lipotropin, and β-endorphin-like material by cultured neonatal rat hypothalamic neurons. *Proc. Natl. Acad. Sci. U.S.A.* 77, 1880–1884.

Liotta, A. S., Advis, J. P., Krause, J. E., McKelvy, J. F., and Krieger, D. T. (1984). Demonstration of *in vivo* synthesis of pro-opiomelanocortin-, β-endorphin-, and α-MSH-like species in the adult rat brain. *J. Neurosci.* 4, 956–965.

Loh, Y. P., and Parish, D. (1984). Proteolytic processing of pituitary prohormones by unique Lys-Arg specific converting enzymes. *In* "7th International Congress of Endocrinology Abstracts," p. 86. Elsevier, Amsterdam.

Lundberg, J. M. (1981). Evidence for coexistence of vasoactive intestinal polypeptide (VIP) and acetylcholine in neurons of rat exocrine glands. Morphological, biochemical, and functional studies. *Acta Physiol. Scand. (Suppl.)* 496, 1–57.

Lundberg, J. M., Hedlund, B., and Bartfai, T. (1982). Vasoactive intestinal polypeptide enhances muscarinic ligand binding in cat submandibular salivary gland. *Nature (London)* 295, 147–149.

McCann, S. M. (1980). Control of anterior pituitary hormone release by brain peptides. *Neuroendocrinology* 31, 355–363.

Mains, R. E., Eipper, B. A., and Ling, N. (1977). Common precursor to corticotropins and endorphins. *Proc. Natl. Acad. Sci. U.S.A.* **74**, 3014–3018.

Matsuishi, T., Yano, E., Inanaga, K., Terasawa, K., Ishihara, O., Shiotsuki, Y., Katafuchi, Y., Aoki, N., and Yamashita, F. (1983). A pilot study on the anticonvulsive effects of a thyrotropin-releasing hormone analog in intractable epilepsy. *Brain Dev.* **5**, 421–428.

Messing, R. B., Jensen, R., Vasquez, J., Martinez, J. L., Spiehler, V. R., and McGaugh, J. L. (1981). Opiate modulation of memory. *In* "Endogenous Peptides and Learning and Memory Processes" (J. L. Martinez, R. A. Jensen, R. B. Messing, H. Rigter, and J. L. McGaugh, eds.), pp. 431–444. Academic Press, New York.

Meyers, C. A., Murphy, W. A., Redding, T. W., Coy, D. H., and Schally, A. V. (1980). Synthesis and biological actions of prosomatostatin. *Proc. Natl. Acad. Sci. U.S.A.* **77**, 6171–6174.

Moran, T. H., and McHugh, P. R. (1982). Cholecystokinin supresses food intake by inhibiting gastric emptying. *Am. J. Physiol.* **242**, R491–R497.

Moroni, F., Cheney, D. L., and Costa, E. (1977). Inhibition of acetylcholine turnover in rat hippocampus by intraseptal injections of β-endorphin and morphine. *Arch. Pharmacol.* **299**, 149–153.

Morrison, J. H., Benoit, R., Magistretti, P. J., and Bloom, F. E. (1983). Immunohistochemical distribution of pro-somatostatin-related peptides in cerebral cortex. *Brain Res.* **262**, 344–351.

Mudge, A. W. (1981). Effect of chemical environment on levels of substance P and somatostatin in cultures sensory neurones. *Nature (London)* **292**, 764–767.

Murphy, M. T., and Lipton, M. J. (1982). Peripheral administration of α-MSH reduces fever in older and younger rabbits. *Peptides* **3**, 775–779.

Myers, R. D., and Tytell, M. (1982). Fever: Reciprocal shift in brain sodium to calcium ratio as the set-point temperature rises. *Science* **178**, 765–767.

Nakanishi, S., Inoue, A., Kita, T., Nakamura, M., Chang, A. C. Y., Cohen, S. N., and Numa, S. (1979). Nucleotide sequence of cloned cDNA for bovine corticotropin-β-lipotropin precursor. *Nature (London)* **278**, 423–427.

Noda, M., Furutani, Y., Takahashi, H., Toyosato, M., Hirose, T., Inayama, S., Nakanishi, S., and Numa, S. (1982). Cloning and sequence analysis of cDNA for bovine adrenal preproenkephalin. *Nature (London)* **295**, 202–206.

Oliveros, J. C., Jandali, M. K., Timsit-Berthier, M., Remy, R., Bengheazi, A., Audibert, A., and Moegland, M. J. (1978). Vasopressin in amnesia. *Lancet* **1**, 42 (letter).

Orlowski, H., and Wilk, S. (1981). A multicatalytical protease complex from pituitary that forms enkephalin and enkephalin-containing peptides. *Biochem. Biophys. Res. Commun.* **101**, 814–822.

Palay, S. L. (1945). Preoptico-hypophyseal pathway in fish. *J. Comp. Neurol.* **82**, 129–144.

Palkovits, M. (1983). Neuroanatomical techniques. *In* "Brain Peptides" (D. T. Krieger, J. B. Martin, and M. J. Brownstein, eds.), pp. 495–546. Wiley, New York.

Patterson, P. H., and Chun, L. L. Y. (1977). The induction of acetylcholine synthesis in primary cultures of dissociated rat sympathetic neuron S. I. Effects of conditioned medium. *Dev. Biol.* **56**, 263–280.

Pecile, A., Guidobono, F., Sibilia, V., and Netti, C. (1984). Calcitonin: A candidate for a neuromodulator of multiple pain inhibiting systems. *In* "7th International Congress of Endocrinology Abstracts," p. 202. Elsevier, Amsterdam.

Pelletier, T., Steinbusch, W. M., and Verhofstad, A. A. J. (1981). Immunoreactive substance P and serotonin present in the same dense-core vesicles. *Nature (London)* **293**, 71–72.

Perry, R. J., Dockray, G. J., Dimaline, E. R., Perry, E. K., Blessed, G., and Tomlinson, B. E. (1981). Neuropeptides in Alzheimer's disease, depression, and schizophrenia. A post mortem analysis of vasoactive intestinal peptide and cholecystokinin in cerebral cortex. *J. Neurol. Sci.* **51,** 465–472.

Pickar, D., Davis, G. C., Schulz, C., Extein, I., Wagner, R., Naber, D., Gold, P. W., van Kammen, D. P., Goodwin, F. K., Wyatt, R. J., Li, C. H., and Bunney, W. E., Jr. (1981). Behavioral and biological effects of acute beta-endorphin injection in schizophrenic and depressed patients. *Am. J. Psychiatry* **138,** 160–166.

Pi-Sunyer, X., Kissileff, H. R., Thornton, J., and Smith, G. P. (1982). C-terminal octapeptide of cholecystokinin decreases food intake in obese men. *Physiol. Behav.* **29,** 627–630.

Pontremoli, S., Melloni, E., Salamino, F., Sparatore, B., Michetti, M., and Horecker, B. L. (1983). Endogenous inhibitors of lysosomal proteinases. *Proc. Natl. Acad. Sci. U.S.A.* **80,** 1261–1264.

Post, R. M., Gold, P., Rubinow, D. R., Ballenger, J. C., Bunney, W. E., Jr., and Goodwin, F. K. (1982). Peptides in the cerebrospinal fluid of neuropsychiatric patients: An approach to central nervous system peptide function. *Life Sci.* **31,** 1–15.

Prange, A. J., Nemeroff, C. B., Lipton, M. A., Breese, G. R., and Wilson, I. C. (1978). Peptides in the central nervous system. *Handb. Psychopharmacol.* **13,** 1–107.

Prasad, C., Jacobs, J. J., and Wilber, J. F. (1980). Immunological blockade of endogenous thyrotropin-releasing hormone produces hypothermic in rats. *Brain Res.* **193,** 580–583.

Renaud, L. P., Blume, H. W., Pittman, Q. J., Lamour, Y., and Tan, A. T. (1979). Thyrotropin-releasing hormone selectively depresses glutamate excitation of cerebral cortical neurons. *Science* **205,** 1275–1277.

Richter, K., Kawashima, E., Egger, R., and Kreil, G. (1984). Bioxynthesis of thyrotropin releasing hormone in the skin of *Xenopus laevis:* Partial sequence of the precursor deduced from cloned cDNA. *EMBO J.* **3,** 617–621.

Robbins, R. J., Mothon, S., and Reichlin, S. (1983). Somatostatin-28 is not the precursor of somatostatin-14 in cerebral cortical cells. *Proc. Endocr. Soc. Meet.* p. 85, #19. (Abstr.)

Robertson, M. (1982). Gene rearrangement and the generation of diversity. *Nature (London)* **297,** 184–186.

Russell, J. T., Brownstein, M. J., and Gainer, H. (1981). Biosynthesis of neurohypophyseal polypeptides: The order of peptide components in pro-pressophysin and pro-oxyphysin. *Neuropeptides* **2,** 59–65.

Sachs, H., and Takabatake, Y. (1964). Evidence for a precursor in vasopressin biosynthesis. *Endocrinology* **75,** 943–948.

Saito, A., Williams, J. A., and Goldfine, I. D. (1981). Alterations in brain cholecystokinin receptors after fasting. *Nature (London)* **289,** 599–600.

Samson, W. K., Lipton, M. J., Zimmer, J. A., and Glynn, J. R. (1981). The effect of fever on central α-MSH concentration in the rabbit. *Peptides* **2,** 419–423.

Sandman, C. A., George, J., Walker, B. B., Nolan, J. D., and Kastin, A. J. (1976). Neuropeptide MSH–ACTH 4-10 enhances attention in the mentally retarded. *Pharmacol. Biochem. Behav.* **5** (Suppl. 1), 23–28.

Scharrer, E., and Scharrer, B. (1940). Secretory cells within the hypothalamus. *Proc. Assoc. Res. Nerv. Ment. Dis.* **20,** 170–194.

Scheller, R. H., Jackson, J. F., McAllister, L. B., Schwartz, J. H., Kandel, E. R., and Axel, R. (1982). A family of genes that codes for ELH, a neuropeptide eliciting a stereotyped pattern of behavior in Aplysia. *Cell* **28,** 707–719.

Scheller, R. H., Jackson, J. F., McAllister, L. B., Rothman, B. S., Mayeri, E., and Axel, R. (1983). A single gene encodes multiple neuropeptides mediating a stereotyped behavior. *Cell* **32,** 7–22.

Schiller, P., Lipton, A., Horrobin, D. G., and Bodansky, M. (1978). Unsulfated C-terminal 7-peptide of cholecystokinin: A new ligand of the opiate receptor. *Biochem. Biophys. Res. Commun.* **4,** 1332–1338.

Schippe, J., and Tilders, F. (1983). A new technique for studying specificity of immunocytochemical procedures: Specificity of serotonin immunostaining. *J. Histochem. Cytochem.* **31**, 12–18.

Schmale, H., Heinsohn, S., and Richter, D. (1983). Structural organization of the rat gene for the arginine vasopressin-neurophysin precursor. *EMBO J.* **2**, 763–767.

Schneider, B. S., Monahan, J. W., and Hirsch, J. (1979). Brain cholecystokinin and nutritional status in rats and mice. *J. Clin. Invest.* **64**, 1348–1356.

Schwartz, J. P., Malfroy, B., and De La Baume, S. (1981). Biological inactivation of enkephalins and the role of enkephalin-dipeptidyl-carboxypeptidase ("enkephalinase") as neuropeptides. *Life Sci.* **29**, 1715–1740.

Smith, G. P., Jerome, C., Cushing, B., Eterno, R., and Simansky, K. J. (1981). Abdominal vagotomy blocks satiety effects of cholecystokinin in rats. *Science* **213**, 136–137.

Snyder, S. J. (1980). Brain peptides as neurotransmitters. *Science* **209**, 976–983.

Tamminga, C. A., Tighe, P. J., Chase, T. N., De Fraites, E. G., and Schaffer, M. H. (1981). Des-tyrosine-γ-endorphin administration in chronic schizophrenics. A preliminary report. *Arch. Gen. Psychiatry* **38**, 167–168.

Tatemoto, K., and Mutt, V. (1978). Chemical determination of polypeptide hormones. *Proc. Natl. Acad. Sci. U.S.A.* **75**, 4115–4119.

Tatemoto, K., Carlquist, M., and Mutt, V. (1982). Neuropeptide Y: A novel brain peptide with structural similarity to peptide Yy and pancreatic polypeptide. *Nature (London)* **296**, 659–660.

Teitelman, G. (1981). Transformation of catecholaminergic precursors into glucagon (A) cells in mouse embryonic pancreas. *Proc. Natl. Acad. Sci. U.S.A.* **78**, 5225–5229.

Teitelman, G., Joh, T. H., and Reis, D. J. (1982). APUD cells of mouse embryonic pancreas originate from catecholamine precursors. *Proc. Endocr. Soc. Meet.* p. 331, #1108. (Abstr.)

Terenius, L. (1975). Effects of peptides and amino acids on dihydromorphine beingin to the opiate receptors. *J. Pharm. Pharmacol.* **27**, 450–452.

Terenius, L., Wahlstrom, A., Lindstrom, L., and Widerlove, E. (1976). Increased CSF levels of endorphins in chronic psychosis. *Neurosci. Lett.* **3**, 157–162.

Van Loon, G. R., and De Souza, E. B. (1978). Effects of β-endorphin on brain serotonin metabolism. *Life Sci.* **23**, 971–978.

Van Wimersma Greidanus, Tj. B., Bohus, B., and de Wied, D. (1975a). The role of vasopressin in memory processes. *Prog. Brain Res.* **42**, 135–141.

Van Wimersma Greidanus, Tj. B., Dogterom, J., and de Wied, D. (1975b). Intraventricular administration of anti-vasopressin serum inhibits memory consolidation in rats. *Life Sci.* **16**, 637–643.

Veale, W. L., Kasting, N. W., and Cooper, K. E. (1981). Arginine vasopressin and endogenous antipyresis: Evidence and significance. *Fed. Proc., Fed. Am. Soc. Exp. Biol.* **20**, 2750–2753.

Wallace, M. M., Bodnar, R. J., Badillo-Martinez, D., Nilaver, G., and Zimmerman, E. A. (1981). Role of neuropeptides in nociceptive processes. *Proc. Soc. Neurosci. Meet.* p. 167, #57.9. (Abstr.)

Weber, E., Evans, C. J., and Barchas, J. D. (1981). Acetylated and nonacetylated forms of beta-endorphin in rat brain and pituitary. *Biochem. Biophys. Res. Commun.* **103**, 982–989.

Weingartner, H., Gold, P., Ballenger, J. C., Smallberg, S. A., Summers, R., Robinow, D. R., Post, R. M., and Goodwin, F. K. (1981). Effects of vasopressin on human memory functions. *Science* **211**, 601–603.

Zingg, H. H., and Patel, Y. C. (1982). Biosynthesis of immunoreactive somatostatin by hypothalamic neurons in culture. *J. Clin. Invest.* **70**, 1001–1009.

Intracellular Mediators of Insulin Action

LEONARD JARETT

Department of Pathology and Laboratory Medicine,
University of Pennsylvania School of Medicine,
Philadelphia, Pennsylvania

FREDERICK L. KIECHLE

Department of Clinical Pathology,
William Beaumont Hospital,
Royal Oak, Michigan

I.	Introduction	51
II.	Subcellular Systems	52
	A. Adipocyte Plasma Membranes and Mitochondria	52
	B. Other Insulin-Sensitive Membrane Systems	55
	C. Other Ligand-Sensitive Membrane Systems	58
III.	Whole Cell and Tissue Studies	60
IV.	Number of Mediators	61
V.	Insulin-Sensitive Enzymes	64
VI.	Physical and Chemical Characteristics of the Mediator	68
VII.	Conclusion	71
	References	72

I. INTRODUCTION

The mechanism of insulin action has been the subject of intensive investigation since the discovery of insulin just over 60 years ago. This quest for fundamental knowledge reflects the importance of diabetes mellitus, one of today's most common and devastating diseases and its control by insulin, a hormone essential for life. Research has led to a general understanding of the action of insulin at the physiological and biochemical levels. Muscle, liver, and adipose tissues are the major target tissues for insulin, although other cells in the body are insulin sensitive. Insulin is the key anabolic hormone regulating the metabolism of carbohydrates, lipids, and proteins. This regulation is brought about by changes in membrane events that occur in seconds, intracellular processes that occur in minutes, and nuclear functions involved in growth that occur in hours. The initial event effecting these metabolic alterations is the interaction of insulin with its receptor on the plasma membrane of responsive cells. Yet the molecular events subsequent to hormone–receptor interaction causing the metabolic alterations are unknown. Several compounds have been proposed as second messengers or intracellular mediators of insulin action; these include cyclic nucleotides, calcium, a fragment of insulin, hydrogen peroxide, and others. None of these substances has proven to be involved. This overall subject has been reviewed extensively (Czech, 1977, 1981; Denton *et al.*, 1981; Goldfine, 1981; Kahn, 1979; Levine, 1982; Smith and Rosen, 1983; Walaas and Horn, 1981).

The interaction of insulin with its receptor may effect rapid generation of a signal or a second messenger system that leads to subsequent reactions. An insulin-sensitive, membrane-associated regulatory process must link this hormone–receptor interaction and the effector system. Therefore, direct effects of insulin should be observable experimentally with subcellular preparations of plasma membranes containing the components and organization necessary for hormone action. Such a plasma membrane preparation, developed in this laboratory, responds to the direct addition of insulin. In this subcellular system direct interaction of insulin with its receptor leads to the generation from the plasma membrane of a new family of mediators potentially accounting for many of the effects of the hormone on diverse metabolic pathways. In this article we review the discovery of these mediators, how they were established as mediators, and what is known of the characteristics and chemical properties of the mediators. Finally, future directions for the field will be discussed. A number of reviews on several aspects of the insulin mediator have been published (Jarett *et al.*, 1981, 1983a,b; Larner, 1982, 1983; Larner *et al.*, 1982a,b; Seals and Czech, 1982).

II. Subcellular Systems

A. Adipocyte Plasma Membranes and Mitochondria

A highly enriched preparation of adipocyte plasma membranes was developed in this laboratory (Jarett, 1974) for the purpose of studying the effects of insulin and other hormones directly on membrane phenomena. Jarett and Smith (1974) showed that the addition of concanavalin A, an insulin-mimetic lectin, and of physiological concentrations of insulin to this plasma membrane preparation rapidly increased the hydrolysis of adenosine triphosphate (ATP) as measured by the release of inorganic phosphate. These data suggested that insulin or concanavalin A activated an Mg^{2+}-ATPase on the plasma membrane in this subcellular system. Since alterations in phosphorylation of proteins are important early events in the regulatory mechanisms involved in metabolic pathways (Krebs and Beavo, 1979) and since insulin is known to alter phosphorylation of adipocyte proteins (Smith and Rosen, 1983), the effect of insulin on phosphorylation of this subcellular plasma membrane preparation from adipocytes was studied.

To study the effect of insulin on membrane phosphorylation, the plasma membrane preparation was modified slightly by omission of ethylenediaminetetraacetic acid (EDTA) during homogenization and fractionation. These studies showed that the addition of physiological concentrations of insulin to this subcellular preparation generated a material from the plasma membrane which dephosphorylated the α-subunit of mitochondrial pyruvate dehydrogenase (PDH) and activated the enzyme. The similarity of this *in vitro* effect to the *in vivo* effect of insulin on this enzyme system (Denton and Hughes, 1978) suggested that the material generated from the plasma membrane could be the putative mediator or second messenger of insulin action.

In the first study (Seals *et al.*, 1978) of this series, [γ-^{32}P]ATP was used to label the plasma membrane preparation with or without insulin. Insulin added directly to the assay mixture containing 50 μM Ca^{2+} and 50 μM Mg^{2+} decreased phosphorylation throughout the incubation from 30 seconds to 10 minutes. The insulin effect was concentration dependent and specific. This direct effect of insulin on the autophosphorylation of plasma membranes was characterized further by electrophoretic analysis of the phosphorylated membrane preparation (Seals *et al.*, 1979a,b). Under the low ionic conditions used (50 μM Mg^{2+} and 50 μM Ca^{2+}), two major and three minor bands of phosphorylation were observed, the major bands being phosphoester phosphoproteins of molecular weight 42,000 and 120,000. Incubations and phosphorylation of the membranes with 5 mM Mg^{2+} increased the number of bands identified to 14 and the magnitude of phosphorylation of the new bands was greater than with the lower Mg^{2+} concentration, actually obscuring some of the phosphorylated bands found under the lower Mg^{2+} concentrations. The phosphorylated bands found in the 5 mM Mg^{2+} condition were similar to those reported by other laboratories (Avruch *et al.*, 1976; Benjamin and Clayton, 1978). Phosphorylated plasma membranes were prepared as well from adipocytes incubated with ^{32}P and compared to the isolated plasma membrane preparations. Some but not all of the bands found in incubations with 50 mM Mg^{2+} were detected. The whole cell patterns resembled those reported by Belsham *et al.* (1980).

In the adipocyte plasma membrane subcellular system using the low Mg^{2+} concentration, insulin rapidly decreased the phosphorylation of the 120,000- and 42,000-Da phosphoproteins. The former was a plasma membrane component and its identity is still unknown. At one stage it was believed that this band was related to the insulin-sensitive Ca^{2+},Mg^{2+}-ATPase identified in adipocyte plasma membranes by Pershadsingh and McDonald (1979). Recent studies have associated the enzyme with a 110,000-Da calcium-sensitive phosphoprotein which contains a rapidly turning over acyl-linkage phosphate bond (Chan and McDonald, 1982), thereby distinguishing it from the 120,000-Da phosphoester phosphoprotein described by Seals *et al.* (1979a,b). The insulin-sensitive phosphoprotein of 42,000 molecular weight proved to be the α-subunit of PDH contained in the mitochondria and contaminating the plasma membrane preparation by 3–10%. Insulin did not affect the phosphorylation of the α-subunit when added directly to purified mitochondrial preparations. The insulin effect, however, was restored upon addition of adipocyte plasma membranes to mitochondria, suggesting that insulin stimulated the generation of a mediator from the plasma membrane that dephosphorylated the α-subunit of PDH in the mitochondria.

Activation of PDH develops upon dephosphorylation of the α-subunit and this enzyme apparently is activated by insulin *in vivo* by this same mechanism (Denton and Hughes, 1978). This suggests that the effect of insulin on the phosphorylated state of the PDH α-subunit in the subcellular system causes concomitant activation of the enzyme system. A subsequent study by Seals and Jarett (1980) showed this to be so. Insulin in a concentration-dependent manner stimulated PDH activity in the subcellular mixture of plasma membrane and mitochondria reaching a maximum stimulation by 50–100 μU/ml. Moreover, concanavalin A and anti-insulin receptor antibody, both insulin-mimetic agents, rapidly stimulated PDH activity when added to the same subcellular mixture of adipocyte plasma membranes and mitochondria. None of these ligands added to mitochondria alone affected PDH activity; thus ligand–plasma membrane interaction is required for generation of the mediator. This study indicated that the mediator was not a piece of the insulin molecule.

At the time these studies with the subcellular system were reported, Larner *et al.* (1979) isolated a low-molecular-weight (1000–1500), acid-stable mediator generated by insulin in rabbit skeletal muscle. This mediator stimulated glycogen synthase by activating glycogen synthase phosphoprotein phosphatase and inhibiting cyclic adenosine 3′,5′-monophosphate (cAMP)-dependent protein kinase. Jarett and

Seals (1979) showed that this material isolated from insulin-treated muscle stimulated PDH in adipocyte mitochondria greater than material from control muscle. The activation of PDH was analogous to the stimulation produced by insulin added to a plasma membrane–mitochondrial mixture suggesting that the insulin-sensitive mediator from adipocyte plasma membrane was similar, if not identical, to the muscle mediator.

The mediator generated from adipocyte plasma membranes was further characterized by two laboratories. In each, the mediator was obtained in a supernatant fraction after centrifugation of plasma membranes in a microfuge. The mediator activity in the supernatant was detected by its ability to stimulate PDH in isolated mitochondria. Seals and Czech (1980) found that insulin increased the amount of mediator compared to control in the supernatant of adipocyte plasma membranes prepared in phosphate buffer. Kiechle et al. (1981) showed that the mediator could be released spontaneously from the plasma membrane without insulin treatment of the membrane. The amount of mediator released spontaneously from the plasma membranes depended on the buffer used to prepare the membranes: Tris–EDTA > Tris alone > phosphate. Insulin stimulation of mediator release was observed only with plasma membranes prepared in phosphate buffer. Regardless of the technique used to prepare the plasma membranes, the final resuspension of membranes prior to study was in phosphate buffer, pH 7.4. The mediator could be depleted from the plasma membranes by repeated centrifugation and washes with phosphate buffer. The supernatant mediator was stable at pH 7.0 and produced linear response curves. In another study Seals and Czech (1981) showed that maximal supernatant activity from insulin treatment was obtained with 100 μU/ml of insulin after 1 minute of treatment of the membranes.

B. Other Insulin-Sensitive Membrane Systems

In Table I are summarized several plasma membrane preparations used to prepare the mediator upon insulin treatment. The adipocyte membrane system has been discussed. Jarett and Kiechle (1981) found that liver plasma membranes would spontaneously release a low-molecular-weight mediator which stimulated PDH in adipocyte and liver mitochondria. The adipocyte mediator was equally effective on liver mitochondrial PDH. Saltiel et al. (1981) reported that insulin treatment of liver plasma membranes increased the amount of mediator as measured by PDH assay with adipocyte or liver mitochondria. Re-

TABLE I

PLASMA MEMBRANE SYSTEMS REPORTED TO PRODUCE INSULIN MEDIATOR AND
CONDITIONS ALTERING MEDIATOR PRODUCTION

Membrane	Condition	Stimulus for mediator production
Adipocyte[a] (rat)	Normal	Insulin, anti-insulin receptor antibody, concanavalin A
	High carbohydrate diet	Insulin
	High fat diet	Not responsive
Liver[b] (rat)	Normal	Insulin, anti-insulin receptor antibody
	High carbohydrate diet	Insulin
	High fat diet	Not responsive
	Diabetes	Not responsive
	Diabetes treated	Insulin
	Fasting	Not responsive
	Fasting–refed	Insulin
Placenta[c] (human)	Normal	Insulin

[a]Begum et al. (1982a,b, 1983b), Jarett and Kiechle (1981), Jarett et al. (1981), Kiechle et al. (1981), Popp et al. (1980), Seals and Czech (1980, 1981), Seals and Jarett (1980), and Seals et al. (1978, 1979a,b).

[b]Amatruda and Chang (1983), Begum et al. (1983a,b), Jarett and Kiechle (1981), and Saltiel et al. (1981, 1982, 1983).

[c]Sakamato et al. (1982).

cently, Sakamoto et al. (1982) found that insulin treatment of human placental plasma membranes produced a low-molecular-weight factor that activated PDH in adipocyte and liver mitochondria.

A series of reports indicates that the physiological state of the animal influences the production of mediator from the membranes by insulin. Begum et al. (1982a,b, 1983a) have shown that diet affects the insulin-dependent generation of the mediator from adipocyte and liver plasma membranes. A high carbohydrate diet did not affect insulin or concanavalin A-induced generation of the mediator from either membrane source, whereas a high fat diet prevented insulin and concanavalin A stimulation of mediator production. It is not clear whether this effect of high fat diet is due to decreased insulin binding to the membranes or a true defect in the ability of the membranes to produce the mediator. Amatruda and Chang (1983) showed that hepatocyte plasma membranes from diabetic or fasted animals released no mediator of PDH activity after insulin stimulation. Treatment of the diabetic rat or refeeding the fasted animal restored the ability of insulin to stimulate mediator release. The binding of insulin to hepatocyte membranes was normal to increased in these altered states. These data support the concept that alterations at or near the plasma membrane can be responsible for or accompany the insulin resistance of liver of fasting or diabetic rats.

An exciting new approach for studying the insulin mediator has been reported by Zhang et al. (1983). This group has shown that mediator generated by insulin from adipocyte plasma membranes as described by Kiechle et al. (1981) can be added to isolated adipocytes and mimic insulin action. The mediator lowered hormonally elevated cAMP levels, stimulated lipogenesis, and inhibited hormonally induced lipolysis. The adipocyte is permeable, therefore, to the mediators and these findings add to the list of insulin-sensitive, physiologically relevant systems that the mediator can affect. These several systems other than PDH will be discussed in Section V.

Rosen et al. (1981) have described another subcellular system that responds to the addition of insulin. Addition of physiological concentrations of insulin to 3T3-L1 adipocytes rapidly increased phosphorylation of ribosomal protein S6 and this effect was mimicked by adding antibody to the insulin receptor. A particulate fraction derived from cells incubated with insulin catalyzed the transfer of ^{32}P from [γ-^{32}P]ATP into ribosomal protein S6 in vitro. The direct addition of insulin or anti-insulin receptor antibody to the particulate fraction, containing ribosomes, ribosome-associated enzymes, and insulin receptors, stimulated the incorporation of ^{32}P from [γ-^{32}P]ATP into ribosomal protein S6. This phosphorylation was increased with increasing concentrations of insulin and showed a time course similar to that found with intact cells. It is not clear whether the insulin mediator that activates PDH is responsible for this insulin effect on ribosomal protein S6.

Recently, another subcellular system approach has been developed to study the mechanism of insulin action on nuclear function. First, Schumm and Webb (1981) reported that insulin added directly to nuclear preparations increased the efflux of mRNA from isolated nuclei. Second, Purrello et al. (1982) showed that insulin activated nuclear envelope nucleoside triphosphatase, an enzyme located at or near the nuclear pore complex. These findings suggest that regulation of this enzyme may be a mechanism by which insulin controls mRNA metabolism. Finally, this same group has shown that insulin (Purrello et al., 1983a), insulin receptor antiserum, and the lectins (Purrello et al., 1983b), concanavalin A and phytohemagglutinin, decrease the ^{32}P incorporation into nuclear envelope proteins. They have suggested that this phosphorylation may regulate the nucleoside triphosphatase. All of the ligands that decrease the liver nuclear envelope phosphorylation showed biphasic dose–response curves with insulin, providing the maximum effect at 10^{-11} M. Possibly related to these findings, Horvat (1980) has shown that a low-molecular-weight molecule from cytosol of liver perfused with insulin stimulated nuclear RNA polymerase activity.

C. Other Ligand-Sensitive Membrane Systems

Since the description of the adipocyte subcellular systems that respond to the direct addition of insulin, there have been other plasma membrane subcellular systems developed, which, in response to specific ligand treatment, generate mediators that may be related to the insulin-generated mediator (Table II). The prolactin system has been studied extensively. Houdebine's laboratory has developed a membrane preparation from mammary gland or other tissues containing prolactin receptors that respond to the hormone with release of a factor that specifically stimulates β-casein gene transcription in isolated mammary nuclei (Teyssot et al., 1981, 1982; Houdebine et al., 1983a). Human growth hormone and ovine placental lactogen also stimulated the mammary gland membranes to produce significant quantities of mediator. Insulin was the only other hormone tested that affected this system and that effect was small. The mediator is generated by anti-prolactin receptor antibody, by the Fab_2 fragment but not the Fab_1 fragment (Teyssot et al., 1982; Houdebine et al., 1984). The production of the mediator was inhibited by colchicine and related drugs (Teyssot

TABLE II
Other Plasma Membrane Systems Generating Mediators Potentially
Related to the Insulin Mediator

Ligand	Tissue	Response
Prolactin, anti-prolactin receptor antibody, growth hormone and insulin[a]	Lactating mammary gland membranes	Increase β-casein gene transcription in isolated mammary nuclei
Insulin-antagonistic growth hormone fragment (C-terminal end)[b]	Liver and adipocyte membranes	Decrease pyruvate dehydrogenase and acetyl-CoA carboxylase activity
Concanavalin A, phytohemagglutin[c]	Lymphocyte membranes	Increase pyruvate dehydrogenase activity

[a]Houdebine et al. (1983, 1984), Martel et al. (1983), Servely et al. (1982), and Teyssot et al. (1981, 1982).
[b]Bornstein et al. (1983).
[c]Beachy et al. (1981).

et al., 1982; Houdebine *et al.*, 1983a), by sodium butyrate (Martel *et al.*, 1983), and by phorbol esters (Houdebine *et al.*, 1984). This mediator is low in molecular weight similar to the insulin mediator, as will be discussed later. The prolactin mediator stimulates a nuclear phosphatase which apparently is involved in activating gene transcription (Houdebine *et al.*, 1984). Blockage of mediator action on the phosphatase prevents the mediator stimulation of β-casein gene transcription. The action of the prolactin mediator on a phosphoprotein phosphatase is similar to the actions of the insulin mediator on glycogen synthase phosphoprotein phosphatase and PDH phosphoprotein phosphatase, as will be discussed in Section V. This prolactin mediator was recently tested in our laboratory and was found to stimulate PDH activity and to inhibit adenylate cyclase activity, similar to the insulin mediator (unpublished observations).

The putative prolactin mediator induces β-casein mRNA synthesis in monolayers of mammary epithelial cells (Servely *et al.*, 1982). The amount required for gene transcription in cultured cells was severalfold greater than required to stimulate isolated nuclei. The mediator had no effect on mammary gland explants. Thus, it appears that the prolactin mediator does not act as a cell-to-cell messenger. It is most likely that the prolactin messenger is produced, acts, and is degraded within each stimulated cell. The same process is probably true for the insulin mediator. However, the addition of putative mediators to intact cells permits investigation of mediator-induced alterations of processes which require an intact cell to measure.

Bornstein's laboratory (1983) has reported that the C-terminal fragment of growth hormone, which has insulin-antagonistic activity, produces a low-molecular-weight mediator in liver or adipocyte plasma membranes that inhibits acetyl-CoA carboxylase activity. Beachy *et al.* (1981) have shown that the mitogenic lectins, concanavalin A and phytohemagglutin, stimulated PDH activity in rat mesenteric lymphocytes. Wheat germ agglutinin, a nonmitogenic lectin, did not alter the activity of this enzyme. Preliminary experiments from this group have shown that lymphocyte plasma membranes treated with concanavalin A or phytohemagglutinin released a soluble factor that stimulated PDH activity in either lymphocyte or adipocyte mitochondria. These data suggest that mitogenic transmembrane signaling in lymphocytes may be similar to the mechanism used by insulin in its target cells. Thus, the use of responsive subcellular membrane preparations have proved useful for studying the mechanism by which insulin and other ligands control metabolic pathways in response to ligand–receptor interactions.

III. Whole Cell and Tissue Studies

To substantiate that this low-molecular-weight material generated from the plasma membrane by insulin represents the mediator of insulin action, additional experimental evidence was required. First, the mediator should be ubiquitous in cellular or tissue distribution and the amount or activity of the material must be altered by insulin in a manner consistent with the known effects of insulin on that cell or tissue type. Second, the mediator should control insulin-sensitive enzymes or systems in a manner analogous to insulin in intact cells. This section will review the various cell types studied.

There is a summary in Table III of the cell or tissue systems producing the mediator and the manner in which insulin affects the amount or activity of the mediator. Larner *et al.* (1979) were the first to extract the mediator from intact tissue, muscle, and to show that insulin treatment of rabbits with insulin increased the amount of mediator extracted. They injected rabbits with or without insulin, freeze-clamped the skeletal muscle, and extracted it in a boiling, acid buffer containing EDTA and a reducing agent. The extract was chromatographed on Sephadex G-25 and eluted at an MW of 1000–1500. The mediator was identified as an inhibitor of cAMP-dependent protein kinase and a stimulator of glycogen synthase phosphoprotein phosphatase. Jarett and Seals (1979) showed that this same material stimulated PDH activity in adipocyte mitochondria. Macaulay in Jarett's laboratory has treated rats with insulin and found an increased amount of mediator from both skeletal muscle and liver (unpublished observations). After

TABLE III

Intact Cell Systems Wherein Insulin Modulates
the Amount or Activity of Mediator

Source	Response to insulin
Adipocytes (rat)[a]	Increase
Muscle (rabbit and rat)[b]	Increase
Liver (rat)[c]	Increase
H$_4$ hepatoma (rat)[d]	Increase
IM-9 (human)[e]	Decrease

[a]Kiechle *et al.* (1980).
[b]Larner *et al.* (1979), Jarett and Seals (1979), and Macaulay and Jarett (1984).
[c]Macaulay and Jarett (1984).
[d]Parker *et al.* (1982).
[e]Jarett *et al.* (1980).

acid extraction and ultrafiltration a 500- to 2000-Da mediator was identified that stimulated PDH and low K_m cAMP phosphodiesterase and inhibited adenlyate cyclase. Previously, Kiechle *et al.* (1980) had shown that treatment of rat adipocytes with insulin increased the amount or activity of an acid-stable, low-molecular-weight material. This mediator stimulated PDH and low K_m cAMP phosphodiesterase activity. The addition of insulin to insulin-sensitive H4-II-E-C3' hepatoma cells produced a concentration-dependent increase in the amount of acid extractable low-molecular-weight mediator as determined by PDH and low K_m cAMP phosphodiesterase activity (Parker *et al.*, 1982).

Generation of the mediator in IM-9 cultured human lymphocytes was investigated (Jarett *et al.*, 1980). There have been extensive studies on binding of insulin to receptors on IM-9 lymphocytes, but no reports of a biological response of this cell to insulin. A low-molecular-weight material was extracted from the IM-9 lymphocytes which stimulated PDH activity. In contrast to other cells or tissues, however, insulin treatment of IM-9 lymphocytes significantly reduced the amount or activity of the material in the Sephadex G-25 fraction that stimulated PDH activity. Recently, Parker and Jarett (unpublished observations) generated data which explain this earlier finding. They found that insulin treatment of IM-9 lymphocytes increased the amount of a low-molecular-weight material similar in size and properties to the stimulator of PDH, but which inhibited the enzyme activity and blocked the stimulatory mediator. Insulin had little effect on the production of the PDH stimulator. The ability of insulin to stimulate production of at least two mediators with differing activity will be discussed in detail in Section IV.

Thus studies with intact cells and tissues showed that there is an insulin-sensitive, low-molecular-weight material produced similar in size and affect on insulin-sensitive enzymes to the mediator obtained from plasma membrane preparations. The variety of enzymes and systems affected and the common properties of the mediator from various sources will be covered in Sections V and VI.

IV. Number of Mediators

In the previous discussion we described the putative second messenger of insulin action as a single entity. There is, however, direct and indirect evidence for the existence of more than one mediator, perhaps a family of related compounds.

Indirect evidence for more than one mediator can be found in the

TABLE IV
BIPHASIC RESPONSES TO INSULIN AND OTHER LIGANDS

System	Effect	Ligand
Liver[a]	Calcium uptake in liver mitochondria	Insulin
Skeletal muscle[b]	Glycogen synthase phosphatase	Insulin
Adipocyte subcellular system[c]	Pyruvate dehydrogenase	Insulin, concanavalin A, anti-insulin receptor antibody
Adipocyte plasma membranes[d]	Pyruvate dehydrogenase	Insulin
Liver plasma membranes[e]	Pyruvate dehydrogenase Acetyl CoA carboxylase	Insulin
Nuclei[f]	Transport of mRNA	Insulin
	Nuclear envelope nucleoside triphosphate	Insulin
	Phosphorylation of nuclear envelope proteins	Insulin, phytohemagglutinin, concanavalin A, anti-insulin receptor antibody

[a]Gainutdinov et al. (1978) and Turakolov et al. (1977, 1979).
[b]Chen et al. (1980) and Larner et al. (1979, 1982b).
[c]Seals and Jarett (1980).
[d]Seals and Czech (1980, 1981).
[e]Saltiel et al. (1981, 1982, 1983).
[f]Purrello et al. (1982, 1983a,b).

biphasic or bell-shaped response detected in some test systems to increasing concentrations of insulin or insulin-mimetic agents (Table IV). Turakulov et al. (1977, 1979) reported that insulin treatment of rats produces an increase in low-molecular-weight material and an insulin-dependent cytoplasmic regulator in the cytosol of liver that effects a biphasic response in calcium uptake by mitochondria (Turakulov et al., 1977). A twofold increase in the concentration of this factor was required to inhibit the oxidation of pyruvate and succinate in liver mitochondria, perhaps by inhibiting substrate transport in the mitochondria (Turakulov et al., 1979). This inhibition was not biphasic. These two actions of the factor appear to be independent of each other.

Mediator generated from diverse sources alters the activity of insulin-sensitive enzymes in a biphasic dose–response relationship upon addition of insulin or insulin-mimetic ligands (Table IV). Larner et al.

(1979) found a biphasic response in glycogen synthase phosphatase activity with increasing concentration of a low-molecular-weight fraction from rabbit skeletal muscle. Seals and Jarett (1980) reported that the direct addition of insulin, concanavalin A, or anti-insulin receptor antibody to the adipocyte subcellular system composed of mitochondria and plasma membranes also activated PDH in a biphasic manner. Seals and Czech (1981) showed that the supernatant obtained from adipocyte plasma membranes incubated in increasing concentrations of insulin produced a biphasic stimulation of PDH when added to isolated adipocyte mitochondria. Saltiel *et al.* (1981, 1983) have observed the same phenomenon—activition of PDH and acetyl-CoA carboxylase using the supernatant from a crude preparation of liver plasma membranes incubated with increasing concentrations of insulin.

A similar biphasic response has been observed for several processes after binding of insulin or insulin-mimetic agents to the nuclear envelope. Increasing concentrations of insulin produce a biphasic response on efflux of mRNA from isolated nuclei (Schumm and Webb, 1981), and in stimulation of an enzyme, nucleoside triphosphatase, located near the nuclear pore (Purrello *et al.*, 1982). Insulin (Purrello *et al.,* 1983a) as well as insulin-mimetic agents, such as concanavalin A, hemagglutinin, and anti-insulin receptor antibody (Purrello *et al.,* 1983b), decrease phosphorylation of the isolated nuclear envelope in a biphasic manner. The relationship between these nuclear phenomena and the generation of a low-molecular-weight mediator is unknown.

Direct evidence for the existence of more than one mediator has been published by two laboratories. Chen *et al.* (1980) have separated the low-molecular-weight mediator from the skeletal muscle of insulin-treated rabbits into two fractions by high voltage electrophoresis. One fraction stimulated the activity of glycogen synthase phosphoprotein phosphatase and inhibited the activity of cAMP-dependent protein kinase. The other fraction produced the opposite effect, i.e., it inhibited glycogen synthase phosphoprotein phosphatase activity and stimulated cAMP-dependent protein kinase. Although these effects were concentration dependent, the biphasic response was not observed. Saltiel *et al.* (1982, 1983) have shown that ethanol precipitation of mediator generated from liver plasma membranes separated the material into an ethanol-insoluble fraction that activates PDH and acetyl-CoA carboxylase and an ethanol-soluble material that inhibited PDH, acetyl-CoA carboxylase, and basal or hormonally stimulated adenylate cyclase. Both the stimulatory and the inhibitory activities showed a monophasic dose–response, suggesting that the relative ratio of the two counteracting substances may be responsible for the biphasic response observed in crude extracts. These two substances must have similar structural properties since both the inhibitor and stimulator of PDH coelute on a HPLC molecular sieve column.

In view of these findings, it is possible that insulin treatment of IM-9 lymphocytes only stimulated the generation of inhibitor of PDH (Jarett *et al.*, 1980). These cells are the only system studied to date wherein insulin reduces the amount and/or activity of mediator. It appears that insulin affects only production of the inhibitory substances (see Section III). In contrast, in H_4 hepatoma cells (Parker *et al.*, 1982), insulin did not produce a biphasic curve but simply increased mediator activity to a maximum, even at high insulin concentrations, suggesting that only an activating material was generated. Perhaps these two cell lines will provide sufficient quantities of both the inhibitor and stimulator to permit further chemical identification.

V. Insulin-Sensitive Enzymes

Modulation of enzyme systems was examined to further substantiate the proposal that the low-molecular-weight, acid-stable material extracted from various cell types represents the mediator of insulin action. The enzymes studied included such insulin-sensitive intracellular processes as calcium transport, and glucose or lipid metabolism (Table V). The activity of these enzymes may be altered by insulin in intact cells or by the mediator of insulin action through dephosphorylation (glycogen synthase, PDH, Ca^{2+},Mg^{2+}-ATPase), phosphorylation (acetyl-CoA carboxylase), or some other mechanism (low K_m cAMP phosphodiesterase and adenylate cyclase). Larner *et al.* (1979) showed that the mediator from skeletal muscle inhibited the activity of cAMP-dependent protein kinase and stimulated the activity of phosphoprotein phosphatase with glycogen synthase was used as a substrate. Dephosphorylation causes activation of glycogen synthase as observed upon insulin treatment of intact cells. The mediator did not alter the activity of several cAMP-independent protein kinases.

This laboratory, as well as others (Seals and Czech, 1980; Saltiel *et al.*, 1981; Amatruda and Chang, 1983; Sakamoto *et al.*, 1982; Begum *et al.*, 1982a,b, 1983a), have used PDH as the major biological assay for the mediator. Pyruvate dehydrogenase is a multienzyme complex composed of three major enzymes: pyruvate decarboxylase, lipoate acetyltransferase, and lipoamide dehydrogenase (Randle *et al.*, 1979). The activity of this complex is regulated by the degree of phosphorylation of the α-subunit of pyruvate decarboxylase (Schuster *et al.*, 1975). The

TABLE V
ENZYME SYSTEMS AFFECTED BY THE INSULIN-SENSITIVE MEDIATOR

Enzyme	Effect	
cAMP-dependent protein kinase[a]	Decrease	
Glycogen synthase phosphoprotein phosphatase[b]	Increase	
cAMP-independent protein kinase[c]	No effect	
Pyruvate dehydrogenase[d]	Increase	
cAMP-independent kinase[d]	No effect	
phosphatase[d]	Increase	
Low K_m cAMP phosphodiesterase[e]	Increase	
High K_m cAMP phosphodiesterase[f]	No effect	
Ca^{2+},Mg^{2+}-ATPase (adipocyte plasma membrane)[g]	Increase	
Acetyl CoA carboxylase[h]	Increase[i]	Decrease[j]
Adenylate cyclase[k]	No effect[i]	Decrease[j]
Pyruvate dehydrogenase[k]	Increase[i]	Decrease[j]

[a]Larner et al. (1979).
[b]Larner et al. (1979).
[c]Larner et al. (1979).
[d]Jarett et al. (1981, 1983b), Kiechle et al. (1980, 1981), and Popp et al. (1980).
[e]Kiechle and Jarett (1981).
[f]Kiechle and Jarett (1981).
[g]McDonald et al. (1981).
[h]Saltiel et al. (1983).
[i]Ethanol-insoluble residue from insulin-treated liver plasma membranes.
[j]Ethanol-soluble material from insulin-treated liver plasma membranes.
[k]Saltiel et al. (1982).

phosphorylated form of the enzyme is inactive; the dephosphorylated form is active (Reed, 1974; Schuster et al., 1975). Three serines are phosphorylated on the α-subunit. The activities of the PDH complexes in pig heart (Sugden et al., 1979), bovine heart, and kidney (Yeaman et al., 1978) mitochondria correlate with the state of phosphorylation of the first site. Therefore, the residual enzyme activity is inversely proportional to the degree of phosphorylation at the first serine residue. The heavily phosphorylated form may be activated more slowly than the lightly phosphorylated form (Reed, 1981; Randle, 1981). The activity of the enzyme complex is controlled by a cAMP-independent protein kinase and phosphoprotein phosphatase (Denton and Hughes, 1978). The mediator of insulin action could alter PDH activity through changes in phosphorylation of the α-subunit by increasing phosphatase activity, by decreasing kinase activity, or by both. A series of studies were performed with or without addition of ATP, sodium fluoride, a known inhibitor of the PDH phosphatase (Hucho et al., 1972), or dichloroacetic acid, an inhibitor of the kinase (Whitehouse et al., 1974).

These studies were performed with adipocyte subcellular system (Popp *et al.*, 1980) and the partially purified mediator from adipocytes (Kiechle *et al.*, 1980), hepatoma cells (Parker *et al.*, 1982), adipocyte plasma membranes (Kiechle *et al.*, 1981), or liver plasma membranes (Jarett and Kiechle, 1981). With each the increase in PDH activity was attributable to activation of the PDH phosphatase and not to affects on PDH kinase. This conclusion is based on three findings: (1) The mediator activated PDH in the absence of ATP, the substrate for the kinase, (2) this activation by mediator was inhibited by NaF even with added ATP, and (3) the mediator activated PDH even with added dichloroacetic acid. The mechanism by which the mediator activates the phosphatase is unknown.

These studies on PDH as well as those by other groups have been performed using non-intact, broken mitochondria, raising questions of the physiological significance of the findings. That is, would the mediator work on intact functional mitochondria as they exist in cells. Parker and Jarett (unpublished observations) have completed a set of studies using intact liver mitochondria with respiratory ratios greater than four. Insulin mediator from liver membranes, hepatoma cells, liver, and muscle stimulated PDH activity, providing evidence that the mediator could be functioning in cells on intact mitochondria.

The earlier studies (Seals and Jarett, 1980; Jarett and Seals, 1979; Seals and Czech, 1980) and many of the subsequent studies (Begum *et al.*, 1982a,b, 1983a; Saltiel *et al.*, 1981) that used PDH in assays for mediator activity reported stimulations of only up to 30%. This limit in activity has several causes. First, no attempts were made to prevent dephosphorylation of the enzyme complex during isolation, so that the control enzyme was already in a dephosphorylated, highly active state allowing little further stimulation. Second, experiments performed with added ATP cause competition between increased dephosphorylation and stimulation of enzyme activity on the one hand and rephosphorylation and inactivation on the other. The result was that the mediator established a new equilibrium of phosphorylation and dephosphorylation with modest increases in activity. Kiechle *et al.* (1980, 1981) addressed this problem as follows. The isolated mitochondria were incubated with ATP, to phosphorylate and inactivate PDH. The mitochondria were washed, stored frozen, and subsequently used for assay in the absence of ATP. Thus the PDH complex starts in a form that is only 10–15% active, allowing for marked stimulation. Subsequent studies by our laboratory have found stimulations from 2- to 10-fold depending on the amount of mediator tested. In many cases the mediator would evoke maximum activity.

Another enzyme system is the insulin-sensitive high-affinity Ca^{2+}-

stimulated Mg^{2+}-dependent ATPase (Ca^{2+},Mg^{2+}-ATPase) found in the plasma membrane of rat adipocytes, which may represent an enzymatic basis for a calmodulin-sensitive plasma membrane Ca^{2+} transport system (Pershadsingh et al., 1981; Pershadsingh and McDonald, 1980). Treatment of adipocytes or adipocyte plasma membranes with physiologic concentrations of insulin, up to 100 μU/ml, decreased enzyme activity and decreased the phosphorylation of a phosphoprotein with an MW of 110,000. This phosphoprotein has been identified as Ca^{2+},Mg^{2+}-ATPase (Pershadsingh and McDonald, 1979, 1981; Chan and McDonald, 1982). The mediator from adipocyte plasma membranes stimulated the activity of Ca^{2+},Mg^{2+}-ATPase fourfold and more than doubled Ca^{2+} transport (McDonald et al., 1981). The mediator altered both enzyme and transport systems opposite to the effect observed with physiologic concentrations of insulin. The explanation for this phenomenon is not known.

Acetyl-CoA carboxylase is activated by phosphorylation by an insulin-stimulated cAMP-independent protein kinase (Witters, 1981; Brownsey and Denton, 1982). This kinase phosphorylates sites distinct from those phosphorylated by the cAMP-dependent protein kinase activated by glucagon or epinephrine; the latter causes inhibition of enzyme activity. Saltiel et al. (1983) have shown that the mediator generated by insulin from liver plasma membranes activates acetyl-CoA carboxylase.

Insulin treatment of hepatocytes (Loten et al., 1978) or adipocytes (Loten and Sneyd, 1970; Makino and Kono, 1980) increased the activity of the low K_m cAMP phosphodiesterase found in the microsomal fraction. This enzyme also is activated by insulin in the plasma membranes of adipocytes (Macaulay et al., 1983a). The enzyme system, as it exists in the microsomal membrane fraction of the adipocyte, was stimulated by the addition of the mediator from several sources (Parker et al., 1982; Kiechle and Jarett, 1981). The mediator increased the V_{max} of the enzyme but did not affect K_m. The low K_m cAMP phosphodiesterase in liver plasma membranes has been reported to be activated by phosphorylation (Marchmont and Houslay, 1981). In our laboratory no effect was found on the adipocyte microsomal or plasma membrane enzymes by phosphorylation. Therefore, at this time low K_m cAMP phosphodiesterase from adipocytes appears to be regulated by a mechanism other than phosphorylation. The mediator from diverse sources was without effect on the high K_m cAMP phosphodiesterase in adiopcytes microsomes. This finding is consistent with the insensitivity of the enzyme to insulin in intact cellular systems (Loten et al., 1978; Loten and Sneyd, 1970).

Insulin has been reported to inhibit both the basal and hormonally stimulated adenylate cyclase in hepatocytes and adipocytes (Torres *et al.*, 1978; Illiano and Cuatrecasas, 1972). Saltiel *et al.* (1982, 1983) have shown that the ethanol-soluble fraction of mediator released from liver plasma membranes inhibits basal as well as hormonally stimulated enzyme. The ethanol residue that activates PDH and acetyl-CoA carboxylase did not affect adenylate cyclase activity. The mechanism controlling activity of this enzyme does not seem to involve phosphorylation.

The recent work by Zhang *et al.* (1983) has shown that the insulin mediator probably regulates key enzymes involved in lipogenesis, antilipolysis, and lowering of cAMP of intact adipocytes. These investigators added insulin-generated mediator from adipocyte plasma membrane to adipocytes and found elevated cyclic AMP levels to be lowered, stimulated lipolysis to be suppressed, and lipogenesis to be stimulated. The enzymes affected are unknown, but this approach provides an interesting method for studying insulin-sensitive metabolic pathways not accessible in a test tube and for confirming mediator actions in intact cells.

Initially, it appeared that the primary function of the mediator of insulin action was to modify the state of phosphorylation and, therefore, the activity of the several regulatory enzymes. The mediator appeared to alter phosphorylation by modulating the activity of phosphatase and kinase enzymes. However, it is evident that some insulin-sensitive enzymes are not regulated by phosphorylation–dephosphorylation mechanism. Therefore, the mediator(s) may alter enzyme activity by fulfilling a cofactor function for specific phosphatases, kinases, or other coenzymes or by direct allosteric effects.

VI. PHYSICAL AND CHEMICAL CHARACTERISTICS OF THE MEDIATOR

The insulin mediators have yet to be purified and chemically identified. The mediators from diverse tissues share several characteristics including: low molecular weight (1000–3000), acid stability, thermostability, isoelectric point of 4.0–5.0, and elution from anion-exchange resins at high salt concentration. Since the mediators are derived from plasma membranes, they must be generated from membrane components or their derivatives, such as proteins, glycoproteins, glycolipids, phospholipids, proteolipids, fatty acids, prostaglandins, and leukotrienes.

Early studies suggested that the mediators might be peptides (Larner *et al.*, 1979, 1982a; Kiechle *et al.*, 1980, 1981). This observation was based on the fact that the mediator copurified with a peak of absorbance at 230 nm and ninhydrin positivity. There was no correlation between the amount or activity of the mediator and the absorbance, attributable to the impure nature of the material. Some investigators have been able to destroy mediator activity with protease (trypsin) digestion (Sakamoto *et al.,* 1982; Seals and Czech, 1980) but others have found no effect or only partial inactivation with protease digestion (Jarett *et al.,* 1983a,b; Larner, 1983). Several investigators report that addition of inhibitors of arginine-specific proteases to plasma membranes prevents generation of the mediator by insulin. Seals and Czech (1980) have proposed that after insulin binds to its receptor a membrane bond protease is activated which cleaves the mediator at an arginine residue. Muchmore *et al.* (1982) have shown that inhibition by protease blockers of insulin effects on adipocytes may be secondary to decreased cellular ATP. Originally, we found no evidence that a peptide structure was necessary for biological activity of the mediator. These studies had been based on use of proteolytic enzymes, dansylation, treatment with fluorescamine, and high-pressure liquid chromatography. Recently, with the mediator from the skeletal muscle of insulin-treated rats, S. L. Macaulay in this laboratory (unpublished observations) has found that trypsin causes little effect on mediator activity, whereas chymotrypsin has a greater effect, and pepsin the greatest effect on activity. Complete inactivation, however, was not obtained. These data indicated that the mediator contains amino acids which, however, are not totally required for biological activity. Several investigators have found amino acids in partially purified preparations of the mediator. Gainutdinov *et al.,* (1978) reported an amino acid composition for the insulin-dependent cytoplasmic regulator consisting of 42 amino acids: aspartic acid, 3; threonine, 1; serine, 7; glutamic acid, 6; proline, 4; glycine, 6; alanine, 3; valine, 1; isoleucine, 1; leucine, 1; tyrosine, 1; phenylalanine, 1; histidine, 1; lysine, 5; and arginine, 1. They also reported that the compound contains sugar residues and organic phosphorus. Larner *et al.* (1982a) reported a provisional amino acid composition of Phe, Lys, Glu, Asp, Gly, Leu, Ser for the mediator extracted from insulin-treated skeletal muscle. Seals (1983) has also reported the presence of a total of 32 amino acids in mediator preparations from insulin-treated and control adipocyte plasma membranes. Seals identified 16 different amino acids. Whether they represent the essential structural components of the mediators or only a part of them must await further experimentation.

Initially, we could not substantiate that common sugars or amino sugars were part of the mediator structure, based on the inability of the material to bind to a variety of immobilized lectins. However, Begum et al. (1983a) have shown that both neuraminidase and β-D-galactoside treatment inactivates the mediator generated by liver plasma membranes. These several tests for composition (carbohydrate or amino acid) have been assessed by biological activity. When greater quantities of purified mediator are available, direct chemical analysis must be applied to confirm these initial results.

The above data led us to consider other membrane components, such as phospholipids and their derivatives as potential mediators. The existence of a phospholipid-sensitive, calcium-dependent protein kinase (protein kinase C) with a wide tissue distribution (Kaibuchi et al., 1981; Wrenn et al., 1980; Kuo et al., 1980) suggests that there may be a direct relationship between phospholipids and phosphorylation. Farese et al. (1982) showed that insulin treatment of adipocytes increased the content of several phospholipids. Walaas et al. (1981) reported that insulin increased the phosphorylation of a muscle sarcolemmal proteolipid with a MW of 3600. Wasner (1980, 1981) found that insulin increased the amount of a low-molecular-weight compound called cAMP antagonist, which may contain PGE_1, phosphate, and inositol as structural components. This compound inhibits adenylate cyclase and protein kinases, and activates phosphoprotein phosphatases and PDH. A preliminary report from Begum et al. (1983b) showed that indomethacin, an inhibitor of prostaglandin synthesis, prevented mediator generation from liver plasma membrane by insulin. This inhibitory effect of indomethacin was reversed by the addition of prostaglandin E_2. Perhaps, the mediator is generated upon activation of a membrane-bound phospholipase A_1 or A_2 as suggested by others (Bereziat et al., 1978; Dietze, 1982).

We have investigated the role of phospholipids and related compounds in insulin action. The mediator prepration from adipocyte plasma membranes before and after gel filtration contains at least 10 phospholipids. The addition of aqueous dispersions of these phospholipids to assays for PDH and low K_m cAMP phosphodiesterase demonstrated specific effects. Phosphatidylserine and phosphatidylinositol 4-phosphate were found to specifically stimulate and inhibit, respectively, PDH activity while other phospholipids were without effect (Kiechle and Jarett, 1983). Similarly, phosphatidylserine and phosphatidylcholine stimulated and phosphatidylinositol 4-phosphate inhibited the low K_m cAMP phosphodiesterase activity of adipocyte microsomal (endoplasmic reticulum) and plasma membrane preparations (Macaulay et al., 1983a,b). The high K_m enzyme was unaffected by these same phospholipids. These initial studies suggest that phosphatidylserine and phosphatylinositol 4-phosphate could be physiologically counterregulatory for enzyme activity. Although Farese *et al.* (1983a,b) have shown that the insulin-induced increase in phosphatidylserine in adipose tissue precedes PDH, a requirement for a second messenger, it seems unlikely that phosphatidylserine alone represents the mediator for insulin action. However, phospholipids may be secondarily involved in certain insulin-sensitive enzymes, such as PDH and low K_m cAMP phosphodiesterase.

VII. Conclusion

The data presented in this review support the contention that the low-molecular-weight material released from the plasma membrane, after insulin interacts with its receptor, is, in fact, the mediator of many of the actions of insulin. The mediator can be produced in subcellular systems as well as intact cells and acts on a variety of insulin-sensitive enzymes. It appears that the mediator is part of a new family of messenger compounds that may account for the action of other hormones, such as prolactin, as well as insulin. The chemical nature of the mediator is as yet unknown, but certainly complex.

The next few years should be exciting as the insulin mediator is purified and identified, the mode of generation of the mediator is determined, and the mechanism by which the mediator acts is unraveled. These projects will not easily be accomplished for several reasons. First, until recently, the quantity of mediator available had been rate limiting. Second, the presence of several mediators requires careful separations and determination of actions of each class. Third, the chemical composition seems complex, possibly being peptide, sugar, phospholipid, and/or prostaglandin. The importance of the problem, the availability of appropriate tools, and the increasing number of investigators working on the problem, however, assure success.

These studies on the insulin mediator are potentially important for clinical as well as basic research toward understanding the postreceptor defects of insulin resistance in obesity and type II diabetes (noninsulin-dependent diabetes mellitus). These conditions might be caused by abnormal release or metabolism of the mediator. Data presented in this review suggest that these defects do exist. Further studies in man and experimental anaimals are needed to support or refute this hypothesis.

ACKNOWLEDGMENTS

The authors wish to thank our colleagues K. L. Kelly, J. O. Macaulay, S. L. Macaulay, J. C. Parker, C. Penn, and J. Smith, without whom this work would not have been accomplished. We thank Dana Kelly-Carson for typing the manuscript. The work was supported by NIH Grant AM 28144 and a grant from the Reynolds Foundation. Dr. Kiechle is a Hartford Fellow.

REFERENCES

Amatruda, J. M., and Chang, C. L. (1983). Insulin resistance in the liver in fasting and diabetes mellitus: The failure of insulin to stimulate the release of a chemical modulator of pyruvate dehydrogenase. *Biochem. Biophys. Res. Commun.* **112**, 35–41.

Avruch, J., Fairbanks, G., and Crapo, L. M. 1976). Regulation of plasma membrane protein phosphorylation in two mammalian cell types. *J. Cell. Physiol.* **89**, 815–826.

Beachy, J. C., Goldman, D., and Czech, M. P. (1981). Lectins activate lymphocyte pyruvate dehydrogenase by a mechanism sensitive to protease inhibitors. *Proc. Natl. Acad. Sci. U.S.A.* **78**, 6256–6260.

Begum, N., Tepperman, H. M., and Tepperman, J. (1982a). Effect of high fat and high carbohydrate diets on adipose tissue pyruvate dehydrogenase and its activation by a plasma membrane-enriched fraction and insulin. *Endocrinology* **110**, 1914–1921.

Begum, N., Tepperman, H. M., and Tepperman, J. (1982b). Effects of high carbohydrate and high fat diets on rat adipose tissue pyruvate dehydrogenase response to concanavalin A and spermine. *Endocrinology* **111**, 1491–1497.

Begum, N., Tepperman, H. M., and Tepperman, J. (1983a). Effects of high fat and high carbohydrate diets on liver pyruvate dehydrogenase and its activation by a chemical mediator released from insulin-treated liver particulate fraction: Effect on neuraminidase treatment on the chemical mediator activity. *Endocrinology* **112**, 50–59.

Begum, N., Tepperman, H. M., and Tepperman, J. (1983b). Effect of indomethacin and prostaglandin E$_2$ on insulin-generation of pyruvate dehydrogenase activator by liver and adipocyte plasma membranes. *Diabetes* **32**, 32A.

Belsham, G. J., Denton, R. M., and Tanner, M. J. A. (1980). Use of a novel rapid preparation of fat cell plasma membranes employing Percoll to investigate the effects of insulin and adrenaline on membrane protein phosphorylation within intact fat cells. *Biochem. J.* **192**, 457–467.

Benjamin, W. B., and Clayton, N.-L. (1978). Action of insulin and catecholamines on the phosphorylation of proteins associated with the cytosol, membranes and "fat cake" of rat fat cells. *J. Biol. Chem.* **253**, 1700–1709.

Bereziat, G., Wolf, C., Colard, O., and Polonovski, J. (1978). Phospholipases of plasmic membranes of adipose tissue. Possible intermediaries for insulin action. *Adv. Exp. Biol. Med.* **101**, 191–199.

Bornstein, J., Ng, F. M., Heng, D., and Wong, K. P. (1983). Metabolic actions of pituitary growth hormone I. Inhibition of acetyl CoA carboxylase by human growth hormone and a carboxy terminal part sequence acting through a second messenger. *Acta Endocrinol.* **103**, 479–486.

Brownsey, R. W., and Denton, R. M. (1982). Evidence that insulin activates fat-cell acetyl-CoA carboxylase by increased phosphorylation at a specific site. *Biochem. J.* **202**, 77–86.

Chan, K. M., and McDonald, J. M. (1982). Identification of an insulin-sensitive calcium-stimulated phosphoprotein in rat adipocyte plasma membranes. *J. Biol. Chem.* **257**, 7443–7448.

Chen, K., Galasko, G., Huang, L., Kellogg, J., and Larner, J. (1980). Studies on the insulin mediator. II. Separation of two antagonistic biologically active materials from fraction II. *Diabetes* **29**, 659–661.

Czech, M. P. (1977). Molecular basis of insulin action. *Annu. Rev. Biochem.* **46**, 359–384.

Czech, M. P. (1981). Insulin action. *Am. J. Med.* **70**, 142–150.

Denton, R. M., and Hughes, W. A. (1978). Pyruvate dehydrogenase and the hormonal regulation of fat synthesis in mammalian tissues. *Int. J. Biochem.* **9**, 545–552.

Denton, R. M., Brownsey, R. W., and Belsham, G. J. (1981). A partial view of the mechanism of insulin action. *Diabetologica* **21**, 347–362.

Dietze, G. J. (1982). Modulation of the action of insulin in relation to the energy state in skeletal muscle tissue: Possible involvement of kinins and prostaglandins. *Mol. Cell. Endocrinol.* **25**, 127–149.

Farese, R. V., Larson, R. E., and Sabir, M. A. (1982). Insulin acutely increases phospholipids in the phosphatidate-inositide cycle in rat adipose tissue. *J. Biol. Chem.* **257**, 4042–4045.

Farese, R. V., Farese, R. V., Jr., Sabir, M. A., and Trudeau, W. L. III. (1983a). A relationship between insulin-induced increases in phospholipids and pyruvate dehydrogenase activation in rat adipose tissue. *Clin. Res.* **30**, 877A.

Farese, R. V., Sabir, M. A., Larson, R. E., and Trudeau, W. L. III. (1983b). Insulin treatment acutely increases the concentration of phosphatidylserine in rat adipose tissue. *Biochim. Biophys. Acta* **750**, 200–202.

Gainutdinov, M. K., Turakulov, Y. K., Akhmatov, M. S., and Lavina, J. I. (1978). Isolation of a cytoplasmic regulator mediating the action of hormones on mitochondria. *Khim. Prirod. Soedin.* **1**, 141.

Goldfine, I. D. (1981). Effects of insulin on intracellular functions. *In* "Biochemical Actions of Hormones" (G. Litwack, ed.), Vol. 8, pp. 273–305. Academic Press, New York.

Horvat, A. (1980). Stimulation of RNA synthesis in isolated nuclei by an insulin-induced factor in liver. *Nature (London)* **280**, 906–908.

Houdebine, L. M., Djiane, J., Teyssot, B., Servely, J. L., Kelly, P. A., Delouis, C., Ollivier-Bousquet, M., and Devinoy, E. (1983). Prolactin and casein gene expression in the mammary cell. *In* "Regulation of Gene Expression by Hormones" (K. W. McKerns, ed.), pp. 71–101. Plenum, New York.

Houdebine, L. M., Djiane, J., Teyssot, B., Devinoy, E., Kelly, P. A., Dusanter-Fourt, J., Servely, J. L., and Martel, P. (1984). Preparation and assay of prolactin intracellular relay acting on milk protein genes. *In* "Methods in Enzymology," Vol. 109. Academic Press, New York, in press.

Hucho, F., Randall, D. D., Roche, T. E., Burgett, M. W., Pelley, J. W., and Reed, L. J. (1972). Alpha-keto acid dehydrogenase complexes. XVII. Kinetic and regulatory properties of pyruvate dehydrogenase kinase and pyruvate dehydrogenase phosphatase from bovine kidney and heart. *Arch. Biochem. Biophys.* **151**, 328–340.

Illiano, G., and Cuatrecasas, P. (1972). Modulation of adenylate cyclase activity in liver and fat cell membranes by insulin. *Science* **175**, 906–908.

Jarett, L. (1974). Cell fractionation of adipocytes. *In* "Methods of Enzymology" (S. Fleischer and L. Parker, ed.), Vol. 31, pp. 60–71. Academic Press, New York.

Jarett, L., and Kiechle, F. L. (1981). Generation of a putative second messenger for insulin action from adipocyte and liver membranes. *In* "Current Views on Insulin Receptors" (D. Adreani, R. De Pirro, R. Lauro, J. Olefsky, and J. Roth, eds.), pp. 245–253. Academic Press, New York.

Jarett, L., and Seals, J. R. (1979). Pyruvate dehydrogenase activation in adipocyte mitochondria by an insulin generated mediator from muscle. *Science* **206**, 1407–1408.

Jarett, L., and Smith, R. M. (1974). The stimulation of adipocyte plasma membrane magnesium ion stimulated adenosine triphosphatase by insulin and concanavalin A. *J. Biol. Chem.* **249**, 5195–5199.

Jarett, L., Kiechle, F. L., Popp, D. A., Kotagal, N., and Gavin, J. R. III. (1980). Differences in the effect of insulin on the generation by adipocytes and IM-9 lymphocytes of a chemical mediator which simulates the action of insulin on pyruvate dehydrogenase. *Biochem. Biophys. Res. Commun.* **96**, 735–741.

Jarett, L., Kiechle, F. L., Popp, D. A., and Kotagal, N. (1981). The role of a chemical mediator of insulin action in the control of phosphorylation. *Cold Spring Harbor Conf. Cell Prolif.* **8**, 715–726.

Jarett, L., Kiechle, F L., and Parker, J. C. (1982). Chemical mediator or mediators of insulin action: response to insulin and mode of action. *Fed. Proc., Fed. Am. Soc. Exp. Biol.* **41**, 2736–2741.

Jarett, L., Kiechle, F. L., Parker, J. C., and Macaulay, S. L. (1983a). The chemical mediators of insulin action: Possible targets for postreceptor defects. *Am. J. Med.* **74**, 31–37.

Jarett, L., Kiechle, F. L., Parker, J. C., and Macaulay, S. L. (1983b). Insulin action mediated by plasma membrane components. *In* "The Adipocyte and Obesity: Cellular and Molecular Mechanisms" (A. Angel, C. Hollenberg, and D. Roncari, eds.), pp. 75–84. Raven, New York.

Kahn, C. R. (1979). The role of insulin receptors and receptor antibodies in states of altered insulin action. *Proc. Soc. Exp. Biol. Med.* **162**, 13–21.

Kaibuchi, K., Takai, Y., and Nishizuka, Y. (1981). Cooperative roles of various membrane phospholipids in the activation of calcium-activated, phospholipid-dependent protein kinase. *J. Biol. Chem.* **256**, 7146–7149.

Kiechle, F. L., and Jarett, L. (1981). The effect of an insulin-sensitive chemical mediator from rat adipocytes on low Km and high Km cyclic AMP phosphodiesterase. *FEBS Lett.* **133**, 279–281.

Kiechle, F. L., and Jarett, L. (1983). Phospholipids and the regulation of pyruvate dehydrogenase from rat adipocyte mitochondria. *Mol. Cell. Biochem.* **56**, 99–105.

Kiechle, F. L., Jarett, L., Popp, D., and Kotagal, N. (1980). Isolation from rat adipocytes of a chemical mediator for insulin activation of pyruvate dehydrogenase. *Diabetes* **29**, 852–855.

Kiechle, F. L., Jarett, L., Popp, D. A., and Kotagal, N. (1981). Isolation from rat adipocyte plasma membrane of a chemical mediator which simulates the action of insulin on pyruvate dehydrogenase. *J. Biol. Chem.* **256**, 2945–2951.

Krebs, E. G., and Beavo, J. A. (1979). Phosphorylation-dephosphorylation of enzymes. *Annu. Rev. Biochem.* **48**, 923–959.

Kuo, J. F., Andersson, R. G. G., Wise, B. C., Mackerlova, L., Salomonsson, I., Brackett, N. L., Katoh, N., Shoji, M., and Wrenn, R. W. (1980). Calcium-dependent protein kinase; widespread occurrence in various tissues and phyla of the animal kingdom and comparison of effects of phospholipid, calmodulin, and trifluoperazine. *Proc. Natl. Acad. Sci. U.S.A.* **77**, 7039–7043.

Larner, J. (1982). Insulin mediator-fact or fancy? *J. Cyclic Nucleotide Res.* **8**, 289–296.

Larner, J. (1983). Mediators of postreceptor action of insulin. *Am. J. Med.* **74**, 38–51.

Larner, J., Galasko, G., Cheng, K., DePaoli-Roach, A. A., Huang, L., Daggy, P., and Kellog, J. (1979). Generation by insulin of a chemical mediator that controls protein phosphorylation and dephosphorylation. *Science* **206**, 1408–1410.

Larner, J., Cheng, K., Schwartz, C., Kikuchi, K., Tamura, S., Creacy, S., Dubler, R., Galasko, G., Pullin, C., and Katz, M. (1982a). A proteolytic mechanism for the action of insulin via oligopeptide mediator formation. *Fed. Proc., Fed. Am. Soc. Exp. Biol.* **41**, 2724–2729.

Larner, J., Cheng, K., Schwartz, C., Kikuchi, K., Tamura, S., Creacy, S., Dubler, R., Galasko, G., Pullin, C., and Katz, M. (1982b). Insulin mediators and their control of metabolism through protein phosphorylation. *Recent Prog. Horm. Res.* **38**, 511–556.

Levine, R. (1982). Insulin: The effects and mode of action of the hormone. *Vitam. Horm.* **39**, 145–173.

Loten, E. G., and Sneyd, J. G. T. (1970). An effect of insulin on adipose-tissue adenosine 3′:5′-cyclic monophosphate phosphodiesterase. *Biochem. J.* **120**, 187–195.

Loten, E. G., Assimacopoulos-Jeannet, F. D., Exton, J. H., and Park, C. R. (1978). Stimulation of a low Km phosphodiesterase from liver by insulin and glucagon. *J. Biol. Chem.* **253**, 746–757.

Macaulay, S. L., Kiechle, F. L., and Jarett, L. (1983a). Comparison of phospholipid effects on insulin-sensitive low Km cyclic AMP phosphodiesterase in adipocyte plasma membranes and microsomes. *Biochim. Biophys. Acta* **760**, 293–299.

Macaulay, S. L., Kiechle, F. L., and Jarett, L. (1983b). Phospholipid modulation of low Km cyclic AMP phosphodiesterase activity on rat adipocyte microsomes. *Arch. Biochem. Biophys.* **225**, 130–136.

Macaulay, S. L., and Jarett, L. (1984). Submitted.

McDonald, J. M., Pershadsingh, H. A., Kiechle, F. L., and Jarett, L. (1981). Parallel stimulation in adipocytes of the plasma membrane Ca^{2+}-transport $[Ca^{2+} + Mg^{2+}]$-ATPase system and mitochondrial pyruvate dehydrogenase by a supernatant factor derived from isolated plasma membranes. *Biochem. Biophys. Res. Commun.* **100**, 857–864.

Makino, H., and Kono, T. (1980). Characterization of insulin-sensitive phosphodiesterase in fat cells. II. Comparison of enzyme activities stimulated by insulin and by isoproterenol. *J. Biol. Chem.* **255**, 7850–7854.

Marchmont, R. J., and Houslay, M. D. (1980). Insulin triggers cyclic AMP-dependent activation and phosphorylation of a plasma membrane cyclic AMP phosphodiesterase. *Nature (London)* **286**, 904–906.

Martel, P., Houdebine, L. M., and Teyssot, B. (1983). Effect of sodium butyrate on the stimulation of casein gene expression by prolactin. *FEBS Lett.* **154**, 55–59.

Muchmore, D. B., Raess, B. U., Bergstrom, R. W., and de Haën, C. (1982). On the mechanisms of inhibition of insulin action by small-molecular-weight trypsin inhibitors. *Diabetes* **31**, 976–984.

Parker, J. C., Kiechle, F. L., and Jarett, L. (1982). Partial purification from hepatoma cells of an intracellular substance which mediates the effects of insulin on pyruvate dehydrogenase and low Km cyclic AMP phosphodiesterase. *Arch. Biochem. Biophys.* **215**, 339–344.

Pershadsingh, H. A., and McDonald, J. M. (1979). Direct addition of insulin inhibits a high affinity Ca^{2+}-ATPase in isolated adipocyte plasma membranes. *Nature (London)* **281**, 495–497.

Pershadsingh, H. A., and McDonald, J. M. (1980). A high affinity calcium-stimulated magnesium-dependent adenosine triphosphatase in rat adipocyte plasma membranes. *J. Biol. Chem.* **255**, 4087–4093.

Pershadsingh, H. A., and McDonald, J. M. (1981). $[Ca^{2+} + Mg^{2+}]$-ATPase in adipocyte plasmalemma: Inhibition by insulin and concanavalin A in the intact cell. *Biochem. Int.* **2**, 243–248.

Pershadsingh, H. A., Landt, M., and McDonald, J. M. (1980). Calmodulin-sensitive ATP-dependent Ca^{2+} transport across adipocyte plasma membranes. *J. Biol. Chem.* **255,** 8983–8986.

Popp, D., Kiechle, F. L., Kotagal, N., and Jarett, L. (1980). Insulin stimulation of pyruvate dehydrogenase in an isolated plasma membrane-mitochondrial mixture occurs by activation of pyruvate dehydrogenase phosphatase. *J. Biol. Chem.* **255,** 7540–7543.

Purrello, F., Vigneri, R., Clawson, G. A., and Goldfine, J. D. (1982). Insulin stimulation of nucleoside triphosphatase activity in isolated nuclear envelopes. *Science* **216,** 1005–1007.

Purrello, F., Burnham, D. B., and Goldfine, I. D. (1983a) Insulin regulation of protein phosphorylation in isolated rat liver nuclear envelopes: Potential relationship to mRNA metabolism. *Proc. Natl. Acad. Sci. U.S.A.* **80,** 1189–1193.

Purrello, F., Burnham, D. B., and Goldfine, I. D. (1983b). Insulin receptor antiserum and plant lectins mimic the direct effects on nuclear envelope phosphorylation. *Science* **221,** 462–464.

Randle, P. J. (1981). Phosphorylation–dephosphorylation cycles and the regulation of fuel selection in mammals. *Curr. Top. Cell. Reg.* **18,** 107–129.

Randle, P. J., Hutson, N. J., Kerbey, A. L., and Sugden, P. H. (1979). Regulation of pyruvate dehydrogenase by phosphorylation/dephosphorylation. *Miami Winter Symp.* **16,** 501–520.

Reed, L. J. (1974). Multienzyme complexes. *Acc. Chem. Res.* **7,** 40–46.

Reed, L. J. (1981). Regulation of mammalian pyruvate dehydrogenase complex by a phosphorylation–dephosphorylation cycle. *Curr. Top. Cell. Reg.* **18,** 95–106.

Rosen, O. M., Rubin, C. S., Cobb, M. H., and Smith, C. J. (1981). Insulin stimulates the phosphorylation of ribosomal protein S6 in a cell-free system derived from 3T3-L1 adipocytes. *J. Biol. Chem.* **256,** 3630–3633.

Sakamoto, Y., Kuzuya, T., and Sato, J. (1982). Demonstration of a pyruvate dehydrogenase activator in insulin-treated human placental plasma membrane. *Biomed. Res.* **3,** 599–605.

Saltiel, A., Jacobs, S., Siegel, M., and Cuatrecasas, P. (1981). Insulin stimulates the release from liver plasma membranes of a chemical modulator of pyruvate dehydrogenase. *Biochem. Biophys. Res. Commun.* **102,** 1041–1047.

Saltiel, A. R., Siegel, M. I., Jacobs, S., and Cuatrecasas, P. (1982). Putative mediators of insulin action: Regulation of pyruvate dehydrogenase and adenylate cyclase activities. *Proc. Natl. Acad. Sci. U.S.A.* **79,** 3513–3517.

Saltiel, A. R., Doble, A., Jacobs, S., and Cuatrecasas, P. (1983). Putative mediators of insulin action regulate hepatic acetyl CoA carboxylase activity. *Biochem. Biophys. Res. Commun.* **110,** 789–795.

Schumm, D. E., and Webb, T. E. (1981). Insulin-modulated transport of RNA from isolated liver nuclei. *Arch. Biochem. Biophys.* **210,** 275–279.

Schuster, S. M., Olson, M. S., and Routh, C. A. (1975). Studies on the regulation of pyruvate dehydrogenase in isolated beef heart mitochondria. *Arch. Biochem. Biophys.* **171,** 745–752.

Seals, J. R. (1983). Insulin-dependent intracellular petide that stimulates pyruvate dehydrogenase in isolated mitochondria. *Diabetes* **32,** 57A.

Seals, J. R., and Czech, M. P. (1980). Evidence that insulin activates an intrinsic plasma membrane protease in generating a secondary chemical mediator. *J. Biol. Chem.* **255,** 6529–6531.

Seals, J. R., and Czech, M. P. (1981). Characterization of a pyruvate dehydrogenase activator released by adipocyte plasma membrane in response to insulin. *J. Biol. Chem.* **256**, 2894–2899.

Seals, J. R., and Czech, M. P. (1982). Production by plasma membranes of a chemical mediator of insulin action. *Fed. Proc., Fed. Am. Soc. Exp. Biol.* **41**, 2730–2735.

Seals, J. R., and Jarett, L. (1980). Activation of pyruvate dehydrogenase by direct addition of insulin to an isolated plasma membrane/mitochondria mixture: Evidence for generation of insulin's second messenger in a subcellular system. *Proc. Natl. Acad. Sci. U.S.A.* **77**, 77–81.

Seals, J. R., McDonald, J. M., and Jarett, L. (1978). Direct effect of insulin on the labelling of isolated plasma membranes by [^{32}-P]ATP. *Biochem. Biophys. Res. Commun.* **83**, 1365–1372.

Seals, J. R., McDonald, J. M., and Jarett, L. (1979a). Insulin effect on protein phosphorylation of plasma membranes and mitochondria in a subcellular system from rat adipocytes. I. Identification of insulin-sensitive phosphoproteins. *J. Biol. Chem.* **254**, 6991–6996.

Seals, J. R., McDonald, J. M., and Jarett, L. (1979b). Insulin effect on protein phosphorylation of plasma membranes and mitochondria in a subcellular system from rat adipocytes. II. Characterization of insulin-sensitive phosphorproteins and conditions for observation of the insulin effect. *J. Biol. Chem.* **254**, 6997–7005.

Servely, J. L., Teyssot, B., Houdebine, L. M., Delouis, C., Djiane, J., and Kelly, P. A. (1982). Induction of β-casein mRNA accumulation by the putative prolactin second messenger added to the culture medium of culture mammary epithelial cells. *FEBS Lett.* **148**, 242–246.

Smith, C. J., and Rosen, O. M. (1983). Mechanism of action of insulin. *In* "Diabetes Mellitus: Theory and Practice" (M. Ellenberg and H. Rifkin, eds.), pp. 89–96. Medical Examination Publ., New Hyde Park, New York.

Sugden, P. H., Kerbey, A. L., Randle, P. J., Waller, C. A., and Reid, K. B. M. (1979). Amino acid sequences around the sites of phosphorylation in the pig heart pyruvate dehydrogenase complex. *Biochem. J.* **181**, 419–426.

Teyssot, B., Houdebine, L. M., and Djiane, J. (1981). Prolactin induces the release of a factor from membranes capable of stimulating β-casein gene transcription in isolated mammary nuclei. *Proc. Natl. Acad. Sci. U.S.A.* **78**, 6729–6733.

Teyssot, B., Djiane, J., Kelly, P. A., and Houdebine, L. M. (1982). Identification of the putative prolactin second messenger activating β-casein gene transcription. *Biol. Cell.* **43**, 81–88.

Torres, H. N., Flawia, M. M., Hernaez, L., and Cuatrecasas, P. (1978). Effects of insulin on the adenylyl cyclase activity of isolated fat cell membranes. *J. Membr. Biol.* **43**, 1–18.

Turakulov, Y. K., Gainutdinov, M. K., Lavina, J. I., and Akhmatov, M. S. (1977). Insulin dependent cytoplasmic regulation of Ca^{2+} ion transport in liver mitochondria. *Rep. Acad. Sci. USSR* **234**, 1471–1474.

Turakulov, Y. K., Gainutdinov, M. K., Lavina, I. I., and Akhmatov, M. S. (1979). Regulation of oxidative phosphorylation by adrenalin and insulin: Role of the insulin-dependent cytoplasmic regulator. *Bull. Exp. Biol. Med.* **88**, 1008–1010.

Walaas, O., and Horn, R. S. (1981). The controversial problem of insulin action. *Trends Pharmacol. Sci.* **2**, 196–198.

Walaas, O., Sletten, K., Horn, R. J., Lystad, E., Adler, A., and Alertsen, A. R. (1981). Insulin-dependent protein phosphorylation in membranes. Isolation and characterization of a phosphorylated proteolipid from sacrolemma. *FEBS Lett.* **128**, 137–141.

Wasner, H. K. (1980). Cyclo-AMP-antagonist-der Hormone des Insulins. *Aktuel. Endokrinol. Stoffwechsel* **1**, 207–208.

Wasner, H. K. (1981). Biosynthesis of cyclic AMP antagonist in hepatocytes from rats after adrenalin- or insulin-stimulation. Isolation, purification and prostaglandin E-requirement for its synthesis. *FEBS Lett.* **133**, 260–264.

Whitehouse, S., Cooper, R. H., and Randle, P. J. (1974). Mechanism of activation of pyruvate dehydrogenase by dichloroacetate and other halogenated carboxylic acids. *Biochem. J.* **141**, 761–774.

Witters, L. A. (1981). Insulin stimulates the phosphorylation of acetyl-CoA carboxylase. *Biochem. Biophys. Res. Commun.* **100**, 872–878.

Wrenn, R. W., Katoh, N., Wise, B. C., and Kuo, J. F. (1980). Stimulation by phosphatidylserine and calmodulin of calcium-dependent phosphorylation of endogenous proteins from cerebral cortex. *J. Biol. Chem.* **255**, 12042–12046.

Yeaman, S. J., Hutcheson, E. T., Roche, T. E., Pettit, F. H., Brown, J. R., Reed, L. J., Watson, D. C., and Dixon, G. H. (1978). Sites of phosphorylation on pyruvate dehydrogenase from bovine kidney and heart. *Biochemistry* **17**, 2364–2370.

Zhang, S.-R., Shi, Q.-H., and Ho, R. J. (1983). Cyclic AMP-lowering mediator of insulin: Generation, quantitation and properties. *J. Biol. Chem.* **258**, 6471–6476.

VITAMINS AND HORMONES, VOL. 41

Relaxin

BRUCE E. KEMP[1] AND HUGH D. NIALL

Howard Florey Institute of Experimental Physiology and Medicine,
University of Melbourne,
Parkville, Victoria, Australia

I. Introduction	79
II. Relaxin Genes	80
A. DNA Sequences	80
B. mRNA Sequences and Processing	85
C. mRNA Localization	85
III. Relaxin Covalent Structure	86
A. Processing	88
B. Evolution	93
IV. Synthetic Relaxin	94
A. Summary	94
B. Chemical Synthesis of Porcine Relaxin	94
C. Synthesis of a Human Relaxin	96
D. Synthesis of Relaxin Connecting Peptide Fragments	97
V. Mechanism of Action of Relaxin	97
A. Regulation of Uterine Contractions	97
B. Smooth Muscle Contraction	98
C. Hormonal Regulation of Smooth Muscle Contraction	99
D. Relaxin Effects on Uterine cAMP	103
VI. Relaxin Receptors	106
VII. Medical and Physiological Perspectives	107
A. Physiology of Relaxin in the Human Female	107
B. Physiology of Relaxin in the Human Male	108
C. Relaxin as a Therapeutic Agent	108
References	109

I. Introduction

Relaxin is now well known as a pregnancy-associated polypeptide. Its most important targets appear to be components of the reproductive tract, namely, the uterus, the cervix, and pubic symphysis. Further physiological functions for relaxin appear likely in nonpregnant females and possibly males but these are presently less well characterized.

[1]Present address: Department of Medicine, University of Melbourne, Repatriation General Hospital, Heidelberg, Victoria 3081, Australia.

Although the history of relaxin dates to the 1920s (Hisaw, 1926) it was not until the purification of porcine relaxin by Sherwood and O'Byrne (1974) that significant interest in this hormone revived, culminating in the determination of the primary structure (Schwabe *et al.*, 1977; James *et al.*, 1977) of porcine relaxin.

Many aspects of the physiology (Porter, 1979, 1982; Bryant-Greenwood, 1982), history (Bryant-Greenwood, 1982; Kroc, 1982; Steinetz and Kroc, 1981), bioassay (Steinetz *et al.*, 1983), radioimmunoassay (Steinetz, 1982; Bryant-Greenwood, 1982), and protein sequencing of relaxin (Schwabe *et al.*, 1978; Bryant-Greenwood, 1982) have been reviewed previously. There have also been a number of conferences devoted to relaxin over the last 4 years (Anderson, 1982; Steinetz *et al.*, 1982; Bryant-Greenwood *et al.*, 1981; Bigazzi *et al.*, 1983) and these are cited under the editors of the conference proceedings.

In this article we review the most recent findings including the discovery of a gene for human relaxin and advances in our understanding of the mechanism of action of relaxin on smooth muscle. We have tried to complement previous reviews and have not attempted an exhaustive citation of the literature particularly that prior to the availability of purified relaxin in 1974 (Sherwood and O'Byrne, 1974).

II. Relaxin Genes

A. DNA Sequences

Like most polypeptide hormones, relaxin belongs to a family of structurally related molecules representing the products of structurally related genes. As discussed in more detail below, relaxins, insulins, and insulin-like growth factors (IGFs) share certain features of primary, secondary, and (probably) tertiary structure. Hence it seems probable that the genes coding for these three hormones in contemporary organisms have evolved through a series of gene duplications from a common ancestral gene, as an example of divergent evolution. Thus there is considerable interest in determining the number and structure of relaxin genes in a range of species wide enough to shed further light on the evolutionary, structural, and functional relationships of the insulin-related gene family.

A discussion in detail of the methods for cloning and sequencing relaxin genes is outside the scope of this article. However, the general approaches used in the cloning of relaxin cDNA in the rat (Hudson *et al.*, 1981a) and pig (Haley *et al.*, 1982) were based on (1) amino acid sequence analysis of the peptide hormone, (2) synthesis of oligodeoxyribonucleotide primers complementary to putative mRNA sequences predicted from the amino acid sequences, (3) use of these synthetic DNA fragments as primers with mRNA isolated from rat and pig corpora lutea of pregnancy for the production of radiolabeled relaxin-specific cDNA probes, and (4) the identification of relaxin-specific clones in cDNA clone banks constructed from total pregnancy-derived corpus luteum mRNA. It proved necessary to treat the cloning of rat and pig relaxins as two totally independent projects because the amino acid sequences of the hormones (and by implication, the nucleotide sequences coding for them) were so divergent that one could not expect to use restriction fragments of the rat relaxin cDNA, for example to identify, through cross-hybridization, pig relaxin clones in a pig ovarian cDNA library.

Cloning of human relaxin genes required a different strategy since there was no amino acid sequence information for the human hormone due to the difficulties in obtaining a suitable human tissue source of relaxin. The relaxin (measured by bioassay) concentrations in non-pregnant human tissues and in readily available tissues from pregnant women (e.g., placenta, decidua) are too low to permit isolation (Bryant-Greenwood, 1982; Yamamoto et al., 1981; Bigazzi et al., 1980). The only practical source is the corpus luteum of pregnancy, a tissue available only rarely and in small quantity, normally as the result of an operation for ectopic pregnancy.

We did, however, identify a region of the pig relaxin cDNA (corresponding to amino acids 45–94 of the C peptide) that showed a reasonably high degree of homology (71% at the nucleotide level) with rat relaxin cDNA, and which therefore potentially could represent an area of relative homology between relaxins of different species. A probe constructed from this restriction fragment was used to screen a human genomic library (Maniatis et al., 1978) and two λ clones were identified on the basis of strong hybridization to the probe. One of these was extensively analyzed to provide the complete coding sequence of a putative human relaxin gene, termed human relaxin gene 1 (Hudson et al., 1983; Niall et al., 1983). The second clone was an incomplete version of the first. Southern blot analysis using a probe obtained from human relaxin gene 1 was carried out on human DNA isolated from leukocytes or placental tissue of different unrelated individuals. The results suggested that all subjects studied possessed human relaxin gene 1; in addition some weaker hybridizing DNA fragments were identified, indicating that at least one other relaxin-related gene may exist in the human (Hudson et al., 1983). Subsequently, rescreening of the *Maniatis* human genomic library has confirmed the presence of a second human relaxin gene (gene 2), analysis of which is in progress. Preliminary data indicate that gene 2 codes for a polypeptide signifi-

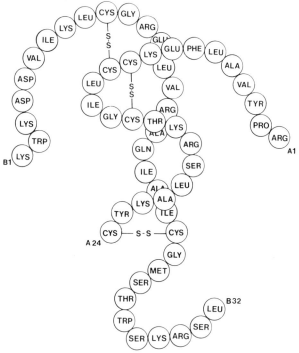

Fɪɢ. 1. Covalent structure of human relaxin (A24,B32) predicted from the nucleotide sequence of gene 1 (Hudson *et al.*, 1983).

cantly different in amino acid sequence to the structure of human relaxin-1 shown in Fig. 1 (Hudson *et al.*, 1984).

These results draw attention to what is now becoming a more frequent problem in molecular and cellular biology: determining whether a particular gene found in genomic (chromosomal) DNA is really a functional gene or a nonfunctional "pseudo-gene." Ultimately, proof resides in identifying in a particular tissue the mRNA and the translated polypeptide coded for by the gene in question. We are currently examining human ovary, placenta, and other reproductive tissues with appropriate probes to detect the sites of relaxin gene expression for relaxin genes 1 and 2. It will also be necessary to examine nonreproductive tissues since one cannot assume that the function of relaxin is confined to the reproductive tract. Although at present these studies are incomplete, there are strong indications that human relaxin gene 1 may be a functional gene. It has an open reading frame, a high degree of homology in the putative coding regions with rat and pig relaxins, and an appropriately positioned consensus sequence for excision of an intron interrupting the C-peptide coding region. More-over Tregear and colleagues have synthesized a relaxin molecule, based on the predicted relaxin gene 1 amino acid sequence, which has relaxin-like biological activity in the rat uterus (Hudson *et al.*, 1983; Tregear *et al.*, 1982) bioassay. These results tell us only that human relaxin gene 1 is a potentially active gene but this falls short of proof. It is now clear, however, that human relaxin gene 2 *is* a functional gene since it is expressed in human corpus luteum tissue during preg-nancy (Hudson *et al.*, 1984), whereas gene 1 does not seem to be ex-pressed under these circumstances. In other recent work, we have found that both human relaxin genes are present on chromosome 9, suggesting an origin by a gene duplication event (Crawford *et al.*, 1984).

The present information on relaxin genes includes cDNA analysis of pig and rat relaxins (from corpus luteum of pregnancy) and partial or complete analysis of the genomic DNA of human relaxin gene 1, human gene 2, a pig relaxin genomic clone (Haley *et al.*, unpublished results), a rat relaxin genomic clone, and a mouse relaxin genomic clone (Cronk *et al.*, unpublished results). The structures obtained are consistent with the overall plan illustrated (for human relaxin gene 1) in Fig. 2. In all species examined so far, the configuration is signal peptide (S) followed by a B chain of about 30 amino acids, a C-peptide of about 105 amino acids, and an A chain of 22–24 amino acids. In the human, pig, mouse, and rat genomic clones, an intron interrupts the

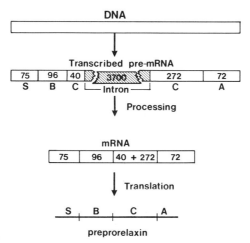

FIG. 2. Schematic illustration of the flow of information from the relaxin gene to the primary peptide hormone product. RNA polymerase transcribes the relaxin gene to give relaxin premessenger-RNA containing a 3700 base intron. After messenger-RNA pro-cessing this serves as a template for translation to yield preprorelaxin (S–B–C–A).

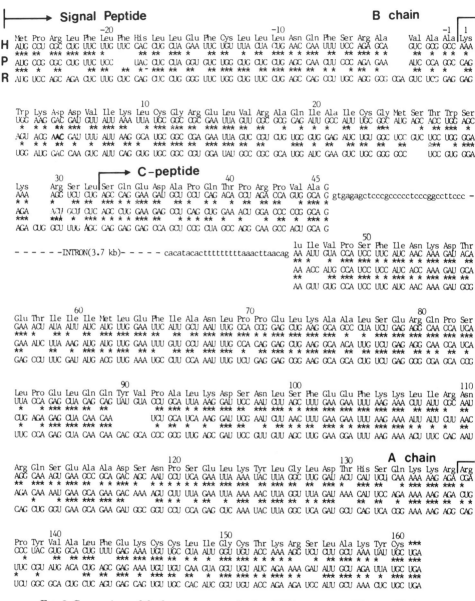

FIG. 3. Comparison of the known preprorelaxin mRNA sequences. Human (H), Pig (P), and Rat (R) sequences are displayed with the corresponding human preprorelaxin amino acid sequence (based on gene 1) on the upper line. A portion of the intron sequence is presented in lower case DNA notation. Nucleotide identities are indicated by asterisks.

coding region at or close to the position shown in Fig. 3. Interestingly, this corresponds almost exactly in position to one of the two introns found in insulin genes (Bell *et al.*, 1980). It is not yet clear whether relaxin genes also have an intron in the 5' untranslated region, where the second insulin gene intron is found. However, conservation of at least one intron site between relaxin and insulin genes provides further support for the concept that they are related through a common ancestral gene.

B. mRNA SEQUENCES AND PROCESSING

In the species for which we have structural information on both relaxin genomic DNA and cDNA (reflecting mRNA), there is complete agreement between the two sequences. The mRNA sequences for human, pig, and rat preprorelaxin are illustrated in Fig. 3. So far there is no evidence of polymorphism or allelic differences in relaxin gene structure, but it is premature to exclude these possibilities. However, in the analysis of rat relaxin cDNA (Hudson *et al.*, 1981a) two different types of clone were identified; they differed in the presence (or absence) of a *Pst*I restriction enzyme cleavage site, which in turn resulted from an insertion/deletion of three nucleotides from the C-peptide region exactly at the site of the intron. It seems likely that this heterogeneity of rat relaxin mRNA is produced by variable excision of the intron in a manner analogous to that described for the human growth hormone gene (Wallis, 1980). Variable processing of pre-mRNA in this way provides a means of generating more than one polypeptide product from a single gene. In this particular case it seems unlikely that the event, which would result in formation of two rat preprorelaxins differing only in a single amino acid (alanine) in the C-peptide, is of any biological significance. It probably reflects a lack of absolute specificity in the intron excision mechanism.

C. mRNA LOCALIZATION

A recently developed technique (Hudson *et al.*, 1981b) for the localization of specific mRNAs in sections of whole tissue, termed "hybridization histochemistry," has been applied to ovaries from pregnant rats (Hudson *et al.*, 1981a). Using a high specific activity ^{32}P-labeled probe, we have identified high levels of relaxin mRNA in the cells of the corpora lutea, with no significant labeling of other tissues (Hudson *et al.*, unpublished results). In more recent studies we have demonstrated the time course of the appearance of relaxin mRNA during pregnancy in the rat. The rat relaxin mRNA appears simultaneously in all corpora lutea on about day 7 of pregnancy, and disappears promptly after parturition (within about 24 hours). This technique promises to be very valuable in identifying the sites of relaxin biosynthesis in other species, including the human. The recent report (Evans *et al.*, 1983) that relaxin is a theca cell rather than a granulosa cell product in porcine preovulatory follicles is of particular interest and further studies should be carried out to confirm this at the level of mRNA localization.

III. Relaxin Covalent Structure

The amino acid sequences of porcine rat and human preprorelaxins are known from predictions based on nucleotide sequences, and, in addition, independently derived amino acid sequences for porcine and rat relaxins have been determined by standard peptide sequence analysis of the native hormones (James *et al.*, 1977; Schwabe *et al.*, 1977;

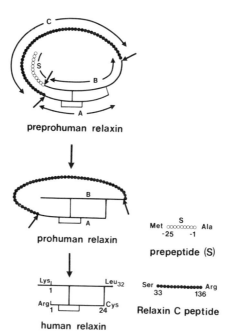

Fig. 4. Schematic summary of the processing of the preproform of human relaxin to the native hormone with the successive removal of the signal peptide (S) and the connecting (C) peptide by proteolytic cleavage.

John *et al.*, 1981a). There is complete agreement between the two sources of data where they overlap. The structural plan of the preprorelaxins is illustrated (for the human hormone) in Fig. 4. The similarity to preproinsulin is obvious, but here are some important distinctions. One of the most striking is the large size of the C-peptide region. It is unclear whether the C-peptide has functions additional to its presumed role in aligning the A and B chains correctly in the precursor molecule to favor correct disulfide bond pairing and correct folding of the relaxin chains. It is interesting that the C-peptide is marginally better conserved than the A and B chains when rat, pig, and human sequences are compared (Fig. 5). In addition, there is good conservation of the distribution and relative numbers of hydrophobic, uncharged polar, acidic, and basic residues between the different C-peptides. Unlike the insulin C-peptide, which has a limited array of amino acids and is rich in glutamic acid, proline, and glycine, the relaxin C-peptides contain all the amino acids except tryptophan, with internal basic residues which could represent subsites for further processing. This variety, in combination with a reasonable level of conser-

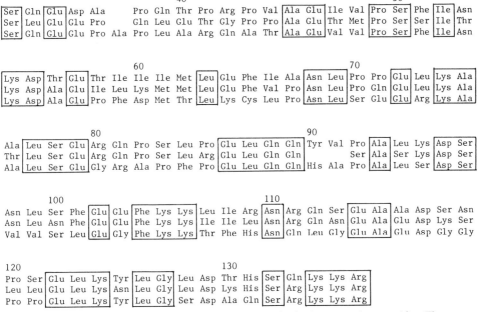

FIG. 5. Comparison of the amino acid sequences of relaxin connecting peptides. The sequences for human (H), rat (R), and pig (P) were deduced from the corresponding nucleotide sequences. Residues common to the three sequences are boxed.

vation of structure between species, is suggestive of a biological function. Thus it would seem justifiable to look for a biological function of the C peptide, or fragments thereof, but at present there is no direct evidence for or against this.

A. Processing

Processing represents another area of difference between relaxin and insulin. Proinsulin is converted to insulin by enzymes that cleave at pairs of basic residues at either end of the C-peptide region. A carboxypeptidase B-like enzyme removes the basic residues then left attached to the carboxyl terminus of the insulin B chain. Prorelaxin contains a cluster of basic amino acids at the C-peptide–A chain junction which may direct cleavage at this site (Fig. 3). However, there are no basic residues at the point of cleavage of B chain from C-peptide. Both pig and rat relaxin B chains end in a leucine residue (John *et al.*, 1981a,b) which is immediately followed by a serine residue in the prohormone (Fig. 3). It would require an enzyme with a chymotryptic-like specificity to cleave this leucine–serine bond to generate relaxin from its precursor. The same leucine–serine sequence is found in human prorelaxin, though here there is also a pair of basic residues nearby which could perhaps be the site of processing. Isolation of intact native human relaxin (from human corpora lutea of pregnancy) will be required to settle this point. Overall it seems likely that, just as insulin and relaxin have evolved by a gene duplication, so too have the enzymes responsible for their precursor processing. It seems also likely that the enzymes that process prorelaxin will be coordinately expressed in the corpus luteum of pregnancy, with the "switch-on" of the relaxin gene.

The first comparison to be made is between the known members of the insulin gene family—insulin itself, relaxin, and IGF_1. The striking similarity is in the number and disposition of disulfide bridges, which are identically spaced in all four hormones (Fig. 6). The additional sequence homology is small, and largely confined to residues which are known to be buried in the hydrophobic core of the insulin structure as determined by X-ray crystallography (Blundell *et al.*, 1972). This observation provided the basis for construction of possible three-dimensional models of relaxin based closely on the insulin coordinates. It was

---

FIG. 6. Amino acid sequences for human relaxin (gene 1), insulin, and IGF_1. Residues are numbered with respect to the insulin sequence. Residues common to the three sequences are boxed (see text).

A CHAIN

	-4	-3	-2	-1	1	2	3	4	5	6	7
Relaxin	Arg	Pro	Tyr	Val	Ala	Leu	Phe	Glu	Lys	Cys	Cys
Insulin					Gly	Ile	Val	Glu	Gln	Cys	Cys
IGF$_1$					Gly	Ile	Val	Asp	Glu	Cys	Cys

	8	9	10	11	12	13	14	15	16	17	18
	Leu	Ile	Gly	Cys	Thr	Lys	Arg	Ser	Leu	Ala	Lys
	Thr	Ser	Ile	Cys	Ser	Leu	Tyr	Gln	Leu	Glu	Asn
	Phe	Arg	Ser	Cys	Asp	Leu	Arg	Arg	Leu	Glu	Met

	19	20	21	22	23	24	25	26	27	28	29
	Tyr	Cys									
	Tyr	Cys	Asn								
	Tyr	Cys	Ala	Pro	Leu	Lys	Pro	Ala	Lys	Ser	Ala

B CHAIN

	-3	-2	-1	1	2	3	4	5	6	7	8	9
Relaxin	Lys	Trp	Lys	Asp	Asp	Val	Ile	Lys	Leu	Cys	Gly	Arg
Insulin				Phe	Val	Asn	Gln	His	Leu	Cys	Gly	Ser
IGF$_1$				Gly	Pro	Glu	Thr	Leu	Cys	Gly	Ala

	10	11	12	13	14	15	16	17	18	19	20	21
	Glu	Leu	Val	Arg	Ala	Gln	Ile	Ala	Ile	Cys	Gly	Met
	His	Leu	Val	Glu	Ala	Leu	Tyr	Leu	Val	Cys	Gly	Glu
	Glu	Leu	Val	Asp	Ala	Leu	Gln	Phe	Val	Cys	Gly	Asp

	22	23	24	25	26	27	28	29	30
	Ser	Thr	Trp	Ser	Lys	Arg	Ser	Leu	
	Arg	Gly	Phe	Phe	Tyr	Thr	Pro	Lys	Thr
	Arg	Gly	Phe	Tyr	Phe	Asn	Lys	Pro	Thr

RELAXIN B CHAINS

Species	-7	-6	-5	-4	-3	-2	-1	1	2	3	4	5	6	7	8	9	10	11	12	13	14	15	16	17
Human					Lys	Trp	Lys	Asp	Asp	Val	Ile	Lys	Leu	Cys	Gly	Arg	Glu	Leu	Val	Arg	Ala	Gln	Ile	Ala
Pig					PCA	Ser	Thr	Asn	Asp	Phe	Ile	Lys	Ala	Cys	Gly	Arg	Glu	Leu	Val	Arg	Leu	Trp	Val	Glu
Rat	Arg	Val	Ser	Glu	Glu	Trp	Met	Asp	Gln	Val	Ile	Gln	Val	Cys	Gly	Arg	Gly	Tyr	Ala	Arg	Ala	Trp	Ile	Glu
Shark-ST		PCA	Ser	Leu	Ser	Asn	Ala	Gly	Ser	Gly	Ile	Lys	Leu	Cys	Gly	Arg	Gly	Phe	Ile	Arg	Ala	Ile	Ile	Phe
Shark-D					PCA	Asn	Ala	Glu	Pro	Gly	Ile	Lys	Leu	Cys	Gly	Arg	Glu	Phe	Ile	Arg	Ala	Val	Ile	Tyr

Species	18	19	20	21	22	23	24	25	26	27	28	29
Human	Ile	Cys	Gly	Met	Ser	Thr	Trp	Ser	Lys	Arg	Ser	Leu
Pig	Ile	Cys	Gly	Ser	Val	Ser	Trp	Gly	Arg	Thr	Ala	Leu
Rat	Val	Cys	Gly	Ala	Ser	Val	Gly	Arg	Leu	Ala	Leu	
Shark-ST	Ala	Cys	Gly	Gly	Ser	Arg						
Shark-D	Ser	Cys	Gly									

RELAXIN A CHAINS

	-4	-3	-2	-1	1	2	3	4	5	6	7	8	9	10	11	12	13	14	15	16	17	18	19	20
Human	Arg	Pro	Tyr	Val	Ala	Leu	Phe	Glu	Lys	Cys	Cys	Leu	Ile	Gly	Cys	Thr	Lys	Arg	Ser	Leu	Ala	Lys	Tyr	Cys
Pig			Arg	Met	Thr	Leu	Ser	Glu	Lys	Cys	Cys	Gln	Val	Gly	Cys	Ile	Arg	Lys	Asp	Ile	Ala	Arg	Leu	Cys
Rat	PCA	Ser	Gly	Ala	Leu	Leu	Ser	Glu	Gln	Cys	Cys	His	Ile	Gly	Cys	Thr	Arg	Arg	Ser	Ile	Ala	Lys	Leu	Cys
Shark-ST	Ala	Thr	Ser	Pro	Ala	Met	Ser	Ile	Lys	Cys	Cys	Ile	Tyr	Gly	Cys	Thr	Lys	Lys	Asp	Ile	Ser	Val	Leu	Cys
Shark-D	Glu	Gly	Ser	Pro	Gly	Met	Ser	Ser	Lys	Cys	Cys	Thr	Tyr	Gly	Cys	Thr	Arg	Lys	Asp	Ile	Ser	Ile	Leu	Cys

Fig. 7. Comparison of amino acid sequences for relaxin A and B chains. The human sequence was deduced solely from the corresponding nucleotide sequence while the remainder were determined by conventional amino acid sequencing. The sand tiger shark (shark-ST) and dogfish shark (shark-D) sequences were determined by Schwabe and his colleagues (Schwabe, 1983). Residues common to the five sequences are boxed. Residues are numbered with respect to the insulin sequence (Fig. 6).

found that the relaxin side chains could be accommodated without strain in the insulin main chain structure; the models were validated as plausible by use of a computer graphics system (Bedarkar et al., 1977; Isaacs et al., 1978). It must be stressed that these models are hypothetical and direct studies of relaxin structure will be required to confirm or refute them. Unfortunately, to date the crystals of relaxin which have been produced have been small and irregular and unsuitable for crystallographic analysis.

There is however some indirect evidence suggesting that relaxin has indeed an overall configuration somewhat similar to that of insulin. Circular dichroism spectra from pig insulin and pig relaxin are similar, consistent with a similar peptide chain folding (Schwabe and Harmon, 1978; Rawitch et al., 1980; Yu-cang et al., 1982). Moreover the models predict that the homologous sequences between insulin and relaxin will be buried and that the molecular surface will comprise residues that differ. This is consistent with the lack of any overlap in immunological or biological activity between the two hormones.

The second kind of comparison to be made is between relaxins of different species (Fig. 7). It is obvious that relaxins differ a great deal more than insulins; for example, pig and rat relaxins differ in over 50% of amino acid positions, whereas pig and rat insulins differ in only 8%. The shark (Gowan et al., 1981; Schwabe, 1983) and human relaxin sequences differ to a similar degree from one another and from the pig and rat structures. This finding indicates that relaxin structures have been under far less evolutionary pressure for conservation than have insulins. The observed differences between relaxins involve many residues which, on the basis of the above model studies, would be predicted to be on the surface. This would explain the poor immunological crossreactivity between relaxins of different species, and also a number of observed differences in their specific biological activity. Obviously these relaxin receptors (e.g., in mouse or guinea pig) are also capable of detecting some structural differences particularly between shark relaxin (which is totally inactive in the mouse) and the mammalian relaxins (which possess varying degrees of activity in the mouse pubic ligament assay). On the other hand, the finding that all relaxins so far isolated are biologically active in the rat argues for a conserved surface domain interacting with the rat relaxin receptor. Dodson and co-workers (Dodson et al., 1982) have concluded that there is a localized surface region potentially involved in receptor binding including residues B9 (arginine), B13 (arginine), A13 and A14 (lysine or arginine), with possible involvement of hydrophobic residues at A17, B14, and B18. Bedarkar et al. (1982) have made a similar proposal. Both shark relaxins contain serine at A17 and the there is a serine at B18 in the dogfish hormone. This could account for the differences in species specificity noted above for shark versus mammalian relaxins. (The numbering used here is that of the insulin chains, see Figs. 6 and 7.) Improved methods for chemical synthesis of relaxins and the use of recombinant DNA-based expression systems should allow this hypothesis to be tested fairly directly through the design and testing of relaxin analogs differing in these putative receptor-active residues.

B. EVOLUTION

The observed species differences between relaxins suggest, as noted above, that only a relatively limited surface region has been conserved during evolution, with the remainder of the surface being relatively free to undergo mutational change. The amino-terminal sequences of both A and B chains of relaxin seem to be particularly variable. Since nonfunctional regions of proteins seem to mutate quite quickly, the question to be answered is not why relaxins have diverged from one another so much but why insulins have not, seeing that a fairly localized surface region in insulin has been identified as involved in binding to, and activation of, receptors (Blundell and Humbel, 1980). Part of the answer may be in the conservation, in all but a few species, of the property of insulins to form dimers, to coordinate zinc atoms, and to form a hexameric crystalline structure (Blundell *et al.*, 1972). The preservation of these and perhaps other intermolecular interactions may require a high degree of conservation of the insulin surface residues. This is not a satisfying explanation since it is unclear why there is any evolutionary advantage in maintaining insulin stores in the form of ordered, zinc-containing crystals.

The proposal that insulin and relaxin have evolved by a process of divergent evolution involving an early gene duplication seems reasonable to the present authors (Fig. 5). However Schwabe *et al.* (1982) have argued that the observed species differences between rat, pig, and shark relaxins cannot readily be explained by such a simple model. For example, it might be expected that shark relaxin, being found in a more primitive species, should be more "insulin-like" than, say, pig relaxin. This argument of course assumes that the shark is really a "living fossil" whose gene structures and protein sequences reflect the situation that applied when more highly developed organisms diverged from the shark's evolutionary line. Schwabe's argument against the commonly accepted version of gene duplication in relation to relaxin and insulin is to be found in his article (Schwabe *et al.*, 1982) and will not be further discussed here.

IV. SYNTHETIC RELAXIN

A. SUMMARY

One of the major driving forces for the chemical synthesis of relaxin was the need for generating sufficient quantities of pure relaxin to undertake detailed physiological studies of this hormone. The species differences in relaxin amino acid sequences together with the difficulty of obtaining native relaxin, particularly human relaxin, have heightened interest in the chemical approach.

The synthesis of relaxin has proved to be extremely difficult with major problems in the procedure. While considerable progress has been made it now seems likely that the original aim of providing large quantities of pure relaxin will not be met by peptide synthesis alone but rather by application of recombinant DNA technology and expression of relaxin genes in microorganisms. Nevertheless, peptide synthesis has played a very important part in the overall recombinant DNA approach and is likely to continue to contribute to structure–function studies as well as in the preparation of species-specific relaxin antisera and monoclonal antibodies (Lerner *et al.*, 1981; Lerner, 1982).

B. CHEMICAL SYNTHESIS OF PORCINE RELAXIN

The chemical synthesis of relaxin requires the assembly of the A and B chains and their recombination in the correct configuration. Since the porcine relaxin sequence became available first the chemical synthesis strategies for relaxin have been developed using this structure. The individual A and B chains of porcine relaxin contain 22 and 31 residues, respectively. Chemical synthesis of peptides of this length can be difficult enough without the added problem of recombination of the chains to give the correct alignment of disulfide bonds.

Several approaches to these problems have been employed. The solid-phase peptide synthesis methodology of Merrifield has been used as the method of peptide assembly. In the earliest attempts to synthesize porcine relaxin the individual chains were synthesized separately (Tregear *et al.*, 1979). It became apparent that the synthetic B chain of relaxin was extremely insoluble and correspondingly difficult to purify. One of the attempts made to overcome this problem was to synthesize an artificial prohormone containing a three residue (Met–Gly–Met) connecting peptide (Tregear et al., 1979). The methionine-containing connecting peptide could be cleaved using cyanogen bromide to generate the two chain form of relaxin. It was hoped that the artificial prohormone approach would overcome the B chain solubility problems and facilitate A and B chain combination in the correct configuration. The artificial 54-residue prohormone proved to be just as insoluble and difficult to purify as the isolated B chain and this approach was abandoned. Recently the artificial prohormone concept has been revised by Stewart and Bell (1982) in relation to relaxin synthesis by genetically engineered microorganisms. They proposed an acid-sensitive –Asp–Pro–Gly–Asp–Pro artificial connecting peptide.

A significant improvement in the synthesis of the porcine B chain came from the work of Tregear and Yu-cang Du (Tregear et al., 1981, 1982) who found that a major contribution to the insoluble nature of the B chain was due to tryptophan at position 27. The results of circular dichroism (CD) studies of the individual S-sulfonated A and B chains of relaxin indicated that the B chain was over 90% in the β-structure whereas the A chain was unordered (Yu-cang et al., 1982). Significantly the shortened form of the B chain (B1-25) lacking the carboxyl-terminal sequence –Ser–Trp–Gly–Arg–Thr–Ala had a CD spectrum indicative of an unordered structure similar to the A chain of relaxin (Yu-cang et al., 1982). The propensity of the relaxin B-chain (B1-28) to assume a tight β-structure is thought to diminish its capacity to recombine with the A chain. The recombination yields obtained with the short form of the B chain (B25) were much improved over those obtained with the B27 chain. Preliminary studies indicate that the recombined relaxin A22,B25 retains biological activity despite the loss of the carboxyl-terminal peptide (Yu-cang et al., 1982; Tregear et al., 1982). This is in marked contrast to insulin where the carboxyl-terminal portion of the B chain has profound effects on the binding of insulin to its receptor (Steiner, 1977). The current strategy employed for the chemical synthesis of relaxin developed by Tregear and colleagues is illustrated below (Fig. 8). The recombination procedures using S-sulfonation were employed by Schwartz and Katsoyannis (1976) for the preparation of insulin but have been optimized for the recombination of relaxin chains by Tregear and Yu-cang. Although the chemical synthesis of relaxin has not proved to be a significant source of relaxin for physiological studies the knowledge gained in studying the recombination of the isolated chains may yet be vital for effecting the recombination of A and B chains expressed by genetically engineered microorganisms.

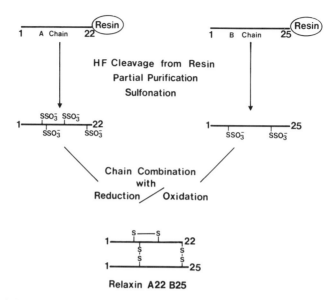

FIG. 8. Schematic representation of the synthetic strategy employed in the chemical synthesis of human relaxin. The A and B chains of relaxin are assembled separately then recombined to yield the two-chain form of the native hormone.

A further problem involved in the synthesis of relaxin has been the assay for biological activity. To date the amounts of synthetic material available have restricted its assessment in most cases to the inhibition of uterine contraction assay. Although more sensitive than the classical interpubic ligament assay (Steinetz *et al.*, 1960) this assay is not as specific. Greater precision can be obtained using the radioimmunoassay, however, this does not necessarily reflect biological activity. To this end a receptor assay would certainly greatly facilitate the quantitative assessment of synthetic relaxin preparations given an appropriate receptor-rich tissue or cell source.

C. SYNTHESIS OF A HUMAN RELAXIN

After the discovery of a human gene for relaxin (Hudson *et al.*, 1983) Tregear and colleagues (Tregear *et al.*, 1982) prepared the corresponding human relaxin (A25,B24). The shortened version of the B chain was used to avoid the anticipated solubility problems due to tryptophan at position 27 (see Section IV,B). By using the same recombination strategies that were developed for porcine relaxin a synthetic human relaxin preparation was obtained with low bioactivity compared to native porcine relaxin (Hudson *et al.*, 1983). It is not yet clear whether the low activity reflects the potency of the human relaxin in the rat uterus bioassay or its chemical integrity.

D. Synthesis of Relaxin Connecting Peptide Fragments

The availability of amino acid sequence information for the connecting peptide has made possible development of appropriate antisera and studies on the biosynthesis, storage, and processing of prorelaxin. In a preliminary report Gorman *et al.* (1983) found that rat C-peptide could be detected in extracts of nonpregnant ovaries at approximately 2 ng/mg. There was an approximate 100-fold rise to 200 ng/mg by late pregnancy. The results indicated that the C-peptide exists in amounts comparable to those for relaxin in the corpora lutea of pregnant rats.

The expectation is that antibodies prepared to synthetic fragments of the C-peptide will yield further valuable information on the processing of prorelaxin. Moreover this work will provide the basis for evaluating the diagnostic potential of human relaxin C-peptide measurements as has been done for the insulin C-peptide (Bonser and Garcia-Webb, 1981).

V. Mechanism of Action of Relaxin

Studies on the mechanism of action of relaxin at the molecular level have been largely limited to the uterus where the relaxin-dependent inhibition of contraction is rapid. Relatively little work has been done on the pubic symphysis and cervix. For this reason our review will concentrate on what is known about the mechanism of action of relaxin on the uterus.

A. Regulation of Uterine Contractions

A brief summary of the regulation of smooth muscle contraction is given below to provide a basis for subsequent discussion of the possible sites of action of relaxin. Relaxin inhibits spontaneous uterine contractions (Krantz *et al.*, 1950; Sawyer *et al.*, 1952; Wiqvist and Paul, 1958) as well as those driven by electrical stimulation (Porter, 1981; Kemp and Niall, 1981), KCl depolarization (St. Louis, 1981), oxytocin, or prostaglandin $PGF_{2\alpha}$ (Porter *et al.*, 1981). In the estrogen-primed rat both longitudinal and circular muscle are sensitive to relaxin.

B. Smooth Muscle Contraction

Unlike skeletal muscle the myosin and actin filaments of smooth muscle are not arranged in regular arrays but rather as more random bundles (Small, 1977). The architecture of smooth muscle cells is also influenced by a cytoskeletal network of intermediate filaments that are not involved directly in the contractile process (Small and Sobieszek, 1980).

In the past 5 years considerable advances have been made in the understanding of the molecular basis of smooth muscle contraction (reviewed by Adelstein and Eisenberg, 1980). Smooth muscle does not contain the troponin calcium regulatory system associated with actin filaments that is characteristic of cardiac and skeletal muscles (Perry and Grand, 1979). In contrast calcium regulates smooth muscle via the myosin thick filament (Adelstein and Eisenberg, 1980). A schematic structure of the smooth muscle myosin and actin filaments is shown in Fig. 9. The myosin globular head region contains the actin binding site, the ATPase site, and the associated myosin light chains. There are two pairs of myosin light chains MLC_1 (M_r = 17,000) and MLC_2 (M_r = 20,000) per pair of myosin heads (Perry, 1975). The smooth muscle myosin light chains from chicken gizzard have been sequenced recently (Maita *et al.*, 1981; Matsada *et al.*, 1981). Skeletal and cardiac muscle also contain tissue-specific myosin light chains (Perry, 1975).

Smooth muscle contraction is accompanied by the reversible phosphorylatin of the myosin light chain MLC_2. This reaction is catalyzed by the myosin light chain kinase (Dabrowska *et al.*, 1977) and reversed by the myosin light chain phosphatase (Aksoy *et al.*, 1976). The myosin

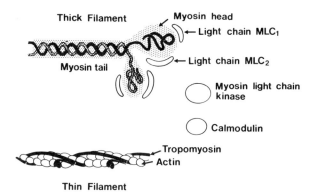

Fig. 9. Diagrammatic representation of the contractile elements of smooth muscle. Phosphorylation of the myosin light chain (MLC_2) stimulates the actin-activated myosin ATPase (see text).

light chain is phosphorylated at a specific residue, serine-19 (Maita *et al.*, 1981). There is now a considerable body of evidence to support the concept that phosphorylation of the smooth muscle myosin light chain is essential for activation of the actin-activated myosin ATPase and generation of contractile force by cross-bridge formation (reviewed by Adelstein and Eisenberg, 1980). Uterine smooth muscle is also regulated by this mechanism since phosphorylation of partially purified ovine uterine myosin increases the actin-dependent ATPase activity (Lebowitz and Cooke, 1979). Moreover, it has been shown that rat myometrial myosin light chain MLC_2 is phosphorylated during spontaneous and carbacol-induced contractions (Janis *et al.*, 1980, 1981).

The calcium controls smooth muscle contraction through myosin light chain kinase which requires both calcium and calmodulin for activity. As expected bovine uterine calmodulin shows sequence homology with calmodulin isolated from other sources (Perry and Grand, 1979). The uterus along with other smooth muscle contains high concentrations of calmodulin which is not limiting; regulation of contraction is primarily dependent on the cellular calcium concentration. It is believed that after elevation of smooth muscle intracellular calcium the calmodulin calcium complex binds the myosin light chain kinase and activates it causing the myosin light chain, MLC_2, to be phosphorylated. Initially it was not clear that all effects of calcium on smooth muscle contraction were effected through calmodulin (Hartshorne, 1982). This question has now been resolved very elegantly by Walsh *et al.* (1983) who showed that a proteolytically modified form of myosin light chain kinase, active without calcium or calmodulin, can activate actin-dependent myosin ATPase producing contraction in skinned muscle fibers. This study convincingly excludes the possibility of calcium acting at other sites for the initiation of contraction and indicates that the myosin light chain kinase is the focal point for the calcium-dependent regulation of smooth muscle contraction.

C. Hormonal Regulation of Smooth Muscle Contraction

A number of hormones influence smooth muscle contraction. In the uterus, acetylcholine, oxytocin, angiotensin, and prostaglandins stimulate contraction whereas β-adrenergic agonists and relaxin cause relaxation.

The β-adrenergic agonists stimulate cAMP production by the myometrium (Korenman and Krall, 1977). Initially it was thought that cAMP caused relaxation of the uterus principally by lowering intracellular calcium (Korenman and Krall, 1977; Marshall and Kroeger,

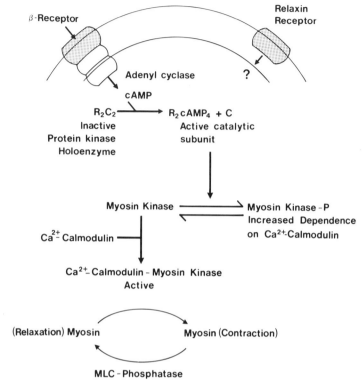

FIG. 10. Hormonal regulation of uterine contractions. The regulatory cascade is shown commencing with β-adrenergic stimulation of the adenylate cyclase, activation of the cAMP-dependent protein kinase (R_2C_2), phosphorylation, and inhibition of the myosin light chain kinase due to increased dependence on calcium and calmodulin (see text).

1973; Scheid *et al.*, 1979). These earlier ideas may now need revision as a result of the findings of Adelstein and colleagues (Adelstein *et al.*, 1978) who found that the smooth muscle myosin light chain kinase is a substrate for the cAMP-dependent protein kinase. Phosphorylation of the myosin light chain kinase by this enzyme inhibits it by increasing the dependence of the myosin light chain kinase for calmodulin (Conti and Adelstein, 1981). This exciting finding provided an interesting model to explain how hormones acting through cAMP can cause relaxation in smooth muscle (Fig. 10). It is another example of a protein phosphorylation regulatory cascade analogous to the classical system for the β-adrenergic control of skeletal muscle glycogenolysis (Krebs, 1972).

Work in several laboratories supports the scheme proposed by Adelstein *et al.* (1981). Mrwa *et al.* (1979) found that cAMP inhibited pig carotid artery actomyosin ATPase and Silver and Di Salvo (1979) reported that cAMP also inhibited myosin light chain phosphorylation in bovine aortic actomyosin. More direct support has come from elegant work by Kerrick and colleagues (Kerrick *et al.*, 1981) using skinned muscle fibers. In these studies addition of the cAMP-dependent protein kinase catalytic subunit strongly inhibited tension development in the smooth muscle fibers but not in skeletal muscle or scallop adductor muscle fibers. The skinned muscle fiber study also provides evidence supporting the idea that the inhibition of smooth muscle contraction by the cAMP-dependent protein kinase is exerted through myosin light chain kinase since addition of excess calmodulin reverses the effect of the cAMP-dependent protein kinase. It should be recognized that these conclusions are based on the assumption that the skinned fibers reflect quantitatively and qualitatively the properties of intact fibers.

The cAMP-dependent protein kinase phosphorylates the smooth muscle myosin light chain kinase on two sites in the absence of bound calmodulin (Conti and Adelstein, 1981) whereas in the presence of bound calmodulin only one of these sites is phosphorylated (see Fig. 11). The increased dependence of the myosin light chain kinase for calcium-calmodulin after phosphorylation correlates only with phosphorylation of the site sensitive to calmodulin.

These observations suggest that phosphorylation and inactivation of myosin light chain kinase may occur predominantly in the relaxed state when intracellular calcium is low. Experiments with skinned chicken gizzard fibers, however, indicate that cAMP-dependent protein kinase can elicit relaxation at maximal Ca^{2+}-activated tension (Kerrick *et al.*, 1981). The order of events is important in considering whether inactivation of the myosin light chain kinase is the major target for hormone regulation or is secondary to changes in calcium. At present it is not known whether protein kinases other than the cAMP-dependent protein kinases can phosphorylate the myosin light chain kinase and alter dependence on calcium-calmodulin.

Recently Nishikori *et al.* (1983) reported that relaxin inhibited uterine myosin light chain phosphorylation and myosin light chain kinase in uteri from estrogen-primed rats. This is the only study wherein effects of relaxin at the molecular level can be related in some detail to the biological action, inhibition of uterine contraction. Nishikori *et al.* (1983) reported that relaxin caused a shift in the ED_{50} value for calcium from 82 to 260 nM and for calmodulin from 2.2 to 25 nM. The changes in calmodulin and calcium dependence of the uterine myosin

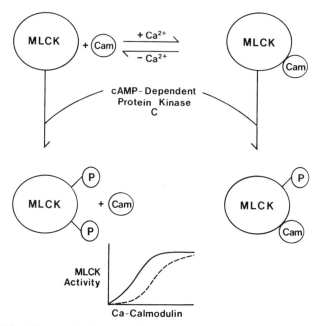

F<small>IG</small>. 11. The influence of calcium and calmodulin on the phosphorylation of the myosin light chain kinase by the cAMP-dependent protein kinase. In the absence of bound calmodulin (Cam) the myosin light chain kinase (MLCK) is phosphorylated (P) at two sites causing an increase in enzyme activity dependence on calmodulin (- - -). Phosphorylation stimulated by calmodulin is effected at one site with no change in calmodulin dependence (see text).

light chain kinase in response to relaxin thus are analogous to results of phosphorylation by cAMP-dependent protein kinase (Fig. 10). This suggests that relaxin may control uterine myosin light chain kinase through a regulatory cascade similar to that for the β-adrenergic system (see Fig. 9). At present it is not known whether cAMP and the cAMP-dependent protein kinase are involved in the relaxin response (see below).

The only other smooth muscle system in which the hormonal regulation of the myosin light chain kinase has been examined thus far is in the trachea. Carefully controlled experiments by Miller *et al.* (1983) revealed that isoproterenol did not change the sensitivity of the myosin light chain kinase to calcium or calmodulin even though isoproterenol stimulated phosphorylase *a* formation and relaxed the trachea. The tracheal myosin light chain kinase could be inhibited *in vitro* with addition of exogenous cAMP-dependent protein kinase indicating that all the components of the system were present. These findings (Miller *et al.*, 1983) imply that hormonal regulation of smooth muscle relaxation mediated by cAMP may not depend exclusively on phosphorylation and inactivation of the myosin light chain kinase. Further studies on the effect of relaxin on the uterine myosin light chain kinase are required to extend the interesting observations made by Nishikori *et al.* (1983). It will be necessary to prove whether relaxin indeed modulates enzyme activity through phosphorylation and to identify the protein kinase responsible (see below relaxin effects on cAMP). To this end it will be important to satisfy the general criteria set forth by Krebs and Beavo (1979), to prove phosphorylation is the molecular basis for control of enzyme activity. For the uterus, one must show (1) significant rates of stoichiometric phosphorylation and dephosphorylation of purified uterine myosin light chain kinase *in vitro* with the appropriate kinase and phosphatase; (2) the relationship between the degree of myosin light chain phosphorylation and changes in the calcium calmodulin dependence of the enzyme; (3) phosphorylation and dephosphorylation of the uterine myosin light chain kinase *in vivo* with accompanying changes in the calcium and calmodulin dependence; and (4) a relationship between the degree of phosphorylation of the uterine myosin light chain kinase and the post receptor events after binding of relaxin.

D. Relaxin Effects on Uterine cAMP

The earliest report that relaxin may alter tissue cAMP levels was that of Braddon (1978) who found that relaxin elevated cAMP in the public symphysis. Subsequently Sanborn *et al.* (1980a) reported that relaxin elevated uterine cAMP levels. The rise in cAMP was slow reaching a maximum after 20 minutes in contrast to the very rapid rises in cAMP observed in response to isoproterenol in the uterus (Koreman and Krall, 1977). The effect of relaxin on uterine cAMP levels has also been studied by Judson *et al.* (1980). These authors observed a more rapid time course than Sanborn *et al.* (1980d) with a significant rise in cAMP within 30 seconds and reaching a maximum at 5 minutes. Their results are more consistent with the idea of cAMP mediating the effect of relaxin on the uterus than those of Sanborn *et al.* (1980d). In both studies high levels of 3-isobutyl-1-methylxanthine were needed to enhance the relaxin-dependent increase in cAMP levels (Sanborn *et al.*, 1980d; Judson *et al.*, 1980). The relatively small increase in myometrial cAMP content elicited by relaxin compared to isoproterenol does not necessarily mean that cAMP is not a mediator for relaxin. It is now clear from studies in other systems that only a very small rise in cAMP is necessary to maximally activate the cAMP-dependent protein kinase (Partridge et al., 1982).

The effects of relaxin on uterine contractions and uterine cAMP concentration were insensitive to β blockade with propranolol (Sanborn et al., 1980d; Judson et al., 1980) indicating that relaxin was not acting via the β receptor. Furthermore the effect of relaxin was not altered by pretreatment of animals with reserpine or bretylium tosylate to deplete or augment uterine stores of catecholamine (Sanborn et al., 1981), respectively. It was claimed in a preliminary report that preincubation of uterine strips with the α-antagonist phentolamine or the prostaglandin synthesis inhibitors indomethacin or tranylcypromine did not alter the relaxin-dependent increase in uterine cAMP levels (Sanborn et al., 1980b). In the above studies the endometrium was separated from the myometrium so that endometrial contributions (Harbon et al., 1978) can be excluded.

The evidence at hand would therefore favor the concept that the relaxin-dependent increase in uterine cAMP is a direct effect of relaxin and not the consequence of release by another hormone. This raises the question whether cAMP is an essential intracellular mediator for relaxin or whether the changes in cAMP are secondary to other events.

Originally Sutherland et al. (1968) proposed a set of criteria that should be met before cAMP could be accepted as the intracellular mediator of a given hormone. These criteria have been incompletely met for relaxin and there remains a real possibility that the effects of cAMP are peripheral to the true mechanism of action of the hormone.

In a preliminary report Sanborn et al. (1980c) claimed that relaxin stimulated uterine adenylate cyclase. It is unfortunate that this study has not been followed up as it is one of the key Sutherland criteria needed before cAMP can be accepted as a mediator for relaxin. If relaxin were able to stimulate adenylate cyclase then the cAMP generated would lead to activation of the cAMP-dependent protein kinase and triggering of the regulatory pathway illustrated in Fig. 10. A further Sutherland criterion is that cAMP must mimic the effect of the hormone. While cAMP can inhibit uterine contractions (Mitznegg et al., 1970) it is questionable whether this provides any further insight into the action of relaxin since cAMP acts as a mediator for the β-adrenergic inhibition of uterine contractions (Sanborn et al., 1980d).

We have observed that relaxin activates the uterine cAMP-dependent protein kinase (Kemp, 1981) and the time course of activation is similar to that observed by Judson *et al.* (1980) for cAMP. The measurement of cAMP-dependent protein kinase activation is, however, subject to a number of artifacts including postextraction activation (Flockhart and Corbin, 1982). Thus while the observed activation of the cAMP-dependent protein kinase is consistent with a cAMP-mediator model for relaxin it does not address the central question any better than the measurements of cAMP.

Another criterion of Sutherland was that phosphodiesterase inhibitors should potentiate effects of the hormone. At concentrations of 10^{-4} M the phosphodiesterase inhibitor 3-isobutyl-1-methylxanthine will itself cause relaxation of the myometrium and this is accompanied by an increase in cAMP as assessed by activation of the cAMP-dependent protein kinase (Kemp and Niall, unpublished results). Again the cAMP mediation of the β-adrenergic effects on the uterus complicates the interpretation of these in addressing the mechanism of action of relaxin.

Since evidence in support of cAMP acting as a mediator for relaxin is presently equivocal it is useful to consider whether the rise in cAMP may be a secondary effect. It is known that the uterus contains a calcium-calmodulin-dependent phosphodiesterase (Kroeger *et al.,* 1977). Thus, any hormone that lowered uterine intracellular calcium could potentially inhibit phosphodiesterase and thereby elevate cAMP levels. At present it is not clear what effect relaxin has on uterine calcium fluxes. However, if relaxin were to lower the myometrial intracellular calcium concentrations then this would fit well with its muscle relaxing function as well as providing an explanation for the cAMP results. Research is urgently needed in this area and it may help elucidate the putative role of cAMP in mechanisms of relaxin's action. There is also a precedent for a secondary effect of relaxin on cAMP content. Prostaglandins PGE_2 and PGI_2 raise myometrial cAMP levels (Vesin *et al.,* 1979) even though these prostaglandins can cause the myometrium to contract (Chamley *et al.,* 1977). Prostaglandin $PGF_{2\alpha}$ on the other hand does not alter cAMP content yet promotes myometrial contractions. Thus a rise in cAMP can be associated with either contraction or relaxation. Since cAMP alone elicits relaxation of the isolated uterus (Mitznegg *et al.,* 1970) the rise in cAMP caused by some prostaglandins is almost certainly a secondary effect and clearly not an obligatory component of the contractile response.

Several lines of evidence implicate cAMP as a potential mediator of the action of relaxin. At present the evidence is equivocal and it is possible that the increase in cAMP produced by relaxin is secondary and not an obligatory component of its mechanism of action.

VI. Relaxin Receptors

Relaxin receptors have been difficult to study due to low abundance. There is presently no continuous cell culture line with characterized relaxin receptors that could be used as a convenient model system. There have been a number of studies at the whole animal and tissue level; however, the most significant progress at the molecular level has been made by Bryant-Greenwood and associates who have partially characterized the rat myometrial relaxin receptor (Mercado-Simmen et al., 1980, 1982b).

The binding of [^{125}I]iodorelaxin to a particulate preparation of the rat uterus exhibited a curvilinear Scatchard plot with a high affinity K_a of $10^{10} M^{-1}$. Thus far the ligand in binding studies, [^{125}I]iodorelaxin, has not been fully characterized chemically. The preparations of porcine relaxin have required ^{125}I labeling by the Bolton–Hunter method on lysine residues and were not purified by ion-exchange chromatography. Nevertheless several interesting findings have emerged. The rat relaxin receptor is under hormonal control by estrogen and the receptor concentration rises dramatically after estrogen administration. These findings fit well with the known estrogen dependence for inhibition of myometrial contraction by relaxin. Bryant-Greenwood and her colleagues (Mercado-Simmen et al., 1982a) have found that the number of relaxin receptors rises sharply during gestation at around day 15 reaching a peak at day 17 and then declining toward parturition in the rat. Similar abrupt changes in the mouse pubic symphysis were observed many years ago between day 15 and 20 of pregnancy (Hall and Newton, 1946). In the light of the uterine relaxin receptor studies it would seem likely that the pubic symphysis relaxin receptors will be under similar hormonal control.

Relaxin receptor studies are clearly at an early stage and new developments are likely to emerge soon. Thus far no structural studies have been reported. Cross-linking experiments with radiolabeled relaxin may provide information on the subunit number and size of the relaxin receptor as has been obtained for the insulin receptor. In view of the discoveries that several important polypeptide hormones including insulin (Petruzzelli et al., 1982), epidermal growth factor (Carpenter et al., 1979), and platelet-derived growth factor (Ek and Heldin, 1982) activate tyrosine protein kinases, it would seem appropriate to test relaxin for such effects.

VII. Medical and Physiological Perspectives

The first point of interest in relaxin as a potential therapeutic agent in clinical medicine took place in the 1950s, with support from some pharmaceutical firms (namely Warner-Lambert and Ciba-Geigy). This led to clinical trials (McCarthy *et al.*, 1957; Eichner *et al.*, 1958; Kupperman *et al.*, 1958) with what we now know, in retrospect, to be highly impure preparations of porcine relaxin, probably consisting of no more than 10% relaxin and 90% unrelated ovarian peptides. Not surprisingly, the results of these trials were equivocal, and were not pursued. When highly purified porcine relaxin became available in 1974 (Sherwood and O'Byrne, 1974) there was a renewed interest in possible clinical applications. Limited clinical trials have now been carried out in two centers (MacLennan *et al.*, 1980; Evans *et al.*, 1983b) to evaluate porcine relaxin applied topically to the cervix as a cervical softening agent in conjunction with the induction of labor. Promising results have been obtained in a double blind trial, indicating that relaxin is capable of improving the cervical score, shortening the duration of labor, and possibly decreasing the need for intervention by cesarean section (MacLennan *et al.*, 1980). Although the results were not statistically superior to those obtained with topical prostaglandin preparations, it seems likely that relaxin may be a more acceptable form of treatment since prostaglandins could have untoward effects on other target organs. Since human relaxin is now known to differ markedly in structure from porcine relaxin this sort of study needs to be repeated with the homologous hormone. Thus, it is premature at present to reach any definite conclusion as to the efficacy of relaxin therapy.

A. Physiology of Relaxin in the Human Female

Interesting studies have been published (Szlachter *et al.*, 1982; Thomas *et al.*, 1980) in which levels of relaxin in normal and abnormal pregnancy and in the nonpregnant state have been reported. So far these have all been based on a heterologous radioimmunoassay (porcine relaxin antibody and tracer), and it is difficult to assess how accurately results reflect true concentrations of the very different human relaxin molecule(s). Thus, the first need is for a homologous and highly sensitive radioimmunoassay. This should not be far off, since human relaxin(s) for use as antigens can now be produced either by chemical synthesis (Tregear *et al.,* 1982) or by recombinant DNA procedures (Hudson *et al.,* 1983). Clearly, since there are at least two different human relaxin genes, it may be necessary, if both are expressed, to develop at least two separate radioimmunoassays. This may require the use of monoclonal antibodies specific for each of the two human relaxins so far identified (at the level of genomic DNA sequences). Radioimmunoassays for human C-peptides as noted above will be of great interest. Monitoring concentration of human relaxin C-peptide may prove the best index of endogenous relaxin secretion, and would be the only approach in situations where exogenous relaxin is being given therapeutically.

B. Physiology of Relaxin in the Human Male

Relaxin has been identified in human seminal fluid (Loumaye *et al.,* 1980) and despite earlier reports of relaxin localization in the testis (Dubois and Dacheux, 1978) it seems likely that it is of prostatic origin (Essig *et al.,* 1982a). A role in maintaining sperm motility has been suggested (Essig *et al.,* 1982b) and local effects in the female reproductive tract of relaxin in the ejaculate cannot be excluded. Again, the availability of a specific radioimmunoassay for human relaxin will be useful in furthering studies of relaxin in this context.

C. Relaxin as a Therapeutic Agent

There is a major need to understand the role of relaxin in human reproduction as the basis of any possible therapeutic use. The physiological studies needed should now be possible, through the availability of purified, human relaxin(s) produced by recombinant DNA technology. There would now seem to be no justification for the continued clinical experimentation with porcine relaxin, since there is clearly a risk of antibody formation. Since relaxin may well have a role in ovulation (Bryant-Greenwood, 1982) and may have other, as yet unknown, effects it would be prudent at least to minimize the risk of immunization by using the homologous hormone. Possible clinical uses of relaxin include (1) facilitation of parturition (via effects on pelvic ligaments and on cervical softening) and (2) prevention of premature labor (via inhibition of myometrial contraction). A highly speculative use of relaxin would be in the treatment of connective tissue diseases (e.g., rheumatoid arthritis, scleroderma, or ankylosing spondylitis). It is beyond the scope of this article to discuss any of these possible uses more fully, but it should be pointed out that there is presently no evidence that relaxin might improve the clinical picture in generalized connective tissue disorders. Nevertheless, one can confidently look forward to an intensive study of relaxin physiology in man over the next few years with newly available tools, and there is at least a possibility that some therapeutic utility will emerge.

ACKNOWLEDGMENTS

We are grateful to those colleagues who provided preprints of their work and thank Kati Bromley and Charlene Kalny for the preparation of figures and for typing the manuscript, respectively. We are grateful to Virginia Kemp for assisting in proofreading.

REFERENCES

Adelstein, R. S., and Eisenberg, E. (1980). Regulation and kinetics of the actin-myosin ATP interaction. *Annu. Rev. Biochem.* **49**, 921–933.

Adelstein, R. S., Conti, M. A., Hathaway, D. R., and Klee, C. B. (1978). Phosphorylation of smooth muscle myosin light chain kinase by the catalytic subunit of the adenosine 3':5'-monophosphate dependent protein kinase. *J. Biol. Chem.* **253**, 8347–8350.

Adelstein, R. S., Pato, M. D., and Conti, M. A. (1981). The role of phosphorylation in regulating contractile proteins. *Adv. Cyclic Nucleotide Res.* **14**, 361–373.

Aksoy, M. O., Williams, D., Sharkey, E. M., and Hartshorne, D. J. (1976). A relationship between Ca^{2+} sensitivity and phosphorylation of gizzard actomyosin. *Biochem. Biophys. Res. Commun.* **69**, 35–41.

Anderson, R. R. (1982). Relaxin: Advances in experimental medicine and biology. *Proc. Midwest Conf. Endocrinol. Metab. 15th, 1979* **143.**

Bedarkar, S., Turnell, W. G., Blundell, T. L., and Schwabe, C. (1977). Relaxin has conformational homology with insulin. *Nature (London)* **270**, 449–451.

Bedarkar, S., Blundell, T., Cowan, L. K., McDonald, J. K., and Schwabe, C. (1982). On the three-dimensional structure of relaxin. *Ann. N.Y. Acad. Sci.* **380**, 22–33.

Bell, G. I., Pictet, R. L., Rutter, W. J., Cordell, B., Tischer, E., and Goodman, H. M. (1980). Sequence of the human insulin gene. *Nature (London)* **284**, 26–32.

Bigazzi, M., Greenwood, F. C., and Gasparri, F. (eds.) (1983). "Biology of Relaxin and its Role in the Human." Excerpta Medica, Amsterdam.

Bigazzi, M., Nardi, E., Bruni, P., and Petrucci, F. (1980). Relaxin in human decidua. *J. Clin. Endocrinol. Metab.* **51**, 939–941.

Blundell, T. L., and Humbel, R. E. (1980). Hormone families: Pancreatic hormones and homologous growth factors. *Nature (London)* **287**, 781–787.

Blundell, T. L., Dodson, G. G., Hodgkin, D. C., and Mercola, D. A. (1972). Insulin: The structure in the crystal and its reflection in chemistry and biology. *Adv. Protein Chem.* **26**, 279–402.

Bonser, A. M., and Garcia-Webb, P. (1981). C-peptide measurement and its clinical usefulness: A review. *Ann. Clin. Biochem.* **18**, 200–206.

Braddon, S. A. (1978). Relaxin-dependent adenosine 3',5'-monophosphate concentration changes in the mouse pubic symphysis. *Endocrinology* **102**, 1292–1299.

Bremel, R. D., Sobieszek, A., and Small, J. V. (1977). Regulation of actin-myosin interactions in vertebrate smooth muscle. *In* "The Biochemistry of Smooth Muscle" (N. L. Stephens, ed.), pp. 533–549. Univ. Park Press, Baltimore, Maryland.

Bryant-Greenwood, G. D. (1981). Relaxin: Evidence for its actions as a local hormone. *In* "Relaxin" (G. D. Bryant-Greenwood, H. D. Niall, and F. C. Greenwood, eds.), pp. 199–203. Elsevier, Amsterdam.

Bryant-Greenwood, G. D. (1982). Relaxin as a new hormone. *Endocr. Rev.* **3,** 62–90.

Bryant-Greenwood, G. D., Niall, H. D., and Greenwood, F. C. (1981). Proceedings of a workshop on the chemistry and biology of relaxin. *In* "Relaxin" (G. D. Bryant-Greenwood, H. D. Niall, and F. C. Greenwood, eds.). Elsevier, Amsterdam.

Carpenter, G., King, L., and Cohen, S. (1979). Rapid enhancement of protein phosphorylation in A-431 cell membrane preparations by epidermal growth factor. *J. Biol. Chem.* **254,** 4884–4891.

Chamley, W. A., Bagoyo, M. M., and Bryant-Greenwood, G. D. (1977). *In vitro* response of relaxin-treated rat uterus to prostaglandins and oxytocin. *Prostaglandins* **14,** 763–769.

Conti, M. A., and Adelstein, R. S. (1981). The relationship between calmodulin binding and phosphorylation of smooth muscle myosin kinase by the catalytic subunit of 3':5' cAMP-dependent protein kinase. *J. Biol. Chem.* **256,** 3178–3181.

Crawford, R. J., Hudson, P., Shine, J., Niall, H. D., Eddy, R. L., and Shows, T. B. (1984). Two human relaxin genes are on chromosome 9. *EMBO J.* (in press).

Dabrowska, A., Aromatorio, D., Sherry, J. M. F., and Hartshorne, D. J. (1977). Composition of the myosin light chain kinase from chicken gizzard. *Biochem. Biophys. Res. Commun.* **78,** 1263–1272.

Dodson, G. G., Eliopoulos, E. E., Isaacs, N. W., McCall, M. J., Niall, H. D., and North, A. C. T. (1982). Rat relaxin: Insulin-like fold predicts a likely receptor binding region. *Int. J. Biol. Macromol.,* **4,** 399–405.

Dubois, M. P., and Dacheux, J. L. (1978). Relaxin, a male hormone? Immunocytological localization of a related antigen in the boar testis. *Cell Tissue Res.* **187,** 201–214.

Eichner, E., Herman, I., Kritzer, L., Platock, G. M., and Rubinstein, L. (1958). The effects of relaxin on term and premature labour. *Ann. N.Y. Acad. Sci.* **75,** 1023–1032.

Ek, B., and Heldin, C. H. (1982). Characterization of a tyrosine-specific kinase activity in human fibroblast membranes stimulated by platelet-derived growth factor. *J. Biol. Chem.* **257,** 10486–10492.

Essig, M., Schoenfeld, C., D'Eletto, R., Amelar, R., Dubin, L., Steinetz, B. G., O'Byrne, E. M., and Weiss, G. (1982a). Relaxin in human seminal plasma. *Ann. N.Y. Acad. Sci.* **380,** 224–230.

Essig, M., Schoenfeld, C., Amelar, R. D., Dubin, L., and Weiss, G. (1982b). Stimulation of human sperm motility by relaxin. *Fertil. Steril.* **38,** 339–343.

Evans, G., Wathes, D. C., King, G. J., Armstrong, D. T., and Porter, D. G. (1983). Changes in relaxin production by the theca during the preovulatory period of the pig. *J. Reprod. Fertil.* **69,** 677–683.

Evans, M. I., Dougan, M-B., Moawad, A. H., Evans, W. J., Bryant-Greenwood, G., and Greenwood, F. C. (1983). Ripening of the human cervix with porcine ovarian relaxin. *Am. J. Obstet. and Gynec.* **147** (4), 410–414.

Flockhart, D., and Corbin, J. (1982). Regulatory mechanisms in the control of protein kinases. *Crit. Rev. Biochem.* **13,** 133–186.

Gorman, J. G., Thorley, B., Walsh, J. R., Tregear, G. W., and Niall, H. D. (1983). Analysis of relaxins, prorelaxin and c-peptide levels in rat corpus luteum by region specific radioimmunoassay. *Endocr. Soc. Meet. San Antonio, June 8–14* Abstr. No. 50.

Gowan, L. K., Reinig, J. W., Schwabe, C., Bedarkar, S., and Blundell, T. L. (1981). On the primary and tertiary structure of relaxin from the Sand Tiger Shark. *FEBS Lett.* **129**, 80–82.

Haley, J., Hudson, P., Sca lon, D., John, M., Cronk, M., Shine, J., Tregear, G., and Niall, H. (1982). Porcine relaxin molecular cloning and cDNA structure. *DNA* **1**, 155–162.

Hall, K., and Newton, W. H. (1946). The normal course of separation of the pubes in pregnant mice. *J. Physiol. (London)* **104**, 348–352.

Harbon, S., Vesin, M. F., Khac, L. D., and Leiber, D. (1978). Cyclic nucleotides in the regulation of rat uterus contractility. *In* "Molecular Biology and Pharmacology of Cyclic Nucleotides" (G. Folco and R. Paoletti, eds.), pp. 279–296. Elsevier, Amsterdam.

Hartshorne, D. J. (1982). The contractile apparatus of smooth muscle and its regulation by calcium. *In* "Vascular Smooth Muscle: Metabolic, Ionic and Contractile Mechanisms" (M. F. Crass and C. D. Barnes, eds.), pp. 135–161. Academic Press, New York.

Hisaw, F. L. (1926). Experimental relaxation of the pubic ligament of the guinea pig. *Proc. Soc. Exp. Biol. Med.* **23**, 661–663.

Hudson, P., Haley, J., Cronk, M., Shine, J., and Niall, H. D. (1981a). Molecular cloning and characterization of cDNA sequences coding for rat relaxin. *Nature (London)* **291**, 127–131.

Hudson, P., Penschow, J., Shine, J., Ryan, G., Niall, H., and Coghlan, J. (1981b). Hybridization histochemistry: Use of recombinant DNA as a homing probe for tissue localization of specific mRNA populations. *Endocrinology* **108**, 353–356.

Hudson, P., Haley, J., John, M., Cronk, M., Crawford, R., Haralambidis, J., Tregear, G., Shine, J., and Niall, H. (1983). Structure of a genomic clone encoding biologically active human relaxin. *Nature (London)* **301**, 628–631.

Hudson, P., John, M., Crawford, R., Haralambidis, J., Scanlon, D., Gorman, J., Tregear, G., Shine, J., and Niall, H. (1984). Relaxin gene expression in human ovaries and the predicted structure of a human preprorelaxin by analysis of cDNA clones. *EMBO J.* (in press).

Issacs, N., James, R., Niall, H., Bryant-Greenwood, G., Dodson, G., Evans, A., and North, A. C. T. (1978). Relaxin and its structural relationship to insulin. *Nature (London)* **271**, 278–281.

James, R., Niall, H., Kwok, S., and Bryant-Greenwood, G. (1977). Primary structure of porcine relaxin and homology with insulin and related growth factors. *Nature (London)* **267**, 544–546.

Janis, R. A., Moats-Stuats, B. M., and Gualtieri, R. T. (1980). Protein phosphorylation during spontaneous contraction of smooth muscle. *Biochem. Biophys. Res. Commun.* **96**, 265–270.

Janis, R. A., Barany, K., Barany, M., and Sarmiento, J. G. (1981). Association between myosin light chain phosphorylation and contraction of rat uterine smooth muscle. *Mol. Physiol.* **1**, 3–11.

John, M. J., Walsh, J. R., Borjesson, B. W., and Niall, H. D. (1981a). Limited sequence homology between porcine and rat relaxins: Implications for physiological studies. *Endocrinology* **108**, 726–729.

John, M. J., Walsh, J. R., James, R. J., Kwok, S., Bryant-Greenwood, G. D., Bradshaw, R. A., and Niall, H. D. (1981b). Heterogeneity of porcine relaxin. *In* "Relaxin" (G. D. Bryant-Greenwood, H. D. Niall, and F. C. Greenwood, eds.), pp. 17–18, Elsevier, Amsterdam.

Judson, D. G., Pay, S., and Bhoola, K. D. (1980). Modulation of cyclic AMP in isolated rat uterine tissue slices by porcine relaxin. *J. Endocrinol.* **87**, 153–159.

Kemp, B. E. (1981). Activation of rat uterine cAMP-dependent protein kinase by relaxin. *Endocr. Soc. Annu. Meet., 63rd, June* 17–19, *Cincinnati* Abstr. No. 371.

Kemp, B. E., and Niall, H. D. (1981). Use of the electrically stimulated rat uterus preparation in the bioassay of relaxin. *In* "Relaxin" (G. D. Bryant-Greenwood, H. D. Niall, and F. C. Greenwood, eds.), pp. 339–340. Elsevier, Amsterdam.

Kerrick, W. G. L., Hoar, P. E., Cassidy, P. S., Bolles, L., and Malencik, D. A. (1981). Calcium-regulatory mechanisms. *J. Gen. Physiol.* **77**, 177–190.

Korenman, S. G., and Krall, J. F. (1977). The role of cyclic AMP in the regulation of smooth muscle cell contraction in the uterus. *Biol. Reprod.* **16**, 1–17.

Krantz, J. C., Bryant, H. H., and Carr, C. J. (1950). The action of aqueous corpus luteum extract upon uterine activity. *Surg. Gynecol. Obstet.* **90**, 372–375.

Krebs, E. G. (1972). Protein kinases. *Curr. Top. Cell. Regul.* **5**, 99–133.

Krebs, E. G., and Beavo, J. A. (1979). Phosphorylation–dephosphorylation of enzymes. *Annu. Rev. Biochem.* **48**, 923–959.

Kroc, R. L. (1982). Relaxin—a perspective. *Ann. N.Y. Acad. Sci.* **380**, 1–5.

Kroeger, E. A., Teo, T. S., Ho, H., and Wang, J. H. (1977). Relaxants, cyclic adenosine 3':5'-monophosphate, and calcium metabolism in smooth muscle. *In* "The Biochemistry of Smooth Muscle" (N. L. Stephens, ed.), pp. 643–652. Univ. Park Press, Baltimore, Maryland.

Kupperman, H. S., Rosenberg, D., and Cutler, A. (1958). Relaxin in dysmenorrhoea and its effect in vitro upon musclar contractions. *Ann. N.Y. Acad. Sci.* **75**, 1003–1010.

Lebowitz, E. A., and Cooke, R. (1979). Phosphorylation of uterine smooth muscle myosin permits action activation. *J. Biochem.* (Tokyo) **85**, 1489–1494.

Lerner, R. A. (1982). Tapping the immunological repertoire to produce antibodies of predetermined specificity. *Nature (London)* **299**, 592–596.

Lerner, R. A., Sutcliffe, J. G., and Shinnick, T. M. (1981). Antibodies to chemically synthesized peptides predicted from DNA sequences as probes of gene expression. *Cell* **23**, 309–310.

Loumaye, E., DeCooman, S., and Thomas, K. (1980). Immunoreactive relaxin-like substances in human seminal plasma. *J. Clin. Endocrinol. Metab.* **50**, 1142–1143.

McCarthy, J. J., Erving, H. W., and Laufe, L. E. (1957). Preliminary report on the use of relaxin in the management of threadened premature labour. *Am. J. Obstet. Gynaecol.* **74**, 134–138.

MacLennan, A. H., Green, R. C., Bryant-Greenwood, G. D., and Greenwood, F. C. (1980). Ripening of the human cervix and induction of labour with purified porcine relaxin. *Lancet* **1**, 220–223.

Maita, T., Chen, J., and Matsuda, G. (1981). Amino-acid sequence of the 20,000-molecular weight light chain of chicken gizzard muscle myosin. *Eur. J. Biochem.* **117**, 417–424.

Maniatis, T., Hardison, R. C., Lacy, E., Lauer, J., O'Connell, C., and Quon, D. (1978). Isolation of structural genes from libraries of eucaryotic DNA. *Cell* **15**, 687–701.

Marshall, J. M., and Kroeger, E. A. (1973). Adrenergic influences on uterine smooth muscle. *Philos. Trans. R. Soc. London Ser B* **265**, 135–148.

Matsuda, G., Maita, T., Kato, Y., Chen, J., and Umegane, T. (1981). Amino acid sequences of the cardiac L-2A, L-2B and gizzard 17,000-Mr light chains of chicken muscle myosin. *FEBS Lett.* **135**, 232–236.

Mercado-Simmen, R. C., Bryant-Greenwood, G. D., and Greenwood, F. C. (1980). Characterization of the binding of I^{125}-relaxin to rat uterus. *J. Biol. Chem.* **255**, 3617–3623.

Mercado-Simmen, R. C., Bryant-Greenwood, G. D., and Greenwood, F. C. (1982a). Relaxin receptor in the rat myometrium: Regulation by oestrogen and relaxin. *Endocrinology* **110**, 220–226.

Mercado-Simmen, R. C., Goodwin, B., Veno, M. S., Yamamoto, S. Y., and Bryant-Greenwood, G. D. (1982b). Relaxin receptors in the myometrium and cervix of the pig. *Biol. Reprod.* **26**, 120–128.

Miller, J. R., Silver, P. J., and Stull, J. T. (1983). The role of myosin light chain kinase phosphorylation in β-adrenergic relaxation of trachael smooth muscle. *Mol. Pharmacol.* **24**, 235–242.

Mitznegg, P., Heim, F., and Meythaler, B. (1970). Influence of endogenous and exogenous cyclic 3′,5′-AMP on contractile responses induced by oxytocin and calcium in isolated rat uterus. *Life Sci.* **9**, 121–128.

Mrwa, V., Troschka, M., and Ruegg, J. C. (1979). Cyclic AMP-dependent inhibition of smooth muscle actomyosin. *FEBS Lett.* **107**, 371–374.

Niall, H., Hudson, P., Haley, J., Cronk, M., Crawford, R., Scanlon, D., Haralambidis, J., Tregear, G. W., and Shine, J. (1983). The genes for relaxin. *In* "Biology of Relaxin and its Role in the Human" (M. Bigazzi, F. C. Greenwood, and F. Gasparri, eds.), pp. 32–44. Excerpta Medica, Amsterdam.

Nishikori, K., Weisbrodt, N. W., Sherwood, O. D., and Sanborn, B. M. (1983). Effect of relaxin on rat uterine myosin light chain kinase activity and myosin light chain phosphorylation. *J. Biol. Chem.* **258**, 2468–2474.

O'Byrne, E. M., Brindle, S., Quintavalla, J., Strawinski, C., Tabachnick, M., and Heinetz, B. G. (1982). Tissue distribution of injected I^{125}-labelled porcine relaxin: organ uptake, whole body autoradiography and renal concentration of radiometabolites. *Ann. N.Y. Acad. Sci.* **380**, 187–197.

Partridge, N. C., Kemp, B. E., Livesey, S. A., and Martin, T. J. (1982). Activity ratio measurements reflect intracellular activation of adenosine 3′,5′-monophosphate-dependent protein kinase in osteoblasts. *Endocrinology* **111**, 178–183.

Perry, S. V. (1975). Contractile and regulatory proteins of the myocardium. *In* "Contraction and Relaxation in the Myocardium" (W. G. Nayler ed.), pp. 29–77. Academic Press, New York.

Perry, S. V., and Grand, R. J. (1979). Mechanism of contraction and the specialized protein components of smooth muscle. *Br. Med. Bull.* **35**, 219–226.

Petruzzelli, L. M., Ganguly, S., Smith, C. J., Cobb, M. H., Rubin, C. S., and Rosen, O. M. (1982). Insulin activates a tyrosine specific protein kinase in extracts of 3T3-Li adipocytes and human placenta. *Proc. Natl. Acad. Sci. U.S.A.* **79**, 6792–6796.

Porter, D. G. (1979). Relaxin: Old hormone, new prospect. *In* "Oxford Reviews of Reproduction Biology" (C. A. Finn, ed.), pp. 1–57. Clarendon, Oxford.

Porter, D. (1981). The rat uterine strip test system, *in vitro. In* "Relaxin" (G. D. Bryant-Greenwood, H. D. Niall, and F. C. Greenwood, eds.), pp. 341. Elsevier, Amsterdam.

Porter, D. G. (1982). Unsolved problems of relaxin's physiological role. *Ann. N.Y. Acad. Sci.* **380**, 151–162.

Porter, D. G., Downing, S. J., and Bradshaw, J. M. C. (1981). Inhibition of oxytocin or prostaglandin F2α-driven myometrical activity by relaxin in the rat is oestrogen dependent. *J. Endocrinol.* **89**, 399–404.

Rawitch, A. B., Moore, W. V., and Frieden, E. H. (1980). Relaxin–insulin homology: Predictions of secondary structure and lack of competitive binding. *Int. J. Biochem.* **11**, 357–362.

Sanborn, B. M., Kuo, H. S., Weisbrodt, N. W., and Sherwood, O. D. (1980a). The interaction of relaxin with the rat uterus I. Effect on cyclic nucleotide levels and spontaneous contractile activity. *Endocrinology* **106**, 1210–1215.

Sanborn, B. M., Sherwood, O. D., and Kuo, H. S. (1980b). Evidence against the primary role of catecholamine release or prostaglandin synthesis in the effect of relaxin on uterine cyclic AMP levels. *Endocr. Soc. Annu. Meet. 62nd, Washington, D.C.* Abstr. No. 4.

Sanborn, B. M., Kuo, H. S., Weisbrodt, N. W., and Sherwood, O. D. (1980c). Effect of porcine relaxin on cyclic nucleotide levels and spontaneous contractions of the rat uterus. *In* "Relaxin. Advances in Experimental Medicine and Biology" (R. R. Anderson, ed.), Vol. 143, pp. 273–287. Plenum, New York.

Sanborn, B. M., Heindel, J. J., and Robison, G. A. (1980d). The role of cyclic nucleotides in reproductive processes. *Annu. Rev. Physiol.* **42**, 37–57.

Sanborn, B. M., Weisbrodt, N. W., and Sherwood, O. D. (1981). Evidence against an obligatory role for catecholamine release or prostacyclin synthesis in the effects of relaxin on the rat uterus. *Biol. Reprod.* **24**, 987–992.

Sawyer, W. H., Frieden, E. H., and Marsh, A. C. (1952). In vitro inhibition of spontaneous contractions of the rat uterus by relaxin containing extracts of sow ovaries. *Am. J. Physiol.* **172**, 547–552.

Scheid, C. R., Honeyman, T. W., and Fay, F. S. (1979). Mechanism of β-adrenergic relaxation of smooth muscle. *Nature (London)* **277**, 32–36.

Schwabe, C. (1983). The amino acid sequences of relaxins. *In* "Biology of Relaxin and its Role in the Human" (M. Bigazzi, F. C. Greenwood, and F. Gasparri, eds.), pp. 22–31. Excerpta Medica, Amsterdam.

Schwabe, C., and Harmon, S. J. (1978). A comparative circular dichroism study of relaxin and insulin. *Biochem. Biophys. Res. Commun.* **84**, 373–380.

Schwabe, C., McDonald, J. K., and Steinetz, B. C. (1977). Primary structure of the B chain of porcine relaxin. *Biochem. Biophys. Res. Commun.* **75**, 503–510.

Schwabe, C., Steinetz, B. G., Weiss, G., Segaloff, A., McDonald, J. K., O'Byrne, E., Hochman, J., Carries, B., and Goldsmith, L. (1978). Relaxin. *Recent Prog. Horm. Res.* **34**, 123–211.

Schwabe, C., Gowan, L. K., and Reinig, J. W. (1982). Evolution, relaxin and insulin: A new perspective. *Ann. N.Y. Acad. Sci.* **380**, 6–12.

Schwartz, G., and Katsoyannis, P. G. (1976). Synthesis of human [9-leucine-B] insulin. *Biochemistry* **15**, 4071–4076.

Sherwood, O. D., and O'Byrne, E. M. (1974). Purification and characterization of porcine relaxin. *Arch. Biochem. Biophys.* **160**, 185–196.

Silver, P. J., and DiSalvo, J. (1979). Adenosine 3':5'-monophosphate-mediated inhibition of myosin light chain phosphorylation in bovine aortic actomyosin. *J. Biol. Chem.* **254**, 9951–9954.

Small, J. V. (1977). The contractile apparatus of the smooth muscle cell, structure and composition. *In* "The Biochemistry of Smooth Muscle" (N. I. Stephens, ed.), pp. 379–411. Univ. Park Press, Baltimore, Maryland.

Small, J. P., and Sobieszek (1980). The contractile apparatus of smooth muscle. *Int. Rev. Cytol.* **64**, 241–306.

St. Louis, J. (1981). Relaxin inhibition of KCl-induced uterine contractions *in vitro* on alternative bioassay. *Can. J. Physiol. Pharmacol.* **59**, 507–512.

Steiner, D. F. (1977). Insulin today. *Diabetes* **26**, 322–340.

Steinetz, B. G. (1982). Specificity and reliability of radioimmunoassays, radioreceptor assays and bioassays: Round table discussion summary. *Ann. N.Y. Acad. Sci.* **380**, 51–59.

Steinetz, B. G., and Kroc, R. L. (1981). Relaxin—an historical perspective. *In* "Relaxin" (G. D. Bryant-Greenwood, H. D. Niall, and F. C. Greenwood, eds.), pp. 1–8. Elsevier, Amsterdam.

Steinetz, B. G., Beach, V. L., Kroc, R. L., Stasilli, N. R., Nussbaum, R. E., Nemith, P. J., and Dunn, R. K. (1960). Bioassay of relaxin using a reference standard: A simple and reliable method utilizing direct measurement of interpubic ligament formation in mice. *Endocrinology* **67**, 102–115.

Steinetz, B. G., Schwabe, C., and Weiss, G. (1982). Proceedings of conference held by Kroc Foundation. Relaxin: Structure, Function and Evolution. Jan. 12–16, 1981, Santa Ynez Valley, California. *Ann. N.Y. Acad. Sci.* **380**.

Steinetz, B. G., O'Byrne, E. M., Sarosi, P., and Weiss, C. R. (1983). Bioassay of relaxin: present status and future prospects. *Proc. Int. Conf. Hum. Relaxin, 1st, Florence*, 140–147.

Stewart, A. G., and Bell, L. D. (1982). Recombinant DNA technique for the production of Relaxin. Australian Patent No. 85072–82.

Sutherland, E. W., Robison, G. A., and Butcher, R. W. (1968). Some aspects of the biological role of adenosine 3′,5′-monophosphate (cyclic AMP). *Circulation* **37**, 279–305.

Szlachter, B. N., Quagliarello, J., Jewelewicz, R., Osathanondh, R., Spellacy, W. N., and Weiss, G. (1982). Relaxin in normal and pathogenic pregnancies. *Obstet. Gynecol.* **59**, 167–170.

Thomas, K., Loumaye, E., and Ferin, J. (1980). Relaxin in non-pregnant women during ovarian stimulation. *Gynecol. Obstet. Invest.* **11**, 75–80.

Tregear, G. W., Kemp B., Borjesson, B., Thompson, A., Scanlon, D., Collier, M., John, M., and Niall, H. D. (1979). Approaches to the chemical synthesis of relaxin. *Proc. Am. Peptide Symp. 6th* pp. 445–453.

Tregear, G., Yu-cang, Du, Kemp, B., Borjesson, B., Scanlon, D., and Niall, H. D. (1981). The synthesis of peptides with relaxin activity. *In* "Relaxin" (G. D. Bryant-Greenwood, H. D. Niall, and F. C. Greenwood, eds.), pp. 151–164. Elsevier, Amsterdam.

Tregear, G. W., Yu-cang, Du, Ke-zhen, Wang, Southwell, C., Jones, P., John, M., Gorman, J., Kemp, B., and Niall, H. D. (1982). The chemical synthesis of relaxin. *In* "Biology of Relaxin and its Role in the Human" (M. Bigazzi, F. C. Greenwood, and F. Gasparri, eds.), pp. 42–55. Excerpta Medica, Amsterdam.

Vesin, M. F., Khac, L. D., and Harbon, S. (1979). Prostacyclin as an endogenous modulator of adenosine cyclic 3′,5′-monophosphate levels in rat myometrium and endometrium. *Mol. Pharmacol.* **16**, 823–840.

Wallis, M. (1980). Growth hormone: Deletion in the protein and introns in the gene. *Nature (London)* **284**, 512.

Walsh, M. P., Bridenbaugh, R., Kerrick, W. G., and Hartshorne, D. J. (1983). Gizzard Ca^{2+}-independent myosin light chain kinase: Evidence in favor of the phosphorylation theory. *Fed. Proc., Fed. Am. Soc. Exp. Biol.* **42**, 45–50.

Wiqvist, N., and Paul, K. G. (1958). Inhibition of the spontaneous uterine motility *in vitro* as a bioassay of relaxin. *Acta Endocrinol. (Copenhagen)* **29**, 135–146.

Yu-cang, Du, Minasian, E., Tregear, G. W., and Leach, S. J. (1982). Circular dichroism studies of relaxin and insulin peptide chains. *Int. J. Peptide Protein Res.* **20**, 47–55.

Yamamoto, S., Kwok, S. C. M., Greenwood, F. C., and Bryant-Greenwood, G. D. (1981). Relaxin purification from human placental basal plates. *J. Clin. Endocrinol. Metab.* **52**, 601–604.

Activation of Plasma Membrane Phosphatidylinositol Turnover by Hormones

JOHN N. FAIN

Section of Biochemistry,
Brown University,
Providence, Rhode Island

I.	Introduction	117
II.	Macrophages, Neutrophils, and Mast Cells	122
III.	Brain Synaptosomes	125
IV.	Hepatocytes	129
V.	Adrenal Medulla	135
VI.	Adrenal Glomerulosa Cells	137
VII.	Adrenal Cortex	138
VIII.	Platelets	139
IX.	Blowfly Salivary Glands	144
X.	Conclusion	150
	References	152

I. Introduction

Hawthorne and White (1975) in Volume 33 of this series reviewed the extraction, analysis, and properties of the phosphoinositides as well as their metabolism in a variety of tissues. One section dealt with phosphatidylinositol turnover and plasma membrane activation. In that section Hawthorne and White posed two questions that still remain unanswered: (1) Are phospholipid changes merely secondary consequences of altered cellular metabolism? (2) Is phosphatidylinositol hydrolysis the key response in cellular activation?

This article is concerned with the increased turnover of phosphatidic acid and phosphoinositides observed after interaction of hormones with plasma membrane receptors. Certain changes in phospholipid metabolism after receptor activation involve the methyltransferase enzymes which convert phosphatidylethanolamine to phosphatidylcholine (Hirata *et al.*, 1979). Phospholipid methylation, reviewed by Crews (1982), generally does not occur in response to the same stimulus as phosphoinositide turnover.

The phosphatidylinositol effect was originally described by Hokin and Hokin (1953, 1955a) as a large increase in the incorporation of [^{32}P]orthophosphate into phosphatidylinositol and phosphatidic acid

117

in response to cholinergic stimulation of slices from pigeon pancreas. Amylase secretion is the physiological response to cholinergic stimulation in these slices and initially it was thought that the phosphatidylinositol effect was secondary to the secretory response. Since that time, however, it has been found that the phosphatidylinositol effect is independent of the secretory response.

The increased incorporation of ^{32}P into phosphatidic acid and phosphatidylinositol is not always accompanied by equivalent increases in the uptake of labeled inositol, fatty acid, or glycerol. In some cases turnover of the fatty acids and acylglycerol (derived from glucose metabolism or glycerol in cells with glycerokinase activity) is not seen because the diacylglycerol derived from phosphatidylinositol breakdown is rapidly rephosphorylated to form phosphatidic acid and ultimately phosphatidylinositol. With appreciable breakdown of diacylglycerol, incorporation of labeled fatty acids will also be increased as well as acylglycerol formation.

The increased incorporation of ^{32}P and other precursors into phosphatidic acid and phosphatidylinositol may be a metabolic consequence of an initial breakdown of phosphatidylinositol. Uptake of ^{32}P into phospholipids is relatively easy to measure but difficult to interpret. In mammalian cells it appears to correlate very well with the ability of hormones to elevate intracellular Ca^{2+} and increase phosphoinositide breakdown. However, in the blowfly salivary gland the breakdown of prelabeled phosphoinositides by serotonin is accompanied by an inhibition of ^{32}P or $[^{3}H]$inositol uptake into both phosphatidic acid and phosphatidylinositol (Berridge and Fain, 1979). The divalent cation ionophore A23187 inhibits uptake of label into phosphoinositides without affecting phosphatidylinositol breakdown in salivary glands. These data suggest that elevations in intracellular Ca^{2+} by A23187 and serotonin may inhibit phosphatidylinositol synthesis in blowfly salivary glands.

Phosphatidylinositol synthesis is inhibited by Ca^{2+} in mammalian cells (Jungalwala et al., 1971; Wootton and Kinsella, 1977). CDP-diglyceride inositol transferase, the enzyme which catalyzes the last step in phosphatidylinositol synthesis, is inhibited by Ca^{2+} in rabbit lung (Bleasdale et al., 1979). In cells in which stimuli increase phosphatidylinositol synthesis, there is a concurrent elevation in cytosolic Ca^{2+} which should inhibit not stimulate phosphatidylinositol synthesis. Possibly the site for phosphatidylinositol synthesis in blowfly salivary glands is in equilibrium with the cytosolic Ca^{2+} while in mammalian cells synthesis occurs in compartments not in equilibrium with cytosolic Ca^{2+}. The endoplasmic reticulum, which is the major site for phosphatidylinositol synthesis, may lose Ca^{2+} resulting in removal of an inhibitory constraint on phosphatidylinositol synthesis. Vasopressin and α_1-catecholamines stimulate the release of Ca^{2+} from the endoplasmic reticulum to the cytosol of liver (Exton, 1981; Williamson et al., 1981). Probably Ca^{2+} as well as the level of diacylglycerol are involved in regulating phosphatidylinositol synthesis in the endoplasmic reticulum. In adipocytes the diacylglycerol content is elevated by lipolytic hormones, but phosphatidylinositol synthesis is not increased (Garcia-Sainz and Fain, 1980). Alternatively, the diacylglycerol pools involved in phosphatidylinositol synthesis and degradation are compartmentalized. Clearly, we know little about the regulation of phosphatidylinositol synthesis in intact cells and even less about the mechanisms by which hormones that elevate cytosolic Ca^{2+} are able to accelerate this process.

In some cells breakdown of phosphatidylinositol is accompanied by increases in phosphatidic acid. Salmon and Honeyman (1980) and Putney et al. (1980) suggested that phosphatidic acid functions as a Ca^{2+} ionophore. In blowfly salivary glands there is no detectable synthesis of phosphatidic acid accompanying phosphoinositide breakdown which rules out a primary function of this lipid as a universal Ca^{2+} ionophore (Berridge and Fain, 1979). Furthermore, the formation of phosphatidic acid appears to occur after the breakdown of phosphatidylinositol and the rise in cytosolic Ca^{2+} content. This is true in mast cells (Cockcroft et al., 1980) and hepatocytes (Thomas et al., 1983). However, in our studies using hepatocytes the rapid decreases in phosphoinositides over the first 120 seconds after hormone addition coincided with increases in ^{32}P incorporation into phosphatidic acid (Litosch et al., 1983b).

One problem with determining the role of phosphatidic acid in hormone action is that the breakdown of phosphatidylinositol leads to accumulation of diacylglycerol which is converted to phosphatidic acid. Many of the effects attributed to phosphatidic acid may actually be due to 1,2-diacylglycerol.

Diacylglycerol derived from phosphoinositide breakdown activates the cyclic AMP and calmodulin-insensitive protein kinase C described by Nishizuki (Kishimoto et al., 1980; Takai et al., 1984). The tumor-promoting phorbol esters are structural analogs of diacylglycerol which are able to activate protein kinase C in intact cells (Castagna et al., 1982; Kaibuchi et al., 1983). In hepatocytes three proteins become phosphorylated upon addition of vasopressin but not A23187. The phosphorylation of these three proteins is also effected by phorbol ester (Garrison, 1983). The data of Garrison (1983) and Castagna et al.

(1982) suggest that one result of phosphatidylinositol breakdown is the activation of protein kinase C by diacylglycerol.

Phosphatidylinositol hydrolysis appears to be a key response regulating diacylglycerol availability. In rat hepatocytes (Takenawa *et al.*, 1982) or guinea pig macrophages (Homma *et al.*, 1982), however, there is evidence that the ionophore A23187 increased diacylglycerol accumulation as the result of triacylglycerol degradation. The ionophore had little effect on phosphatidylinositol turnover but increased ^{32}P uptake into phosphatidic acid by hepatocytes (Takenawa *et al.*, 1982).

The growth of literature relating to phosphatidylinositol turnover has been enormous over the past few years. A lot of information is accumulating but it is rather confusing to the novice in the field.

Some of the key events in the phosphatidylinositol story are shown in Table I. While the number of tissues showing the phosphatidylinositol effect increases each year, agreement about the meaning of the effect has not yet been reached. Cockcroft (1981) believes that the phosphatidylinositol effect is probably the result not the cause of Ca^{2+} gating while Michell and Kirk (1982) have defended the hypothesis that phosphatidylinositol breakdown is associated with Ca^{2+} gating in a causal relationship. Michell, however, has abandoned his original idea that phosphatidylinositol breakdown produced cyclic inositol phosphate which he postulated might function as an intracellular second messenger. Michell's new hypothesis is that phosphatidylinositol 4,5-bisphosphate is cleaved to produce inositol 1,4,5-trisphosphate which is now the postulated second messenger (Michell, 1982; Downes and Michell, 1982).

TABLE I

SELECTED EVENTS IN THE PHOSPHATIDYLINOSITOL (PI) STORY

1953. Increased uptake of ^{32}P into PI noted by Hokin and Hokin during enzyme secretion in pancreatic slices

1969. Durell, Garland, and Friedel suggest that PI breakdown is activated by hormones and is responsible for uptake of ^{32}P into PI

1975. Michell suggests that PI breakdown results in diacylglycerol and cyclic inositol formation with the latter linked to gating of Ca^{2+}

1979. Nishizuka and his associates postulate that diacylglycerol activates protein kinase C

1982. Wallace *et al.* demonstrate that vasopressin addition to rat liver plasma membranes increased phosphatidylinositol breakdown

1983. Streb *et al.* provide evidence that inositol trisphosphate derived from breakdown of phosphatidylinositol 4,5-bisphosphate releases Ca^{2+} from the endoplasmic reticulum

---

Several reviews related to phosphatidylinositol turnover are in the proceedings of the symposiums on Ca^{2+} held at the Spring 1983 FASEB meetings in Chicago (Rubin et al., 1984). An entire issue of Cell Calcium (Vol. 3, No. 4/5) in 1982 was devoted to papers and reviews selected by R. H. Michell on inositol phospholipids and cell calcium. Downes and Michell (1982) published a review which emphasized phosphatidylinositol 4-phosphate and phosphatidylinositol 4,5-bisphosphate function. Farese (1983a,b) has emphasized studies on polyphosphoinositide synthesis. Farese divided phosphatidylinositol turnover into three types of effects: (1) breakdown of phosphatidylinositol via a Ca^{2+}-independent mechanism, (2) breakdown of phosphatidylinositol via a Ca^{2+}-dependent mechanism, and (3) stimulation of de novo (net) synthesis of phosphatidic acid, phosphatidylinositol, and polyphosphoinositides. The latter type of effect has been observed with most steroidogenic agents as well as with insulin.

The proceedings of a minisymposium on phosphatidylinositol turnover and cellular function have been published with an excellent introduction by Gil et al. (1983) and presentations by Agranoff (1983), Fain et al. (1983a), Lapetina (1983), and Michell (1983). Michell's review (1975) probably generated the greatest impact because of his suggestion that phosphatidylinositol was involved in Ca^{2+} gating. Reviews by Berridge (1981a) and Fain (1982) suggested that phosphatidylinositol hydrolysis might have a causal relationship to release of intracellular stores of Ca^{2+}.

Irvine et al. (1982), Abdel-Latif (1983), and Hawthorne (1982a,b) have published more neutral reviews on the meaning of phosphatidylinositol turnover, emphasizing the complexities in linking stimulated labeling of phosphatidylinositol with any particular cellular function. Irvine et al. (1982) suggested that stimulated phosphatidylinositol turnover is just one facet of the complex sequence of events evolving from interaction of ligands with the plasma membrane of cells. Whether it is linked solely to one function (elevation of Ca^{2+}) and to that in a causal relationship remains to be proved. They also point out that it is important to show that breakdown of phosphatidylinositol occurs as there are possibilities of isotopic artifacts in studies with labeled precursors.

The pathways involved in phosphoinositide turnover are depicted in Fig. 1. Diacylglycerol is converted to phosphatidic acid which then reacts with cytidine triphosphate (CTP). The activated CDP-diacylglycerol, which could also be designated as CMP-phosphatidic acid, reacts with free inositol to form phosphatidylinositol. The figure indicates that there are kinases and phosphatases involved in the interconver-

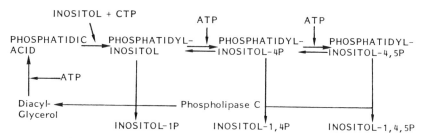

FIG. 1. General pathways of phosphoinositide metabolism.

sion of the three phosphoinositides. The phosphodiesterase cleavage of the three phosphoinositides gives the appropriate inositol phosphate plus diacylglycerol and this enzyme(s) has been referred to as phospholipase C. Hormones appear to stimulate the breakdown of all phosphoinositides via phospholipase C. It is unclear whether there are separate phospholipase C enzymes for each phosphoinositide and whether the hormones increase substrate availability or directly activate the enzymes.

II. MACROPHAGES, NEUTROPHILS, AND MAST CELLS

Macrophages are large leukocytes which can be readily collected in the peritoneal exudate several days after the injection of a foreign substance. The tripeptide formylmethionylleucylphenylalanine (fMLP) stimulates the release of secretory products from cytochalasin B-treated cells. Initially, Cockcroft and Gomperts (1979) thought that stimulus–secretion coupling was linked to phosphatidylinositol turnover and involved the regulation of Ca^{2+} channels in rat peritoneal mast cells. However, a year later Cockcroft et al. (1980) concluded that phosphatidylinositol breakdown and its subsequent resynthesis were not linked in a causal fashion to Ca^{2+} gating. The same group recently demonstrated that the initial site of fMLP stimulated phosphatidylinositol breakdown was the plasma membrane (Bennett et al., 1982). Earlier, Cockcroft et al. (1980) had shown that at least 25% of prelabeled phosphatidylinositol was degraded within 10 seconds after the addition of fMLP and this was accompanied by a 32% increase in labeling of phosphatidic acid.

The confusion about whether Ca^{2+} released from the intracellular membranes causes the phosphatidylinositol breakdown or vice versa may be the result of studies using Ca^{2+} ionophores and Ca^{2+}-free medium. Cockcroft et al. (1981) observed that in neutrophils incubated in Ca^{2+}-free buffer containing 10 μM EGTA and cytochalasin B there was no net change in labeled phosphatidylinositol or secretion of β-glucuronidase 3 minutes after addition of 1–1000 nM fMLP. Addition of Ca^{2+} caused the expected changes in secretion and phospholipids. The effects of the fMLP were mimicked by the divalent ionophore, ionomycin. Homma et al. (1982) and Takenawa et al. (1983) obtained different results using guinea pig macrophages. They confirmed that A23187 mimicked the effects of fMLP on secretion and ^{32}P uptake into both phosphatidic acid and phosphatidylinositol. Secretion was much slower in guinea pig macrophages with the maximal response to fMLP at 5 minutes and to the ionophore at 20 minutes. They used various radiolabels for measurements of phospholipid turnover including [^{14}C]glycerol, [^{3}H]arachidonic acid, and ^{32}P. While both A23187 and fMLP increased turnover of phosphatidic acid and phosphatidylinositol, the mechanisms involved were different. The stimulated breakdown of phosphatidylinositol due to fMLP was via a phosphatidylinositol-specific phospholipase C. In contrast, A23187 increased breakdown of triacylglycerols and activated phospholipase A_2 (Homma et al., 1982). Activation of both pathways increased diacylglycerol formation, fatty acid release, and phosphatidic acid formation. Interestingly, there was little effect of either A23187 or fMLP on the turnover of [^{32}P]- or [^{3}H]arachidonic acid-labeled phosphatidylinositol 4,5-bisphosphate (Homma et al., 1982).

Takenawa et al. (1983) subsequently found that, in macrophages incubated in Ca^{2+}-free media containing 100 μM EGTA, fMLP stimulated a net increase in ^{32}P uptake into phosphatidic acid and phosphatidylinositol. The ionophore A23187 also increased ^{32}P uptake into phosphatidic acid and phosphatidylinositol. However, the addition of fMLP to guinea pig macrophages incubated in the Ca^{2+}-free medium with 100 μM EGTA and 1 μM A23187 increased ^{32}P uptake into both phospholipids to a much greater extent than found without A23187 (Takenawa et al., 1983). These macrophages had previously been incubated for 1 hour in medium containing ^{32}P and therefore changes in ^{32}P lipids represented the net result of phospholipid breakdown and phospholipid synthesis. Possibly, the stimulation of phosphatidic acid and phosphatidylinositol synthesis was so great in Ca^{2+}-free medium that it was difficult to see net breakdown of these phospholipids.

The data of Homma et al. (1982) and Cockcroft et al. (1981) suggest that phosphatidylinositol labeled by incubation with glycerol is preferable for studies on breakdown. When macrophages are prelabeled with [^{14}C]glycerol for 1.5–2 hours and then chased with 10 mM unlabeled glycerol for 20–30 minutes, the subsequent addition of fMLP resulted

in loss of about 25–40% of the [³H]glycerol-labeled phosphatidylinositol by 10 seconds in regular buffer. There was no further
breakdown with prolonged incubation. Future studies should examine
time points from 5 to 300 seconds in Ca^{2+}-free buffer and compare
enzyme secretion, ^{32}P uptake into phospholipids, and breakdown of
glycerol-labeled phosphatidylinositol as well as polyphosphoinositides.

It is of interest to examine critically the three observations which
Cockcroft (1982) claimed ruled out phosphatidylinositol hydrolysis as
being linked to receptor activation in macrophages. The first was that
it took more ligand to give half-maximal activation of phosphatidylinositol hydrolysis than to give the physiological response. Homma et al.
(1982) found this to be true in guinea pig macrophages with respect to
synthesis of phospholipids. However, the dose–response relationships
for breakdown of glycerol-labeled phosphatidylinositol and enzyme secretion were similar in macrophages and neutrophils (Homma et al.,
1982; Cockcroft et al., 1981). The second point of Cockcroft (1982) was
that phosphatidylinositol breakdown lagged behind secretion. What
she actually found was that phosphatidylinositol hydrolysis and enzyme secretion occurred concurrently with maximal effects observed at
the earliest time point (10 seconds). It is true that maximal uptake of
label into phosphatidic acid occurs long after secretion is concluded.
However, phosphatidic acid formation appears to be secondary to an
initial degradation of phosphatidylinositol and thus is not a valid criteria for the onset of phosphatidylinositol response. The third point of
Cockcroft (1982) was that both enzyme secretion and appreciable
breakdown of phosphatidylinositol (at least as measured at 3 minutes)
were abolished in Ca^{2+}-free buffer. This was taken by her to prove
that Ca^{2+} entry is required for phosphatidylinositol breakdown. Takenawa et al. (1983), however, found that Ca^{2+} ionophores produced
effects rather different from those of fMLP in macrophages.

The available data indicate that after fMLP addition to macrophages
or neutrophils there is a rapid breakdown of plasma membrane-bound
phosphatidylinositol which seems to be a unique event linked to receptor activation. In contrast, the effects of elevating Ca^{2+} are rather
different suggesting that intracellular Ca^{2+} probably does not cause
all the initial changes in phosphatidylinositol degradation.

The data of Homma et al. (1982) suggest that the turnover of polyphosphoinositides was little affected by fMLP. Volpi et al. (1983) on the
other hand found that fMLP reduced prelabeled ^{32}P content of phosphatidylinositol 4,5-bisphosphate by 20% within 10 seconds of the addition to rabbit neutrophils. Further studies are warranted using mac-

rophages to discern the role of phosphatidylinositol and polyphospho-inositides in the function of these cells.

III. BRAIN SYNAPTOSOMES

An entire symposium on phospholipids in the nervous system was recently published (Horrocks et al., 1982). Hawthorne and Pickard (1979) and Downes (1982) have reviewed the role of phosphoinositide turnover in the central nervous system.

There is evidence for neurotransmitter induced increases in phosphoinositide turnover in brain in vivo. Lunt and Pickard (1975) found that, in synaptic vesicles isolated from brain after an intraventricular injection of carbachol, there was a 20% breakdown of phosphatidylino-sitol previously labeled in vivo with ^{32}P. Similar results were obtained by Berry et al. (1981) and Soukup et al. (1978). More recently, Soukup and Schanberg (1982) demonstrated that intracisternal injection of norepinephrine increased uptake of labeled precursors (^{32}P and [^{3}H]inositol) into phosphatidylinositol 4,5-bisphosphate, phosphatidylinositol, and phosphatidic acid by 40–80% within 5 minutes. The stimulatory effects of norepinephrine were greater in the cerebellum and brainstem than in the cerebral cortex. Demonstration of a hormone effect on phosphatidylinositol 4,5-bisphosphate labeling required short-term labeling as well as the use of microwave irradiation to prevent brain polyphosphoinositide breakdown.

In vitro studies with brain slices have not been particularly useful. However, Downes (1982) suggested that relatively thick brain slices may be suitable since they contain a greater proportion of morphologically intact neurons. Most studies have been done with brain synaptosomes which are really minicells. Agranoff (1983) has described them as anucleated nerve endings containing integral postsynaptic cholinergic receptors which have resealed into bags containing ATP-generating systems. Downes (1982) suggested that during homogenization some closed vesicles of dendritic origin are formed which are responsible for the phosphoinositide effect. The synaptosome or dendrosome preparations probably contain many different types of closed vesicles but only a small fraction may respond to neurotransmitters with increased phosphoinositide turnover. The effects of cholinergic stimulation are particularly interesting because of the suggestion that age-related memory disturbances may be linked to decreases in central cholinergic function (Bartus et al., 1982).

Hokin and Hokin (1955b) originally reported that acetylcholine increased the incorporation of ^{32}P into phosphatidic acid and phosphatidylinositol in brain slices. Durell and Sodd (1966) suggested that the increased synthesis of phosphatidylinositol observed in brain cell-free systems by Hokin and Hokin (1959) was due to synaptosomes. These are not a truly cell-free system but rather more of a minicell system as noted earlier.

Recently, it has been found that the response to acetylcholine involves activation of muscarinic receptors at postsynaptic sites (Agranoff, 1983; Downes, 1982). Many of the effects of muscarinic cholinergic stimulation can be mimicked by the ionophore A23187 and require the presence of extracellular Ca^{2+}. However, there is no evidence that muscarinic cholinergic stimulation of synaptosomes alters Ca^{2+} influx or efflux (Agranoff, 1983).

Durell and Garland (1969) were the first to report that the breakdown of phosphoinositides in brain synaptosomes was accelerated by acetylcholine. The products of breakdown appeared to be inositol 1-phosphate and inositol 1,4-bisphosphate. Subsequent studies have confirmed these findings (Warfield and Segal, 1978; Berry et al., 1981). Most evidence suggests that the breakdown of phosphatidylinositol is a direct result of receptor activation while some phosphatidylinositol 1,4-bisphosphate breakdown may be secondary to elevations in cytosol Ca^{2+}.

Griffin and Hawthorne (1978) labeled synaptosome phospholipids with ^{32}P and then added A23187 to elevate cytosolic Ca^{2+}. The ionophore had little effect on net labeling of phosphatidylinositol in 10-minute incubations but increased the amount of label in phosphatidic acid and decreased that in the polyphosphoinositides. Addition of EGTA to the medium after 10 minutes with A23187 caused a marked rebound in label present in the polyphosphoinositides but only a small increase in label in phosphatidic acid.

An analysis of the water-soluble breakdown products of phosphoinositide in synaptosomes from rats previously injected intracerebrally with [^{3}H]inositol indicated that A23187 doubled the accumulation of inositol 1,4-bisphosphate, increased slightly the amount of inositol 1-phosphate but had no effect on that of inositol 1,4,5-trisphosphate. The distribution of the polyphosphoinositides was similar to that of Na^+, K^+-ATPase suggesting that they were preferentially located in the plasma membrane. Griffin and Hawthorne (1978) suggested that elevation of synaptosomal Ca^{2+} activated phosphatidylinositol 4,5-phosphate phosphomonoesterase and phosphatidylinositol

4,5-bisphosphate phosphodiesterase, but had little effect on phosphatidylinositol phosphodiesterase (phospholipase C).

Van Rooijen et al. (1983) confirmed that Ca^{2+} activates breakdown of polyphosphoinositides in synaptosomal membrane preparations. The products of breakdown were both inositol bis- and trisphosphates indicating that a phosphodiesterase was involved. Ca^{2+} did not stimulate phosphatidylinositol breakdown.

Warfield and Segal (1978) found that incubation with acetylcholine for 60 minutes decreased the total amount of brain synaptosomal phosphatidylinositol by 22%. In synaptosomes from rats with experimental galactose toxicity, which impairs brain function, the effect of acetylcholine on phosphatidylinositol breakdown was reduced by 50%. The fact that these investigators obtained a net breakdown of phosphatidylinositol may have been due to 1.4 mM Ca^{2+} in the medium which reduced the stimulatory effect of acetylcholine on phosphatidylinositol synthesis. In fact, the total uptake of [³H]inositol into phosphatidylinositol was unaffected by acetylcholine but the specific activity increased due to net breakdown.

Fisher and Agranoff (1981) omitted Ca^{2+} from the medium used for brain synaptosome studies because it decreased uptake of ³²P label into phosphatidylinositol. They did not measure content but rather net uptake of labeled [³H]inositol and [³²P]P$_i$. Acetylcholine increased the net uptake of ³²P into phosphatidylinositol while having no effect on uptake of other precursors. Similar results have been seen in hepatocytes where vasopressin increased the uptake of ³²P but not of inositol into phosphatidylinositol (Tolbert et al., 1980).

Rat brain synaptosomes incorporate [³H]inositol into phosphatidylinositol via an exchange reaction which is accelerated by Mn^{2+} and cytidine monophosphate (CMP) (Berry et al., 1983). CMP was equally active on intact synaptosomes and synaptosomal membranes. The large amount of [³H]inositol incorporation into phosphatidylinositol due to exchange reaction may be related to the failure of acetylcholine to increase labeled inositol accumulation in phosphoinositides of brain synaptosomes under conditions in which ³²P uptake is accelerated.

Fisher and Agranoff (1981) found that in Ca^{2+}-free medium the Ca^{2+} ionophore A23187 increased ³²P uptake into phosphatidylinositol while decreasing uptake of [³H]glycerol and [³H]glucose. The addition of acetylcholine had no effect on the ionophore mediated reduction in [³H]glycerol and [³H]glucose incorporation into phosphatidylinositol but markedly increased [³²P]P$_i$ uptake into phosphatidylinositol. The above studies used a 30 minute uptake with the acetylcholine added at the same time as the label. Acetylcholine or A23187 decreased net accumulation of [^{32}P]P$_i$ in phosphatidylinositol 4-phosphate and phosphatidylinositol 4,5-bisphosphate. In synaptosomes prelabeled with [^{32}P]P$_i$ for 10–20 minutes the addition of A23187 blocked further incorporation of label into both polyphosphoinositides and acetylcholine decreased accumulation of label only when the ionophore was added. The data of Fisher and Agranoff (1981) suggest that acetylcholine has effects on phosphoinositide turnover that are not mimicked by A23187.

Recently Brown and Nahorski (1983) and Berridge et al. (1982) found that acetylcholine addition to brain slices increased the accumulation of inositol 1-phosphate in the presence of 5–10 mM Li$^+$. Allison and Stewart (1971) found that Li$^+$ decreased the concentration of myo-inositol in the cerebral cortex of rats. Sherman et al. (1981) and Allison et al. (1976) found that this was accompanied by a marked increase in the concentration of inositol 1-phosphate. Lithium appears to act primarily by inhibiting the conversion of inositol 1-phosphate to inositol by a phosphatase but it may also stimulate a muscarinic cholinergic response.

Since Sherman et al. (1981) found that the D-enantiomer of inositol 1-phosphate was elevated; the source was phospholipase C-mediated phosphoinositide breakdown. In brain slices incubated with Li$^+$, agonists which increase the accumulation of inositol 1-phosphate include phenylephrine, histamine, serotonin, Substance P, vasopressin, neurotensin, and CCK octapeptide in addition to acetylcholine (Berridge et al., 1982; Brown and Nahorski, 1983; Downes, 1982). Downes (1982) also noted that in slices from the cerebral cortex, corpus striatum, hypothalamus, and hippocampus, but not the cerebellum, there was a 440–700% increase due to carbachol in labeled inositol 1-phosphate accumulation over a 30-minute incubation. These data suggest that phosphoinositide breakdown is a widespread response coupled to a variety of receptors in the brain.

Previous studies were hampered by the fact that in most mammalian cells the breakdown of phosphoinositides releases inositol which is promptly reincorporated into phosphatidylinositol. This process is often markedly reduced by Li$^+$ due to inhibition of inositol 1-phosphate phosphatase. Future studies using 10 mM Li$^+$ may prove most rewarding in the central nervous system.

Another function of phosphoinositide breakdown might be the release of arachidonic acid. Hawthorne and Pickard (1979) pointed out that the arachidonic acid content of phosphoinositides is much higher than in other brain phospholipids. The key role of arachidonic acid release and its conversion to prostaglandins, thromboxanes, and the other biologically active products derived from its metabolism is well established. It is likely that the main physiological source of arachidonic acid release in brain is phosphoinositide breakdown to diacylglycerol followed by diacylglycerol lipase cleavage.

Cohen et al. (1983) have found that muscarinic cholinergic stimulation produced an increased uptake of ^{32}P into phosphatidylinositol in tw mouse neuroblastoma cell lines. These cultured cells should be especially useful in studies on phosphoinositide breakdown since they can be prelabeled by incubation with [^{3}H]inositol and breakdown of all phosphoinositides examined in the presence of 5–10 mM Li$^+$ at short time periods.

We are probably on the brink of an explosive phase of growth in studies relating to phosphoinositide breakdown in the central nervous system. The paucity of our current information is matched only by the difficulty in working with the complex central nervous system. We need model systems which are simpler than those currently available. A broadly based research effort should lead to substantial progress over the next few years. Synaptosomes appear to be particularly promising and better procedures for separation of the various types could be developed. It may soon be possible to confirm the early reports by deScarnatti and Arnaiz (1972) of a direct activation of phosphatidylinositol degradation by addition of acetylcholine to rat brain membranes as has been seen with rat hepatocyte membranes (Wallace et al., 1982b; Harrington and Eichberg, 1983).

IV. HEPATOCYTES

The previous sections on synaptosomes and macrophages demonstrated that there are distinct differences between the increases in phosphoinositide turnover due to calcium ionophores and hormones. In hepatocytes A23187 also increases diacylglycerol accumulation but this is apparently the result of triacylglycerol degradation as well as nonspecific effects of phospholipid breakdown (Takenawa et al., 1982). Vasopression or α_1-adrenoceptor activation leads to breakdown of all phosphoinositides in hepatocytes and there is no effect of A23187 (Billah and Michell, 1979; Tolbert et al., 1980; Prpic et al., 1982; Thomas et al., 1983).

Studies on Ca^{2+} depletion in the medium by the addition of EGTA have produced variable results. It was already clear by 1978 that α_1-adrenoceptor activation of glycogen phosphorylase in rat hepatocytes was not dependent on the influx of extracellular Ca^{2+} (Fain, 1978). Epinephrine is generally agreed to elevate intracellular Ca^{2+} stores which actually results in efflux of Ca^{2+} at high hormone concentrations (Fain, 1978; Exton, 1981; Williamson *et al.*, 1981). Fain *et al.* (1983b) and Billah and Michell (1979) found that the breakdown of phosphatidylinositol was unimpaired by chelation of extracellular Ca^{2+} and readily exchangeable stores of hepatocyte Ca^{2+} with short-term exposure to EGTA. However, our experience is that this is a very deleterious procedure; prolonged incubation of hepatocytes caused loss of response to vasopressin as noted by Thomas *et al.* (1983). Prpic *et al.* (1982) and Rhodes *et al.* (1983) found that isolating, washing, and then incubating hepatocytes in Ca^{2+}-free buffer containing 1 mM EGTA abolished the effects of vasopressin on activation of glycogen phosphorylase, as well as on breakdown of prelabeled phosphatidylinositol and phosphatidylinositol 4,5-bisphosphate. In contrast, Kirk *et al.* (1981b) reported that if 2 mM EGTA was added to hepatocytes incubated with 1 mM Ca^{2+} 15 minutes prior to vasopressin addition, there was a 9% breakdown of phosphatidylinositol 4,5-bisphosphate over the first 60 seconds. There was about 23% breakdown of this lipid if excess Ca^{2+} were present. Thomas *et al.* (1983) found that chelation of extracellular Ca^{2+} by adding 2.5 mM EGTA to buffer containing 1.3 mM Ca^{2+} 90 minutes prior to addition of vasopressin abolished both stimulation of phosphorylase and changes in phosphoinositides. Fain *et al.* (1983b) incubated hepatocytes in buffer containing 1.3 mM Ca^{2+} and then added 2 mM EGTA to chelate Ca^{2+} 10 minutes before vasopressin. They found the same degradation of phosphoinositides at 30 seconds as in buffer without EGTA. This procedure abolishes the stimulation by vasopressin of glycogen phosphorylase (Tolbert *et al.*, 1980). Tolbert *et al.* (1980) also found that the stimulation of ^{32}P uptake into phosphatidylinositol by vasopressin was reduced but not abolished by chelation of extracellular Ca^{2+} as originally reported by Kirk *et al.* (1978). These results indicate that under appropriate conditions vasopressin cannot release enough intracellular Ca^{2+} to activate glycogen phosphorylase but is able to stimulate phosphoinositide turnover. This observation is incompatible with the suggestion that the elevation of Ca^{2+} is responsible for phosphoinositide turnover.

The most convincing evidence that degradation of plasma membrane phosphoinositides is not secondary to elevations in cytosol Ca^{2+} is the finding of direct effects of vasopressin on this process in plasma membrane preparations from rat hepatocytes. Wallace *et al.* (1982b) reported that vasopressin addition to rat liver membranes caused an increase in total phosphatidylinositol degradation. This effect of vasopressin was not dependent on Ca^{2+}. Subsequently, Fain et al. (1983b) found a similar effect on breakdown of labeled phosphatidylinositol in hepatic plasma membranes obtained from rats injected 18 hours previously with myo- [2-^{3}H]inositol. There was a 12% decrease in labeled phosphatidylinositol in membranes incubated with 50 mU/ml of vasopressin in buffer containing 1 mM $CaCl_2$ and 17% breakdown in Ca^{2+}-free buffer containing 0.5 mM EGTA. Wallace et al. (1983) also found an 8% breakdown of total rat hepatic plasma membrane phosphatidylinositol due to norepinephrine.

The direct effect of norepinephrine on phosphatidylinositol degradation in rat liver plasma membranes was independently reported by Harrington and Eichberg (1983). Their results were similar in that Ca^{2+} was not required but they found effects only in the presence of cytosol. The localization and nature of the enzyme activated by hormone remains to be elucidated. There is a hepatic cytosolic phospholipase C which acts on exogenous phosphatidylinositol in the presence of appreciable amounts of Ca^{2+} (Dawson et al., 1980). The role of Ca^{2+} in vitro might be to neutralize the negative charge on phosphatidylinositol allowing the enzyme to interact with its substrate. In contrast, when phosphatidylinositol is present in the native membrane, there may be no requirement for added Ca^{2+}. The activity of the cytosolic enzyme on phosphatidylinositol appears to be modulated by other phospholipids and diacylglycerol (Dawson et al., 1980; Hofmann and Majerus, 1982).

The site of the initial degradation of phosphatidylinositol due to vasopressin appears to be the plasma membrane. Lin and Fain (1981) found selective degradation of plasma membrane phosphatidylinositol in hepatocytes incubated for only 5 minutes with vasopressin or epinephrine. Phosphatidylinositol was labeled by injection of [^{3}H]inositol into rats 18 hours prior to isolation of hepatocytes. In these studies it was necessary to homogenize the hepatocytes at 5°C and use conditions which minimized activation of lysosomal phospholipases as well as redistribution of phosphatidylinositol through phospholipid transfer proteins.

However, Kirk et al. (1981a) incubated hepatocytes under similar conditions and found 42.8% of the recovered labeled phosphatidylinositol in the microsomal fraction from controls and 41.9% of the label in microsomes from vasopressin-treated cells. Unfortunately, they did not separate the microsomal fraction into the plasma membrane versus endoplasmic reticulum so it was impossible for them to determine whether there was any change in the plasma membrane phosphatidylinositol content. Kirk et al. (1981a) did point out that there may have been rapid phosphatidylinositol exchanges between the various fractions in their homogenates, which may explain their negative results.

The direct activation of hepatocyte phosphatidylinositol breakdown by hormone addition to membranes is difficult to reconcile with the suggestion by Michell et al. (1981) that hormones only increase the degradation of phosphatidylinositol 4,5-bisphosphate. Phosphatidylinositol loss presumably proceeds solely through its phosphorylation to replenish phosphatidylinositol 4,5-bisphosphate. In isolated plasma membranes from rat livers there was so little polyphosphoinositide found that its degradation could not be measured With membranes incubated with [γ-^{32}P]ATP, however, label was incorporated into polyphosphoinositides. The uptake of label was rapid, and reached half-maximal within 10 seconds and near-maximal at 30 seconds (Fain et al., 1983). Vasopressin did not affect the incorporation of [γ-^{32}P]ATP label into polyphosphoinositides. Under the conditions used for measuring polyphosphoinositide formation there was a 6% breakdown of total phosphatidylinositol over 30 minutes with added vasopressin (Fain et al., 1983b).

Michell et al. (1981) first showed that vasopressin rapidly stimulated polyphosphoinositide breakdown in hepatocytes. Rhodes et al. (1983) found a rapid breakdown of polyphosphoinositides but claimed that it was secondary to an elevation in Ca^{2+}. Kirk (1982) proposed that polyphosphoinositide breakdown is the primary event in hormone action and that loss of phosphatidylinositol proceeds by phosphorylation to phosphatidylinositol 4,5-bisphosphate. Our group (Fain et al., 1983; Litosch et al., 1983b) and Thomas et al. (1983) found that hormones directly accelerate the breakdown of all phosphoinositides in hepatocytes.

Fain et al. (1983b) found that in hepatocytes prelabeled with either [^{3}H]inositol or ^{32}P for 45 minutes there was an appreciable degradation of all phosphoinositides in response to vasopressin. The hormone response was maximal at 30 seconds and the decrease in phosphatidylinositol and polyphosphoinositides ranged from 10 to 36% with 1.4 mM Ca^{2+} and from 20 to 60% with 2 mM EGTA added to the cells 10 minutes prior to addition of hormone (Fain et al., 1983b). By 120 seconds this effect had disappeared as uptake of label was increased sufficiently to balance the breakdown of labeled phosphoinositides.

Litosch et al. (1983) found that in hepatocytes previously incubated with ^{32}P or [^{3}H]inositol for 60 minutes, there was near-maximal breakdown of phosphatidylinositol and phosphatidylinositol 4,5-bisphosphate within 30 seconds after vasopressin addition. The percentage disappearance of ^{32}P label at 30 seconds was 10% for phosphatidylinositol, 15% for phosphatidylinositol 4-phosphate, and 40% for phosphatidylinositol 4,5-bisphosphate. With [^{3}H]inositol label, phosphatidylinositol lost approximately five times as much label as did phosphatidylinositol 4,5-bisphosphate over the first 30 seconds. These results indicated that the hormone-sensitive pool of hepatocyte phosphoinositides could be labeled *in vitro* with both [^{3}H]inositol and ^{32}P, but the rate of phosphatidylinositol breakdown appeared similar to that of phosphatidylinositol 4,5-bisphosphate.

Measurements of total phospholipid content 30 seconds after the addition of vasopressin indicated that despite loss of 30–50% of the labeled phosphatidylinositol 4,5-bisphosphate the total content increased by 40% (Litosch et al., 1983). The increase in content appears due to a marked increase in synthesis of phosphatidylinositol 4,5-bisphosphate using a pool of ATP which equilibrates poorly with [^{32}P]ATP. These data indicate that vasopressin increases phosphatidylinositol conversion to phosphatidylinositol 4,5-bisphosphate as well as its degradation.

In hepatocytes, α_1-adrenergic agonists and vasopressin stimulate degradation of all phosphoinositides and increase intracellular free Ca^{2+} concentration. Elevations in cytosolic Ca^{2+} are probably caused by release of Ca^{2+} from intracellular sites (Blackmore et al., 1978; Chen et al., 1978; Althaus-Salzman et al., 1980; Malbon et al., 1980) and possibly the entry of Ca^{2+} via receptor-regulated channels. The signal generated by hormones which trigger intracellular Ca^{2+} mobilization is probably inositol 1,4,5-trisphosphate derived from breakdown of phosphatidylinositol 4,5-bisphosphate.

Streb et al. (1983) reported that inositol 1,4,5-trisphosphate addition to permeabilized pancreatic acinar cells resulted in the release of Ca^{2+} from intracellular stores thought to be the endoplasmic reticulum. These findings have been extended to hepatocytes where an effect of inositol trisphosphate on Ca^{2+} release was seen by Joseph et al. (1984) and Burgess et al. (1984). These data suggest that breakdown of phosphatidylinositol 4,5-bisphosphate induced by ligands results in the formation of inositol 1,4,5-trisphosphate which releases Ca^{2+} from the endoplasmic reticulum. Whether this compound is also involved in entry of Ca^{2+} as well as its release from the plasma membrane and/or mitochondria remains to be established.

The resynthesis of phosphatidic acid and phosphatidylinositol may be a consequence of intracellular Ca^{2+} mobilization as well as increased diacylglycerol content. Release of Ca^{2+} from the endoplasmic reticulum could relieve an inhibitory constraint on phospholipid syn-

thesis resulting in a stimulated uptake of ^{32}P into phosphatidylinositol. The stimulated resynthesis of phosphatidylinositol is found only
with ^{32}P label not with [^{3}H]inositol. Although there is appreciable
incorporation of [^{3}H]inositol into hepatocyte phosphatidylinositol,
there is no further stimulation of [^{3}H]inositol uptake with vasopressin
or α_1-adrenergic activation. This suggests that labeled inositol does
not equilibrate with the pool of inositol used for the compensatory
resynthesis of [^{32}P]phosphatidylinositol seen in the presence of vasopressin. Alternatively, [^{3}H]inositol may be incorporated into phosphoinositides via an exchange process at such a high rate that the
stimulatory effects of hormones are masked. In liver the uptake of
[^{3}H]inositol into phosphoinositides is greatly enhanced by Mn^{2+}
(Tolbert et al., 1980). Whether the exchange reaction is catalyzed via a
separate enzyme or is a reversal of the last step in the synthesis of
phosphatidylinositol involving the reaction of CDP-diacylglycerol with
inositol is unclear (Takenawa et al., 1977; Berry et al., 1983).

Vasopressin does not stimulate ^{32}P or [^{3}H]inositol incorporation into
polyphosphoinositides (Tolbert et al., 1980). These results were crit-
icized by Michell et al. (1981) because the measurements were made
after an hour incubation with ^{32}P. However, similar results were obtained at earlier time periods. In hepatocytes incubated with ^{32}P for
only 5 minutes most of the inositol lipid label is in phosphatidylinositol
4,5-bisphosphate and addition of vasopressin results in a transient loss
of label (Litosch et al., 1983). These data suggest that the metabolic
regulation of phosphatidylinositol synthesis differs from that of phosphatidylinositol 4,5-bisphosphate.

In addition to breakdown of phosphatidylinositol, the addition of
vasopressin or α_1-catecholamine agonists to isolated rat liver plasma
membranes causes release of labeled $^{45}Ca^{2+}$ and increased membrane
fluidity (Burgess et al., 1983). A fourth effect of vasopressin and α_1-
catecholamine agonists on hepatocyte plasma membranes is inhibition
of the Ca^{2+},Mg^{2+}-ATPase activity (Lin et al., 1983). After incubation of
rat hepatocytes with vasopressin, the activity of Ca^{2+},Mg^{2+}-ATPase in
plasma membranes was decreased by 15–30%. The effect of vasopressin
on the activity of this enzyme did not require extracellular calcium and
maximal inhibition was found after only 15 seconds exposure to vasopressin. The concentration of vasopressin needed for half-maximal
inhibition of this enzyme in hepatocytes was approximately 6 nM (Lin et
al., 1983). These findings indicate that the high affinity Ca^{2+},Mg^{2+}-
ATPase of hepatocyte plasma membranes could be involved in the
elevation of cytoplasmic calcium due to vasopressin and α_1-catechol-
amine agonists.

The effects of vasopressin and α_1-catecholamine stimulation on rat

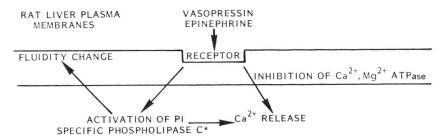

FIG. 2. Outline of vasopressin and α_1-catecholamine action on rat hepatocyte plasma membranes. *Although breakdown of prelabeled phosphatidylinositol 4,5-bisphosphate is seen at 30 seconds, there is a stimulation of total accumulation.

hepatocyte plasma membranes are summarized in Fig. 2. The key questions remaining to be resolved are the relationship between the four effects depicted in Fig. 2. It is possible that the hormone receptor complex causes the release of Ca^{2+} bound to the receptor or closely associated proteins and this increases the access of phosphatidylinositol or phosphatidylinositol 4,5-bisphosphate to enzymes which liberate diacylglycerol and inositol phosphates. Probably the hormone–receptor complex activates a membrane-bound phospholipase C resulting in breakdown of the membrane-bound phosphoinositides which results in liberation of bound intracellular stores of Ca^{2+} as well as increased influx of Ca^{2+}.

The question of whether it is phosphatidylinositol 4,5-bisphosphate that is degraded is difficult to resolve. Michell (1982) and Berridge (1983) are convinced that only phosphatidylinositol 4,5-bisphosphate is degraded. Possibly hormones increase the degradation of any phosphoinositide which is readily accessible on the plasma membrane. Much more of the phosphatidylinositol 4,5-bisphosphate than of phosphatidylinositol which is readily labeled may be present in the plasma membrane, so a greater fraction of it is degraded during the first few seconds after hormone addition. The resulting increase in inositol trisphosphate is apparently able to release Ca^{2+} from the endoplasmic reticulum. At later periods the breakdown of phosphatidylinositol occurs with the liberation of diacylglycerol but no messenger for Ca^{2+} release. Thus the relative proportions of the two messengers may change with time and an additional site for regulation may be the ATP-dependent formation of the polyphosphoinositides.

V. ADRENAL MEDULLA

Hokin et al. (1958) were the first to find that the acetylcholine-stimulated secretion of epinephrine by guinea pig adrenal medullary slices was accompanied by increased incorporation of ^{32}P into phosphatidylinositol. The adrenal medulla has proven interesting because the role of phosphatidylinositol hydrolysis in this tissue does not appear to be regulation of calcium entry. In chromaffin cell cultures, Fisher et al. (1981) observed that acetylcholine increased catecholamine release and Ca^{2+} entry via nicotinic receptors and activation of these receptors did not affect phosphatidylinositol turnover. In contrast, muscarinic activation did not stimulate catecholamine release but did increase phosphatidylinositol labeling (Fisher et al., 1981). Similar results were obtained in the bovine adrenal medulla by Adnan and Hawthorne (1981) and reviewed by Hawthorne and Swilem (1982).

Azila and Hawthorne (1982) found that KCl depolarization of perfused bovine adrenals stimulated catecholamine secretion without affecting phosphatidylinositol turnover. In contrast, the addition of carbachol, even in a Ca^{2+}-free medium, stimulated breakdown of about one-third of prelabeled phosphatidylinositol and phosphatidic acid. The loss of prelabeled phosphatidylinositol in carbachol-stimulated adrenal medulla was not due to specific loss from any particular fraction as determined by the subcellular distribution of label. At least 15 minutes was required, however, to separate the medulla from the cortex and homogenize the tissue and redistribution of label may have occurred. These data suggest that in the adrenal medulla there is an appreciable loss of prelabeled phosphatidylinositol due to muscarinic cholinergic effect linked via receptor activation and not a consequence of Ca^{2+} entry or secretion.

There is evidence that phosphatidylinositol 4-phosphate and 4,5-bisphosphate exist in the chromaffin granules of the adrenal medulla (Buckley et al., 1971; Phillips, 1973; Trifaro and Dworkind, 1975; Lefevre et al., 1976). It might be interesting to compare the breakdown of all three phosphoinositides as well as protein phosphorylation in response to cholinergic activation under conditions where secretion does not occur (Ca^{2+}-free medium). There are several possible results but the most likely finding is that under Ca^{2+}-free conditions there is breakdown of phosphoinositides and phosphorylation of proteins but no secretion. If this occurs, the addition of a Ca^{2+} ionophore along with restoration of medium Ca^{2+} to normal levels might have a much greater effect on secretion in glands preexposed to carbachol. The available data indicate that the changes in phosphoinositide turnover in the adrenal medulla are not likely to be secondary to elevation of cytosol Ca^{2+} or involved in Ca^{2+} gating. Possibly, the breakdown of polyphosphoinositides in the adrenal medullary chromaffin granule aids in fusion of the granule with the plasma membrane either directly or through formation of diacylglycerol. In isolated chromaffin granules as much as 20% of its phosphatidylinositol content can be converted to phosphatidylinositol 4-phosphate with added ATP (Phillips, 1973). Since the site of phosphorylation appears to be the outer (or cytoplasmic) surface of the granule membrane the extent of phosphorylation could contribute to the charge of the chromaffin granule *in vivo*. The addition of ATP to isolated chromaffin granules also causes release of stored amines but not labeled phosphatidylinositol 4-phosphate (Trifaro and Dworkind, 1975).

VI. ADRENAL GLOMERULOSA CELLS

Angiotensin II acts via a cyclic AMP-independent mechanism to stimulate steroidogenesis (aldosterone production) in bovine adrenal glomerulosa cells (Fig. 3). There is a cycloheximide-sensitive step in steroidogenesis that causes increased *de novo* synthesis of phosphatidic acid, phosphatidylinositol, and polyphosphoinositides (see reviews by Farese, 1983a,b). Farese has suggested that the polyphosphoinositides provoke large increases in mitochondrial pregnenolone synthesis, thought to be rate limiting for steroidogenesis.

Elliott *et al.* (1982, 1983) found that in isolated bovine adrenal glomerulosa cells angiotensin II or dibutyryl cyclic AMP stimulated steroidogenesis and reduced the total content of phosphatidylinositol while only angiotensin II increased turnover of phosphatidylinositol.

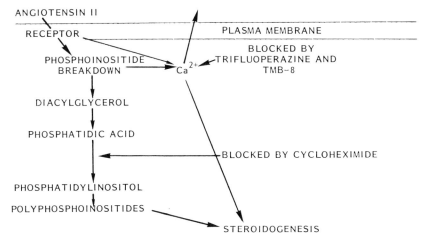

FIG. 3. Regulation of steroidogenesis in adrenal glomerulosa cells by angiotensin II.

JOHN N. FAIN

Steroidogenesis without net increases in phosphatidylinositol as previously observed by Farese *et al.* (1980, 1983) in rat adrenal capsules suggests that *de novo* synthesis of phosphatidylinositol is not a necessary requirement for aldosterone production. Hunyady *et al.* (1982) similarly found that corticotropin, dibutyryl cyclic AMP, prostaglandin E_2, elevated K^+, and angiotensin II stimulated steroidogenesis but only the latter increased ^{32}P uptake into phosphatidylinositol.

Elliott *et al.* (1983) found that incubation of glomerulosa cells with TMB-8 or in Ca^{2+}-free buffer with 0.5 mM EGTA did not abolish the increase in phosphatidylinositol turnover but did block steroidogenesis. The combination of TMB-8 and EGTA, however, blocked phosphatidylinositol turnover due to angiotensin. Elliott *et al.* (1982) also found (as depicted in Fig. 3) that the efflux of prelabeled Ca^{2+} from glomerulosa cells due to angiotensin II was blocked by TMB-8 as well as trifluoperazine but neither agent blocked phosphatidylinositol turnover. In contrast, mepacrine (also known as quinacrine), ouabain, and cycloheximide did not affect either Ca^{2+} flux or phosphatidylinositol turnover but abolished steroidogenesis (Elliott *et al.*, 1982).

VII. ADRENAL CORTEX

The adrenal cortex is interesting because it appears to be a system wherein ACTH, which stimulates cyclic AMP formation, also increases

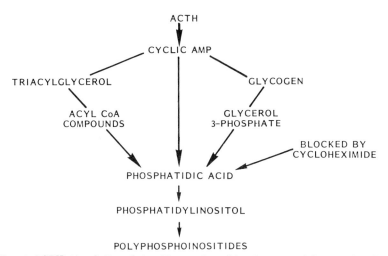

FIG. 4. ACTH stimulation of steroidogenesis and involvement of *de novo* phospholipid synthesis.

the net accumulation of phosphatidic acid, phosphatidylinositol, and polyphosphoinositides. This is an effect distinct from the mechanism whereby hormone-induced increases in cytosolic Ca^{2+} enhance breakdown of plasma membrane phosphatidylinositol. Figure 4 depicts schematically the current view of Farese (1983a,b) that cyclic AMP increases breakdown of triacylglycerol and glycogen, leading to increased steroidogenesis and *de novo* accumulation of phosphoinositides as well as phosphatidic acid via a cycloheximide-sensitive process. Just as in the adrenal glomerulosa cells, the increases in polyphosphoinositides are thought to stimulate pregnenolone synthesis in mitochondria.

VIII. Platelets

Platelets have been extensively investigated since these anucleated cells can be readily obtained from humans or experimental animals. Lloyd *et al.* (1972, 1973) examined the changes in total phosphoinositides and phosphatidic acid as well as turnover of ^{32}P in platelet lipids. They used rabbit platelets stimulated with ADP. The first change detected was an increase in the labeling of phosphatidic acid 7 seconds after ADP addition to platelets previously incubated for 30 minutes with ^{32}P. At 30 seconds there was a 40–70% increase in [^{32}P]phosphatidic acid but only a 12% increase in total phosphatidic acid. There was a 9–16% increase in [^{32}P]phosphatidylinositol 4,5-bisphosphate, a 16–44% increase in phosphatidylinositol 4-phosphate, and little change in labeled phosphatidylinositol. The total content of phosphatidylinositol 4,5-bisphosphate was unchanged 30 seconds after ADP addition. These results first indicated that a very early effect of ADP was to induce the synthesis of a small highly labeled pool of phosphatidic acid.

Broekman *et al.* (1980) measured the changes in phospholipid content 15 and 60 seconds after the addition of thrombin to human platelets. There was a 15% decrease in total phosphatidylinositol at 15 seconds and this was accompanied by a 300% increase in phosphatidic acid. The net increase in phosphatidic acid (assuming that all was synthesized from diacylglycerol generated as a result of phosphatidylinositol breakdown) was equivalent to 42% of the disappearance of phosphatidylinositol. The effects of thrombin on these two phospholipids were blocked by the addition of 3 mM dibutyryl cyclic AMP 5 minutes prior to the addition of thrombin. Broekman *et al.* (1980) noted that in platelets preincubated with 5 mM EGTA to chelate extracellular Ca^{2+} the decrease in phosphatidylinositol and the increase in phosphatidic acid content due to thrombin were unaffected during the first 3 minutes after its addition. However, continued incubation of platelets with thrombin plus EGTA markedly attenuated the changes by 30 minutes. These studies showed that marked decreases in phosphatidylinositol content and increases in phosphatidic acid accumulation develop within 15 seconds after addition of thrombin even in the absence of extracellular Ca^{2+}.

Rittenhouse-Simmons (1979) found that human platelets responded to thrombin with an increase in 1,2-diacylglycerol accumulation within 5 seconds. Maximal increases (30-fold) in diacylglycerol were found at 15 seconds and prior incubation with 2 mM dibutyryl cyclic AMP prevented the accumulation of diacylglycerol. The results of Broekmann et al. (1980) suggested that the diacylglycerol was derived from breakdown of phosphatidylinositol since that was the only phospholipid that decreased in content during the first 15 seconds after thrombin addition. Bell and Majerus (1980) found a 45% drop in human platelet phosphatidylinositol within 10 seconds of thrombin addition. Since there is an appreciable amount of diacylglycerol kinase in human platelets (Call and Rubert, 1973), some of the diacylglycerol formed from phosphatidylinositol may be readily converted to phosphatidic acid.

Diacylglycerol derived from phosphatidylinositol is cleaved via a diacylglycerol lipase to release arachidonic acid found in relatively high amounts (Bell et al., 1979). Phosphatidylinositol breakdown may represent a more important source for arachidonic acid release than the phospholipase A_2 pathway. More recently Prescott and Majerus (1983) found that diacylglycerol is preferentially cleaved to give a 2-monoacylglycerol. A transient increase in arachidonoylmonoacylglycerol was noted in thrombin-stimulated platelets.

Some workers, impressed with early rises in phosphatidic acid after thrombin is added to platelets, have postulated that phosphatidic acid is a second messenger (Holmsen et al., 1981; Imai et al., 1982). However, Lapetina (1983) pointed out that the formation of phosphatidic acid may reflect the level of 1,2-diacylglycerol.

Kawahara et al. (1980) found that 1,2-diacylglycerol stimulated protein kinase C resulting in phosphorylation of a protein in platelets with an apparent M_r of 40,000. The properties of protein kinase C have been reviewed by Takai et al. (1984). This kinase is distinct from the cyclic AMP-dependent and Ca^{2+}-calmodulin-activated protein kinases. Elevation of Ca^{2+} content of platelets by the addition of the ionophore A23187 at a concentration of 0.4 μM did not cause an increase in phosphorylation of the protein with an M_r of 40,000 but did stimulate that of a protein with an M_r of 20,000 (Kaibuchi *et al.*, 1983). The stimulation of 5-hydroxytryptamine (5-HT) release from platelets was not increased by 0.4 μM A23187 or a synthetic diacylglycerol alone, but 5-HT release was seen if both were present. In these studies the synthetic diacylglycerol analog added to intact platelets was 1-oleoyl- 2-acetylglycerol but phorbol myristate was equally active (Kaibuchi *et al.*, 1983).

In hepatocytes Fain *et al.* (1984) found that 1 μM A23187 produced little stimulatory effect on glycogen phosphorylase and of 1 μg/ml phorbol myristate was inactive. The combination of ionophore and phorbol gave an activation of glycogen phosphorylase at 2 minutes comparable to that seen with vasopressin. Similar results have been observed with lymphocytes where the phorbol ester, when combined with A23187, mimicked the mitogenic effects of concanavalin A (Mastro and Smith, 1983). These results support the hypothesis of Takai *et al.* (1984) that Ca^{2+} and diacylglycerol work synergistically through phosphorylation of a 20K and 40K protein, respectively, and stimulate platelet aggregation as well as release of 5-HT (Fig. 5).

In rabbit platelets, Ieyasu *et al.* (1982) found that platelet-activating factor (PAF, 1-O-alkyl-2-acetyl-*sn*-glycerol-3-phosphorylcholine) and thrombin increased degradation of [^{32}P]phosphatidylinositol, formation of diacylglycerol, phosphorylation of the 40K protein, and 5-HT release. All these effects were inhibited by prior incubation of platelets

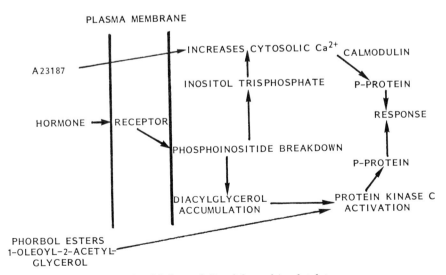

FIG. 5. The role of Ca^{2+} and diacylglycerol in platelet responses.

with prostaglandin E_1 or dibutyryl cyclic AMP each causing increased cyclic AMP content of platelets. It is unclear how elevations in cyclic AMP prevent phosphoinositide breakdown, but the most likely site is inhibition of phosphoinositide-specific phospholipase C activity. Billah *et al.* (1979) found that in horse platelets prelabeled with arachidonic acid, the addition of 2.5 mM deoxycholate increased degradation of labeled phosphatidylinositol and stimulated diacylglycerol accumulation. This effect was virtually abolished by preincubation of platelets for 20 minutes prior to addition of deoxycholate with dibutyryl cyclic AMP in the presence of cyclic AMP phosphodiesterase inhibitors. Earlier, Lapetina *et al.* (1977) found that cyclic AMP inhibited the thrombin-induced release of arachidonic acid in horse platelets, but it did not affect the metabolism of exogenous arachidonic acid. Further studies are needed in this area but it is clear that Ca^{2+} and cyclic AMP are antagonistic signals in platelets.

Fain and Garcia-Sainz (1980) postulated that all α_1 effects of catecholamines are linked to turnover of phosphatidylinositol and elevation of cytosolic Ca^{2+} while α_2 effects are linked to inhibition of adenylate cyclase. Deykin and Snyder (1973), however, found that epinephrine increased phosphatidylinositol turnover in platelets which appear to have only α_2 receptor sites for catecholamines (Hoffman *et al.*, 1979, 1981; Daiguji *et al.*, 1981; Shattil *et al.*, 1981). Wallace *et al.* (1982a) confirmed that epinephrine increased phosphatidylinositol turnover in human platelets but found that the effect was mediated through α_2-adrenoceptor activation. α_2-Catecholamine agonists stimulate human platelet aggregation as does ADP. Probably the inhibition of adenylate cyclase by α_2-catecholamine agonists causes an elevation of cytosolic Ca^{2+} or directly relieves an inhibitory constraint on phosphoinositide turnover. These findings show that just as an increase in cyclic AMP reduces the ability of agents to stimulate phosphatidylinositol turnover, a reduction in basal cyclic AMP may be linked to platelet aggregation and enhanced turnover of phosphatidylinositol.

One of the more intriguing aspects of phosphoinositide metabolism in platelets is the relative importance of polyphosphoinositide versus phosphatidylinositol turnover. Some think that early degradation of phosphatidylinositol 4,5-bisphosphate during the first 5–10 seconds after the addition of thrombin is important; others are more impressed with the later increases in content.

Agranoff *et al.* (1983) found that the addition of thrombin to prelabeled human platelets caused a 30% decrease of labeled phosphatidylinositol 4,5-bisphosphate at 5 or 10 seconds and an increase in inositol 1,4,5-trisphosphate but not inositol 1,4-bisphosphate. This clearly indicates that the cleavage of polyphosphoinositide is, at least partly, via a phosphodiesterase (phospholipase C). By 15 seconds labeled phosphatidylinositol 4,5-bisphosphate had returned to control values. Billah and Lapetina (1982) found a decrease in phosphatidylinositol 4,5-bisphosphate 5–15 seconds after the addition of thrombin, and there was no effect of 1 μM A23187 on loss of label. At 30 seconds, however, there was a 20% increase in labeled phosphatidylinositol 4,5-bisphosphate in the presence of ionophore. Billah and Lapetina (1983) found a 50% drop in labeled phosphatidylinositol 4,5-bisphosphate after addition of PAF to horse platelets which was maximal at 5 seconds and returned to control values by 20–30 seconds. There was a 40% drop in both labeled phosphatidylinositol and phosphatidylinositol 4-phosphate which was maximal at 10 seconds, sustained for 30 seconds, and returned to control values by 120 seconds. Interestingly, the decrease of phosphatidylinositol 4,5-bisphosphate at 10 seconds was observed with concentrations of PAF which had little effect on breakdown of the other phosphoinositides. The addition of prostacyclin, a potent stimulator of adenylate cyclase in platelets, did not affect the initial drop in phosphatidylinositol 4,5-bisphosphate but did prevent the net increase in label found in this lipid at 30 seconds or thereafter.

Shukla and Hanahan (1982) also found in rabbit platelets that PAF increased breakdown of phosphatidylinositol (20% at 15 seconds) and secretion of 5-HT. They found rapid increases in the uptake of ^{32}P from the medium into phosphatidic acid and somewhat slower, but ultimately sixfold larger, increases in the uptake of label into phosphatidylinositol 4,5-bisphosphate after PAF addition.

Imai et al. (1983) found that thrombin increased by about 20% the loss of label from [^{3}H]glycerol-labeled phosphatidylinositol 4,5-bisphosphate at 10 seconds. However, by 30 seconds it had returned to control values and to greater than control by 60 seconds. In platelets prelabeled with [^{3}H]arachidonic acid there was only an increase in labeled phosphatidylinositol 4,5-bisphosphate after thrombin addition. Similar findings were made by Perret et al. (1983) who found a marked elevation in phosphatidylinositol 4,5-bisphosphate at 60 seconds after thrombin addition to human platelets and increases in phosphatidylinositol 4-phosphate by 120 seconds. Probably, the addition of thrombin or PAF causes a rapid decrease in all phosphoinositides in platelets which is often maximal by 10 seconds and is followed by compensatory increases in the synthesis of all the phosphoinositides. The variability in results between different groups may in part reflect different rates of stimulated resynthesis. However, it is clear that breakdown of phosphoinositides is an immediate result of thrombin or PAF interaction with platelet membranes and the elevation in diacylglycerol activates protein kinase C in addition to serving as a precursor for release of arachidonic acid.

Thus the significance of phosphatidic acid formation and the late increases in polyphosphoinositide accumulation remain to be established in platelets. There is little evidence in platelets that all breakdown of phosphatidylinositol is secondary to formation of phosphatidylinositol 4,5-bisphosphate. The first detectable effect of stimuli in platelets is to increase the diacylglycerol content and this is probably due to activation of phospholipase C which preferentially cleaves membrane-bound phosphoinositides.

IX. Blowfly Salivary Glands

Blowfly salivary glands have proven useful as a model system for studies of phosphoinositide metabolism as well as salivary secretion. 5-HT stimulates secretion in the glands and increases cyclic AMP through a 5-HT$_2$ receptor while it stimulates Ca^{2+} flux and phosphoinositide breakdown through a separate 5-HT$_1$ receptor (Fig. 6). Berridge (1981a) and Fain (1982) have reviewed the hormonal regulation of salivary gland secretion and phosphoinositide metabolism by 5-HT. This section is primarily concerned with developments over the past few years.

Fain and Garcia-Sainz (1980) suggested that the effects of hormones on Ca^{2+} and cyclic AMP could be divided into three types. These are outlined in Table II and involve activation of adenylate cyclase which for catecholamines is through β-type receptors. Catecholamines inhibit adenylate cyclase through α_2 receptors and elevate Ca^{2+} through α_1 receptors. It was suggested that activation of adenylate cyclase by 5-HT is through a β type receptor while elevation of Ca^{2+} is through a separate receptor, called α by analogy with catecholamines. Subsequently, Berridge (1981b) and Berridge and Heslop (1981) presented electrophysiological and biochemical evidence for the existence of separate receptors. They named the receptor mediating effects on Ca^{2+} 5-HT$_1$ and on cyclic AMP 5-HT$_2$, by analogy with the naming of receptors for histamine (Table II). Peroutka and Snyder (1979) have also distinguished at least two separate binding sites for 5-HT in brain membranes which they described as 5-HT$_1$ and 5-HT$_2$. This nomenclature appears to be more suitable than α and β which tend to be confused with catecholamine receptors.

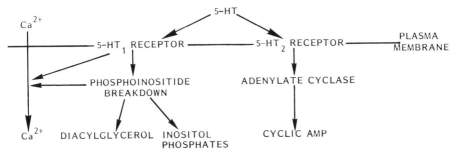

FIG. 6. A model for regulation of cyclic AMP and Ca^{2+} in blowfly salivary glands involving separate receptors for each effect.

The functional correlates of the two 5-HT receptor sites in rat brain are still unclear (Fozard, 1983). However, in blowfly salivary glands Berridge (1981b) found that the depolarizing response to 5-HT is mediated through Ca^{2+} and linked to the 5-HT_1 receptors while the hyperpolarizing response appeared to be linked to cyclic AMP and involve 5-HT_2 receptors. Berridge and Heslop (1981) and Fain et al. (1983a) found that 5-methyltryptamine was equipotent to 5-HT in stimulating phosphatidylinositol breakdown, linked to elevations in Ca^{2+}, but had little effect on adenylate cyclase activation. A compound such as 4-fluoro-α-methyltryptamine was much more active as a stimulator of cyclic AMP accumulation than it was in increasing phosphatidylinositol turnover. Presumably, this analog preferentially stimulates 5-HT_2 receptors. Unfortunately, there is no known compound that is equipotent to 5-HT as an activator of adenylate cyclase but is without effect on phosphatidylinositol breakdown. Although the available 5-

TABLE II

THREE TYPES OF HORMONE EFFECTS ON CYCLIC AMP AND Ca^{2+}

Elevation of cytosolic Ca^{2+} and increased phosphoinositide breakdown	Activation of adenylate cyclase	Inhibition of adenylate cyclase[a]
α_1-Adrenoceptors	β_1- or β_2-Adrenoceptors	α_2-Adrenoceptors
5-HT_1	5-HT_2	5-HT_3
Histamine H-1	Histamine H-2	
Vasopressin V_1	Vasopressin V_2	
Muscarinic cholinergic 1		Muscarinic cholinergic 3
	Dopamine D-2	Dopamine D-3
		Somatostatin

[a]Inhibition of adenylate cyclase appears to involve the N_i protein and is blocked by pertussis toxin.

HT antagonists have some selectivity (Berridge and Heslop, 1981), there is no compound which affects only one response.

There is evidence that a third type of receptor which I call 5-HT$_3$ might be present which inhibits adenylate cyclase activation. Berridge and Heslop (1981) found that 5-chlorotryptamine inhibited the rise in cyclic AMP due to 4-fluoro-α-methyltryptamine. The latter compound had little effect on the increase in phosphatidylinositol breakdown due to 5-chlorotryptamine. Possibly a rise in Ca^{2+} linked to phosphatidyl-inositol breakdown might have inhibited adenylate cyclase, but Litosch et $al.$ (1982b) could find no evidence for Ca^{2+} inhibition of salivary gland adenylate cyclase since Ca^{2+} had exactly the opposite effect of slightly stimulating adenylate cyclase activity. Ca^{2+} did not affect cyclic AMP phosphodiesterase in these glands.

Forskolin is a diterpene that directly activates adenylate cyclase in diverse cell types; it appears to mimic the effects of 5-HT$_2$ receptor activation on cyclic AMP and secretion in blowfly salivary glands without affecting phosphatidylinositol breakdown (Litosch et $al.$, 1982c). The addition of 5-HT to blowfly salivary gland homogenates activates adenylate cyclase activity; 5-methyltryptamine is consider-ably less active than 5-HT (Litosch et $al.$, 1982b).

Some advantages of the invertebrate salivary gland for studies on phosphatidylinositol breakdown as compared to most mammalian sys-tems are (1) the intracellular inositol pool is very small as there does not appear to be an active uptake process resulting in accumulation of inositol against a concentration gradient. Thus the intracellular pool rapidly equilibrates with medium inositol. (2) There is little uptake of labeled inositol into phosphatidylinositol via the so-called exchange reaction to complicate experiments. (3) The synthesis of phosphatidyl-inositol is inhibited by 5-HT whereas in mammalian cells there is such a large stimulation of synthesis that it is difficult to measure break-down of labeled phosphoinositides except at very early time points. The inhibition of phosphatidylinositol synthesis by 5-HT is apparently due to elevations in cytosolic Ca^{2+} since A23187 inhibits synthesis of phos-phatidylinositol without affecting breakdown. (4) The phosphatidyl-inositol synthesized during short-term labeling rapidly equilibrates with the small pool of phosphatidylinositol which is degraded during exposure of 5-HT. (5) In glands previously incubated with 5-HT and allowed to recover during an hour incubation there was no subsequent effect of 5-HT on Ca^{2+} gating unless there was inositol in the medium during the recovery period.

The initial studies of Fain and Berridge (1979a) showed that 5-HT increased the breakdown of prelabeled phosphatidylinositol in blowfly salivary glands via mechanisms which were not mimicked by cyclic AMP or the ionophore A23187. A23187 stimulates phosphatidylino-sitol 4,5-bisphosphate conversion to phosphatidylinositol via a phos-phomonoesterase (Litosch *et al.*, 1984). There is a stimulation by Ca^{2+} of phosphatidylinositol 4,5-bisphosphate but not of phosphatidylinosi-tol degradation in salivary gland homogenates (Litosch *et al.*, 1984). Appreciable breakdown of phosphatidylinositol was also found in ho-mogenates after direct addition of 5-HT under conditions in which the free Ca^{2+} was less than 0.01 μM (Fain *et al.*, 1983a).

It is unclear what the relationship is between $5\text{-}HT_1$ receptor activa-tion of phosphatidylinositide breakdown and the release of bound in-tracellular Ca^{2+} as well as entry of extracellular Ca^{2+}. In blowfly salivary glands, however, it has been possible to show that salivary secretion and Ca^{2+} flux are critically dependent on a small pool of phosphoinositides which appears to be less than 5% of the total cellular phosphoinositides. Fain and Berridge (1979b) found that salivary glands previously exposed to 5-HT for 2 hours and allowed to recover, over a 15-minute incubation in the absence of hormone, did not re-spond to a second addition of 5-HT with regard to salivary secretion and Ca^{2+} gating. If 200 μM inositol was added to the medium during the recovery period, a response to 5-HT could be obtained (Fain and Berridge, 1979b). If only 2 μM inositol was added during a 2-hour recovery period, 0.3 pmol of phosphatidylinositol was resynthesized and there was little Ca^{2+} flux due to 5-HT. Increasing the [^{3}H]inositol concentration to 20 μM led to synthesis of 1.7 pmol of phosphatidylino-sitol and a maximal effect on salivary secretion. Maximal recovery of Ca^{2+} gating required an inositol concentration of 200 μM. There was no recovery of Ca^{2+} gating with added choline or ethanolamine. These results represent the best evidence that continued breakdown of phos-phatidylinositol is linked in some unknown fashion to Ca^{2+} gating and salivary secretion.

Berridge (1983) has suggested that 5-HT increases the breakdown of phosphatidylinositol 4,5-bisphosphate in salivary glands and that all phosphatidylinositol disappearance is secondary to its conversion to this compound. Our data suggest that the hormone-induced break-down of phosphoinositides is not restricted to phosphatidylinositol 4,5-bisphosphate. The regulation of phosphatidylinositol conversion to phosphatidylinositol 4-phosphate and phosphatidylinositol 4,5-bis-phosphate is obscure at the moment. Earlier it was pointed out that an elevation in Ca^{2+} activates a phosphomonoesterase which converts phosphatidylinositol 4,5-bisphosphate to phosphatidylinositol. There is, however, breakdown of phosphatidylinositol 4,5-bisphosphate due to 5-HT involving a phospholipase C type enzyme that functions as a phosphodiesterase causing formation of diacylglycerol and inositol 1,4,5-trisphosphate (Berridge, 1983; Berridge *et al.*, 1983; Litosch *et al.*, 1984). These results indicate that the rise in cytosolic Ca^{2+} is not responsible for all the breakdown of the phosphatidylinositol 4,5-bisphosphate seen after 5-HT addition.

It is possible that phosphatidylinositol newly synthesized in the salivary gland binds in part to the inner surface of the plasma membranes and this fraction is readily phosphorylated to polyphosphoinositides. It is this pool of phosphoinositides which may be broken down first after binding of 5-HT to its receptor. Berridge (1983) found a substantial increase in inositol 1,4,5-trisphosphate and inositol 1,4-bisphosphate accumulation but little increase in inositol 1-phosphate after 5-HT addition unless $1–10$ mM Li^+ was present in the incubation medium to inhibit the phosphatase which cleaves inositol 1-phosphate to inositol (Berridge *et al.*, 1982).

The effects of low concentrations of 5-HT on salivary secretion and Ca^{2+} flux should be potentiated by the presence of Li^+ which increases the level of inositol 1-phosphate (Berridge *et al.*, 1982). Breakdown of phosphatidylinositol 4,5-bisphosphate rather than phosphatidylinositol is more costly from an energy standpoint but the inositol trisphosphate formed serves as a unique second messenger to release Ca^{2+} from the endoplasmic reticulum. Berridge (1983) has also suggested that phosphatidylinositol conversion to polyphosphoinositides is regulated by the availability of ATP. Extrusion of Ca^{2+} from cells presumably occurs via ATP-linked pumps. Under conditions in which ATP is depleted, the conversion of phosphatidylinositol to phosphatidylinositol 4,5-bisphosphate may be reduced. This provides a mechanism by which ATP availability regulates Ca^{2+}. This provocative hypothesis should stimulate much experimentation.

Sadler *et al.* (1984) found that prior exposure of salivary glands for only 30 minutes to as little as 0.1 μM 5-HT doubled phosphatidylinositol 4,5-bisphosphate formation during the first 60 minutes after removal of the hormone if the inositol concentration was 3–5 μM. Total synthesis of phosphoinositides was unaffected and phosphatidylinositol formation was proportionately decreased. A second addition of 5-HT stimulated the same percentage breakdown of prelabeled phosphatidylinositol regardless of whether the glands had been incubated during the recovery period with 3–5 or 30 μM inositol. However, there was little recovery of 5-HT-induced Ca^{2+} gating in glands incubated with 3 μM inositol (Sadler *et al.*, 1984). These data provide further support for the hypothesis that a critical amount of phosphoinositide breakdown is required for Ca^{2+} gating.

Litosch *et al.* (1982a) found that in salivary glands prelabeled with [^{3}H]arachidonic acid there was a selective net release of arachidonic acid from phosphatidylinositol which was accompanied by an elevation of diacylglycerol containing arachidonic acid. The effect was maximal at the earliest time (30 seconds) examined after hormone addition. In Ca^{2+}-free buffer the net disappearance of [^{3}H]arachidonic acid-labeled phosphatidylinositol was markedly reduced as was the accumulation of labeled diacylglycerol, suggesting that in the absence of Ca^{2+} there is substantial resynthesis of diacylglycerol to phosphatidylinositol (Litosch *et al.*, 1982a).

The demonstration of a direct effect of hormones on phosphoinositide breakdown in cell-free systems from blowfly salivary glands (Fain *et al.*, 1983a) and rat hepatocytes (Wallace *et al.*, 1982b; Harrington and Eichberg, 1983) provides two systems in which the question of how hormones regulate phosphoinositide metabolism can be examined. Serotonin effects on phosphatidylinositol breakdown in cell-free systems from blowfly salivary glands do not require Ca^{2+}. The latter finding is difficult to reconcile with the hypothesis of Berridge (1983) that 5-HT stimulates only the breakdown of phosphatidylinositol 4,5-bisphosphate. In cell-free systems from blowfly salivary glands the breakdown of phosphatidylinositol 4,5-bisphosphate was also accelerated by 5-HT and associated with a corresponding increase in inositol phosphates (I. Litosch and J. N. Fain, unpublished results).

Possibly phospholipase C activated by 5-HT in the salivary gland is able to degrade any phosphoinositide. If the labeled pool of polyphosphoinositides were preferentially localized on the inner surface of the plasma membrane, it would then be preferentially hydrolyzed at early time periods after the addition of hormone. In hepatocytes, platelets, and the blowfly salivary gland about one-third of the phosphatidylinositol 4,5-bisphosphate is degraded within the first few seconds after ligand addition. We still do not know how this is accomplished, but it appears to precede most other effects of these ligands. One of the useful features of the blowfly salivary gland is that this breakdown is not accompanied by stimulated resynthesis of phosphatidic acid and phosphoinositides. It is this feature which probably accounts for the desensitization of the salivary gland to 5-HT with regard to Ca^{2+} gating and prevents these glands from becoming overwhelmed with Ca^{2+}.

It is unlikely that phosphatidic acid will prove to be very important in regulation of Ca^{2+} flux and secretion in blowfly salivary glands. The formation of phosphatidic acid is inhibited at early time periods (0.5–5 minutes) after 5-HT addition and only increased at 30 minutes (Litosch *et al.*, 1983a). Similar results were originally reported by Fain and Berridge (1979a). However, in cells such as platelets and hepato-cytes breakdown of phosphatidylinositol is accompanied by rapid in-creases in phosphatidic acid formation which may play some role in the response.

X. Conclusion

It is clear from data accumulated over the past several years that the breakdown of phosphoinositides is accelerated as a result of ligand interactions with membranes as originally suggested by Durell *et al.* (1969). Breakdown of the polyphosphoinositides may be more impor-tant than that of phosphatidylinositol as first pointed out by Haw-thorne and Kai (1970). Michell (1975) postulated that the increase in cyclic inositol phosphate due to stimulation by hormones was involved in Ca^{2+} entry. No evidence for such a function of cyclic inositol phos-phate (the initial product of phosphatidylinositol degradation by phos-pholipase C) has yet been produced. Furthermore, it is now clear that phosphoinositide breakdown is not necessarily linked to gating of Ca^{2+} entry since in hepatocytes and adrenal glomerulosa cells efflux rather than influx of Ca^{2+} appears in response to hormones that in-crease phosphoinositide breakdown. While we do not yet understand very much about the significance of phosphoinositide turnover, the available data are compatible with the view that hormones which di-rectly elevate cytosolic Ca^{2+} by releasing bound intracellular stores and increasing Ca^{2+} influx also rapidly stimulate the breakdown of phosphoinositides.

In nearly all mammalian cells in which hormones elevate cytosolic Ca^{2+} there is an increased incorporation of $[^{32}P]P_i$ into phosphatidic acid and phosphatidylinositol but not into polyphosphoinositides. This was the original finding of the Hokins over 30 years ago and still remains unexplained. It probably involves more than an increase in di-acylglycerol due to phosphoinositide breakdown. In blowfly salivary glands the increased breakdown of phosphoinositides is not accom-panied by an increase in phosphatidic acid or phosphatidylinositol for-mation. The enzymes involved in formation of these phospholipids are inhibited by Ca^{2+} (Wallace and Fain, 1984) so it is difficult to under-stand why all cells do not behave like the blowfly salivary gland. The site of stimulated phosphatidylinositol synthesis upon ligand addition to mammalian cells is probably the endoplasmic reticulum. Ligands stimulate release of Ca^{2+} from the endoplasmic reticulum and this might relieve an inhibitory constraint on phosphatidylinositol synthesis (Fain, 1982). In contrast, in the blowfly salivary gland the site for synthesis of these phospholipids may be in equilibrium with the cytosolic pool of Ca^{2+}.

The list of cells in which phosphoinositide metabolism is influenced by ligands expands each year (Michell, 1982; Farese, 1983a,b; Downes and Michell, 1982). The field has now grown so large that it is difficult for one review to cover all aspects. This article has focused on a small number of cells wherein phosphoinositide breakdown has been extensively examined. With the expansion of data there has been a corresponding proliferation of explanations and the field is currently as active as it is controversial. The data reviewed here suggest that phosphoinositide breakdown is a direct effect of ligand interaction with receptors in the plasma membrane and not secondary to elevations in intracellular Ca^{2+}. This is true even in macrophages and brain synaptosomes where the ability of the divalent cation ionophore A23187 to mimic the effects of ligands on certain aspects of phosphoinositide metabolism has created so much confusion in the past. We hope that within the next few years most of the current controversies will be only faint memories and that we will understand how inadequate are our current views.

The current picture as of the end of 1983 about the meaning of the phosphoinositide breakdown due to hormones is summarized in Table III. The known functions of phosphoinositide breakdown are the liberation of inositol trisphosphate, which is involved in the release of Ca^{2+}

TABLE III

1983 MODEL FOR HORMONAL ACTIVATION OF PHOSPHOINOSITIDE BREAKDOWN

The interaction of Ca^{2+}-mobilizing hormones with receptors activates a membrane-bound phospholipase C which degrades the hormone-sensitive pool of phosphoinositides

The breakdown of phosphatidylinositol-4P and PI generates diacylglycerol which activates C-kinase but no second messenger for Ca^{2+} release. Diacylglycerol also provides a source of free arachidonic acid through the action of diacylglycerol lipase. The arachidonic acid is utilized for synthesis of prostaglandins

The breakdown of phosphatidylinositol 4,5-P_2 generates IP_3 which releases bound calcium from the endoplasmic reticulum

The rate of Ca^{2+} release from endoplasmic reticulum is dependent on IP_3 formation. The amount of IP_3 formation is regulated by phospholipase C activity and the rate of conversion of PI to phosphatidylinositol 4-P and phosphatidylinositol 4,5-P_2. The latter is dependent on ATP availability and maximal rate of the synthetic pathway from intracellular stores, and of diacylglycerol, which activates protein kinase C. Additionally diacylglycerol can serve as a source of arachidonic acid for conversion to prostaglandins and related compounds.

REFERENCES

Abdel-Latif, A. A. (1983). Metabolism of phosphoinositides. *Handb. Neurochem.* **3**, 91–131.

Adnan, N. A. M., and Hawthorne, J. N. (1981). Phosphatidylinositol labelling in response to activation of muscarinic receptors in bovine adrenal medulla *J. Neurochem.* **36**, 1858–1860.

Agranoff, B. W. (1983). Biochemical mechanisms in the phosphatidylinositol effect. *Life Sci.* **32**, 2047–2054.

Agranoff, B. W., Murthy, P., and Seguin, E. B. (1983). Thrombin-induced phosphodiesteratic cleavage of phosphatidylinositol bisphosphate in human platelets. *J. Biol. Chem.* **258**, 2076–2078.

Allison, J. H., and Stewart, M. A. (1971). Reduced brain inositol in lithium-treated rats. *Nature (London) New Biol.* **233**, 267–268.

Allison, N., Blisner, M. E., Holland, W. H., Hipps, P. P., and Sherman, W. R. (1976). Increased brain myo-inositol 1-phosphate in lithium-treated rats. *Biochem. Biophys. Res. Commun.* **71**, 664–670.

Althaus-Salzmann, M., Carafoli, E., and Jakob, A. (1980). Ca^{2+},K^+ redistributions and alpha-adrenergic activation of glycogenolysis in perfused rat livers. *Eur. J. Biochem.* **106**, 241–248.

Azila, N., and Hawthorne, J. N. (1982). Subcellular localization of phospholipid changes in response to muscarinic stimulation of perfused bovine adrenal medulla. *Biochem. J.* **204**, 291–299.

Bartus, R. T., Dean, R. L., III, Beer, B., and Lippa, A. S. (1982). The cholinergic hypothesis of geriatric memory dysfunction. *Science* **217**, 408–417.

Bell, R. L., and Majerus, P. W. (1980). Thrombin-induced hydrolysis of phosphatidylinositol in human platelets. *J. Biol. Chem.* **255**, 1790–1792.

Bell, R. L., Kennerly, D. A., Stanford, N., and Majerus, P. W. (1979). Diglyceride lipase: A pathway for arachidonic release from human platelets. *Proc. Natl. Acad. Sci. U.S.A.* **76**, 3238–3241.

Bennett, J. P., Cockcroft, S., Caswell, A. H., and Gomperts, B. D. (1982). Plasma-membrane location of phosphatidylinositol hydrolysis in rabbit neutrophils stimulated with formylmethionylleucylphenylalanine. *Biochem. J.* **208**, 801–808.

Berridge, M. J. (1981a). Phosphatidylinositol hydrolysis: A multifunctional transducing mechanism. *Mol. Cell. Endocrinol.* **24**, 115–140.

Berridge, M. J. (1981b). Electrophysiological evidence for the existence of separate receptor mechanisms mediating the actions of 5-hydroxytryptamine. *Mol. Cell. Endocrinol.* **23**, 91–104.

Berridge, M. (1983). Rapid accumulation of inositol triphosphate reveals that agonists hydrolyse polyphosphoinositides instead of phosphatidylinositol. *Biochem. J.* **212**, 849–858.

Berridge, M., and Fain, J. N. (1979). Inhibition of phosphatidylinositol synthesis and the inactivation of calcium entry after prolonged exposure of the blowfly salivary gland to 5-hydroxytryptamine. *Biochem. J.* **178**, 59–69.

Berridge, M., and Heslop, J. P. (1981). Separate 5-hydroxytryptamine receptors on the salivary gland of the blowfly are linked to the generation of either cyclic adenosine 3',5'-monophosphate or calcium signals. *Br. J. Pharmacol.* **73**, 729–738.

Berridge, M. J., Downes, C. P., and Hanley, M. R. (1982). Lithium amplifies agonist-dependent phosphatidylinositol responses in brain and salivary glands. *Biochem. J.* **206**, 587–595.

Berridge, M. J., Dawson, R. M. C., Downes, C. P., Heslop, J. P., and Irvine, R. F. (1983). Changes in the levels of inositol phosphates following agonist-dependent hydrolysis of membrane phosphoinositides. *Biochem. J.* **212**, 473–482.

Berry, G., Yandrasitz, J. R., and Segal, S. (1981). Experimental galactose toxicity: Effects on synaptosomal phosphatidylinositol metabolism. *J. Neurochem.* **37**, 888–891.

Berry, G., Yandrasitz, J R., and Segal, S. (1983). CMP-dependent phosphatidylinositol:myo-inositol exchange activity in isolated nerve-endings. *Biochem. Biophys. Res. Commun.* **112**, 817–821.

Billah, M. M., and Lapetina, E. G. (1982). Rapid decrease of phosphatidylinositol 4,5-bisphosphate in thrombin-stimulated platelets. *J. Biol. Chem.* **257**, 12705–12708.

Billah, M. M., and Lapetina, E. G. (1983). Platelet-activating factor stimulates metabolism of phosphoinositides in horse platelets: Possible relationship to Ca^{2+} mobilization during stimulation. *Proc. Natl. Acad. Sci. U.S.A.* **80**, 965–968.

Billah, M. M., and Michell, R. H. (1979). Phosphatidylinositol metabolism in rat hepatocytes stimulated by glycogenolytic hormones. *Biochem. J.* **182**, 661–668.

Billah, M. M., Lapetina, E. G., and Cuatrecasas, P. (1979). Phosphatidylinositol-specific phospholipase C of platelets: Association with 1,2-diacylglycerol-kinase and inhibition by cyclic AMP. *Biochem. Biophys. Res. Commun.* **90**, 92–98.

Blackmore, P. F., Brumley, F. T., Marks, J. L., and Exton, J. H. (1978). Studies on alpha-adrenergic activation of hepatic glucose output. *J. Biol. Chem.* **253**, 4851–4858.

Bleasdale, J. E., Wallis, P., MacDonald, P. C., and Johnston, J. M. (1979). Characterization of the forward and reverse reactions catalyzed by CDP-diacylglycerol: Inositol transferase in rabbit lung tissue *Biochim. Biophys. Acta* **575**, 135–147.

Broekman, M. J., Ward, J. W., and Marcus, A. J. (1980). Phospholipid metabolism in stimulated human platelets. *J. Clin. Invest.* **66**, 275–283.

Brown, E., and Nahorski, S. R. (1983). α_1-Adrenoceptor and muscarinic receptor-stimulated breakdown of inositol phospholipids in rat cortex. *Br. J. Pharmacol.* **78**, 108P.

Buckley, J. T., Lefebvre, Y. A., and Hawthorne, J. N. (1971). Identification of an actively phosphorylated component of adrenal medulla chromaffin granules. *Biochim. Biophys. Acta* **239**, 517–519.

Burgess, G. M., Giraud, F., Poggioli, J., and Claret, M. (1983). α-adrenergically mediated changes in membrane lipid fluidity and Ca^{2+} binding in isolated rat liver plasma membranes. *Biochim. Biophys. Acta* **731**, 387–396.

Burgess, G. M., Godfrey, P. P., McKinney, J. S., Berridge, M. F., Irvine, R. F., and Putney, J. W. (1984). The second messenger linking receptor activation to internal Ca^{2+} release in liver. *Nature (London)* **309**, 63–66.

Call, F. L., and Rubert, M. (1973). Diglyceride kinase in human platelets. *J. Lipid Res.* **14**, 466–474.

Castagna, M., Takai, Y., Kaibuchi, K., Sano, K., Kikkawa, U., and Nishizuka, Y. (1982). Direct activation of calcium-activated, phospholipid-dependent protein kinase by tumor-promoting phorbol esters. *J. Biol. Chem.* **257**, 7847–7851.

Chen, J. L., Babcock, D. F., and Lardy, H. A. (1978). Norepinephrine, vasopressin, glucagon, and A-23187 induce efflux of calcium from an exchangeable pool in isolated rat hepatocytes. *Proc. Natl. Acad. Sci. U.S.A.* **75**, 2234–2238.

Cockcroft, S. (1981). Does phosphatidylinositol breakdown control the Ca^{2+}-gating mechanism? *Trends Pharm. Sci.* **2**, 340–342.

Cockcroft, S. (1982). Phosphatidylinositol metabolism in mast cells and neutrophils. *Cell Calcium* **3**, 337–350.

Cockcroft, S., and Gomperts, B. D. (1979). Evidence for a role of phosphatidylinositol turnover in stimulus-secretion coupling. *Biochem. J.* **178**, 681–687.

Cockcroft, S., Bennett, J. P., and Gomperts, B. D. (1980). Stimulus-secretion coupling in rabbit neutrophils is not mediated by phosphatidylinositol breakdown. *Nature (London)* **288**, 275–277.

Cockcroft, S., Bennett, J. P., and Gomperts, B. D. (1981). The dependence on Ca^{2+} of phosphatidylinositol breakdown and enzyme secretion in rabbit neutrophils stimulated by formylmethionylleucylphenylalanine or ionomycin. *Biochem. J.* **200**, 501–508.

Cohen, N. M., Schmidt, D. M., McGlennen, R. C., and Klein, W. L. (1983). Receptor-mediated increases in phosphatidylinositol turnover in neuron-like cell lines. *J. Neurochem.* **40**, 547–554.

Crews, F. T. (1982). Rapid changes in phospholipid metabolism during secretion and receptor activation. *Int. Rev. Neurobiol.* **23**, 141–163.

Daiguji, M., Meltzer, H. Y., and U'Prichard, D. C. (1981). Human platelet α_2-adrenergic labeling with ^{3}H-yohimbine, a selective antagonist ligand. *Life Sci.* **28**, 2705–2717.

Dawson, R. M. C., Hemington, N., and Irvine, R. F. (1980). The inhibition and activation of Ca^{2+}-dependent phosphatidylinositol phosphodiesterase by phospholipids and blood plasma. *Eur. J. Biochem.* **112**, 33–38.

DeScarnati, O. C., and Arnaiz, G. R. (1972). Acetylcholine stimulation of phosphatidyl-inositol-inositol phosphohydrolase of rat brain cortex. *Biochim. Biophys. Acta* **270**, 218–252.

Deykin, D., and Snyder, D. (1973). Effect of epinephrine on platelet metabolism. *J. Lab. Clin. Med.* **82**, 554–559.

Downes, C. P. (1982). Receptor-stimulated inositol phospholipid metabolism in the central nervous system. *Cell Calcium* **3**, 413–428.

Downes, C. P., and Michell, R. H. (1982). Phosphatidylinositol 4-phosphate and phosphatidylinositol 4,5-bisphosphate lipids in search of a function. *Cell Calcium* **3**, 467–502.

Durell, J., and Garland, J. T. (1969). Acetylcholine-stimulated phosphodiesteratic cleavage of phosphoinositides: Hypothetical role in membrane depolarization. *Ann. N.Y. Acad. Sci.* **165**, 743–754.

Durell, J., and Sodd, M. A. (1966). Studies on the acetylcholine-stimulated incorporation of radioactive inorganic orthophosphate into the phospholipid of brain particulate preparations. *J. Neurochem.* **13**, 487–491.

Durell, J., Garland, J. T., and Friedel, R. O. (1969). Acetylcholine action: Biochemical aspects. *Science* **165**, 862–866.

Elliott, M. E., Alexander, R. C., and Goodfriend, T. L. (1982). Aspects of angiotensin in the adrenal. Key roles for calcium and phosphatidyl inositol. *Hypertension* **4** (Suppl. 2), II52–58.

Elliott, M. E., Farese, R. V., and Goodfriend, T. L. (1983). Effects of angiotensin II and dibutyryl cyclic adenosine monophosphate on phosphatidylinositol metabolism, $^{45}Ca^{2+}$ fluxes, and aldosterone synthesis in bovine adrenal glomerulosa cells. *Life Sci.* **33**, 1771–1778.

Exton, J. H. (1981). Molecular mechanisms involved in α-adrenergic responses. *Mol. Cell. Endocrinol.* **23**, 233–264.

Fain, J. N. (1978). Hormones, membranes and cyclic nucleotides. *In* "Receptors and Recognition Series 6A" (P. Cuatrecasas and M. F. Greaves, eds.), pp. 1–62. Chapman & Hall, London.

Fain, J. N. (1982). Involvement of phosphatidylinositol breakdown in elevation of cytosol

Ca^{2+} by hormones and relationship to prostaglandin formation. *Horiz. Biochem. Biophys.* **6**, 237–276.

Fain, J. N., and Berridge, M. J. (1979a). Relationship between hormonal activation of phosphatidylinositol hydrolysis, fluid secretion and calcium flux in the blowfly salivary gland. *Biochem. J.* **178**, 45–58.

Fain, J. N., and Berridge, M. J. (1979b). Relationship between phosphatidylinositol synthesis and recovery of 5-hydroxytryptamine-responsive Ca^{2+} flux in blowfly salivary glands. *Biochem. J.* **180**, 655–661.

Fain, J. N., and Garcia-Sainz, J. A. (1980). Role of phosphatidylinositol turnover in alpha$_1$ and of adenylate cyclase inhibition in alpha$_2$ effects of catecholamines. *Life Sci.* **26**, 1183–1194.

Fain, J. N., Lin, S.-H., Litosch, I., and Wallace, M. (1983a). Hormonal regulation of phosphatidylinositol breakdown. *Life Sci.* **32**, 2055–2068.

Fain, J. N., Lin, S.-H., Randazzo, P., Robinson, S., and Wallace, M. (1983b). Hormonal regulation of glycogen phosphorylase in rat hepatocytes: Activation of phosphatidylinositol breakdown by vasopressin and alpha$_1$ catecholamines. *In* "Isolation, Characterization and Use of Hepatocytes" (R. A. Harris and N. W. Cornell, eds.), pp. 411–418. Elsevier, Amsterdam.

Fain, J. N., Li, S.-Y., Litosch, I., and Wallace, M. (1984). Synergistic activation of rat hepatocyte glycogen phosphorylase by A23187 and phorbol ester. *Biochem. Biophys. Res. Commun.* **119**, 88–94.

Farese, R. V. (1983a). Phosphoinositide metabolism and hormone action. *Endocr. Rev.* **4**, 78–95.

Farese, R. (1983b). The phosphatidate-phosphoinositide cycle: An intracellular messenger system in the action of hormones and neurotransmitters. *Metabolism* **32**, 628–641.

Farese, R. V., Sabir, M. A., and Larson, R. E. (1980). Potassium and angiotensin II increase the concentrations of phosphatidic acid, phosphatidylinositol, and polyphosphoinositides in rat adrenal capsules *in vitro. J. Clin. Invest.* **66**, 1428–1431.

Farese, R. V., Larsen, R. E., Sabir, M. A., and Gomez-Sanchez, C. E. (1983). Effects of angiotensin-II, K$^+$, adrenocorticotropin, serotonin, cyclic AMP, cyclic GMP, A23187 and EGTA on aldosterone synthesis and phospholipid metabolism in the rat adrenal zona glomerulosa. *Endocrinology* **113**, 1377–1386.

Fisher, S. K., and Agranoff, B. W. (1981). Enhancement of the muscarinic synaptosomal phospholipid labeling effect by ionophore A23187. *J. Neurochem.* **37**, 968–977.

Fisher, S. K., Holz, R. W., and Agranoff, B. W. (1981). Muscarinic receptors in chromaffin cell cultures mediate enhanced phospholipid labeling but not catecholamine secretion. *J. Neurochem.* **37**, 491–497.

Fozard, J. R. (1983). Functional correlates of 5-HT$_1$ recognition sites. *Trends Pharmacol. Sci.* **4**, 288–289.

Garcia-Sainz, J. A., and Fain, J. N. (1980). Effects of insulin, catecholamines, and calcium ions on phospholipid metabolism in isolated white fat cells. *Biochem. J.* **186**, 781–789.

Garrison, J. C. (1983). Role of Ca^{2+}-dependent protein kinases in the response of hepatocytes to α-agonists, angiotesin II and vasopression. *In* "Isolation, Characterization and Use of Hepatocytes" (R. A. Harris and N. W. Cornell, eds.), pp. 551–559. Elsevier, Amsterdam.

Gill, D. W., Brown, S. A., Seeholzer, S. H., and Wildey, G. M. (1983). Minisymposium: Phosphatidylinositol turnover and cellular function. *Life Sci.* **32**, 2043–2406.

Griffin H. D., and Hawthorne, J. N. (1978). Calcium-activated hydrolysis of phosphatidyl-myo-inositol 4-phosphate and phosphatidyl-myo-inositol 4,5-bisphosphate in guinea pig synaptosomes. *Biochem. J.* **176**, 541–551.

Harrington, C. A., and Eichberg, J. (1983). Norepinephrine causes α_1-adrenergic receptor-mediated decrease of phosphatidylinositol in isolated rat liver plasma membranes supplemented with cytosol. *J. Biol. Chem.* **258**, 2087–2090.

Hawthorne, J. N. (1982a). Is phosphatidylinositol now out of the calcium gate? *Nature (London)* **295**, 281–282.

Hawthorne, J. N. (1982b). Inositol phospholipids. *In* "Phospholipids" (J. N. Hawthorne and B. Ansell, eds.), Chap. 7, pp. 263–278. Elsevier, Amsterdam.

Hawthorne, J. N., and Kai, M. (1970). Metabolism of phosphoinositides. *Handb. Neurochem.* **3**, 491–508.

Hawthorne, J. N., and Pickard, M. R. (1979). Phospholipids in synaptic function. *J. Neurochem.* **32**, 5–14.

Hawthorne, J. N., and Swilem, A. F. (1982). Phosphatidylinositol metabolism in the adrenal medulla. *Cell Calcium* **3**, 351–358.

Hawthorne, J. N., and White, D. A. (1975). Myo-inositol lipids. *Vita. Horm.* **33**, 529–573.

Hirata, F., Strittmatter, W. J., and Axelrod, J. (1979). Beta-adrenergic receptor agonists increase phospholipid methylation, membrane fluidity, and beta-adrenergic receptor adenylate cyclase coupling. *Proc. Natl. Acad. Sci. U.S.A.* **76**, 368–372.

Hoffman, B. B., De Lean, A., Wood, C. L. Schocken, D. D., and Lefkowitz, R. J. (1979). Alpha-adrenergic receptor subtypes: Quantitative assessment by ligand binding. *Life Sci.* **24**, 1739–1746.

Hoffman, B. B., Mullikin-Kilpatrick, D., and Lefkowitz, R. J. (1980). Heterogeneity of radioligand binding to α-adrenergic receptors. *J. Biol. Chem.* **255**, 4645–4652.

Hofmann, S. J., and Majerus, P. W. (1982). Modulation of phosphatidylinositol-specific phospholipase C activity by phospholipid interactions, diglycerides and calcium ions. *J. Biol. Chem.* **257**, 14359–14364.

Hokin, M. R., and Hokin, L. E. (1953). Enzyme secretion and the incorporation of ^{32}P into phospholipids of pancreas slices. *J. Biol. Chem.* **203**, 967–977.

Hokin, L. E. and Hokin, M. R. (1955a). Effects of acetylcholine on the turnover of phosphoryl units in individual phospholipids of pancreas slices and brain cortex slices. *Biochim. Biophys. Acta* **18**, 102–110.

Hokin, L. E., and Hokin, M. R. (1955b). Effects of acetylcholine on phosphate turnover in phospholipids of brain cortex *in vitro*. *Biochim. Biophys. Acta* **16**, 229–237.

Hokin, L. E., and Hokin, M. R. (1959). The mechanism of phosphate exchange in phosphatidic acid in response to acetylcholine. *J. Biol. Chem.* **234**, 1387–1390.

Hokin, M. R., Benfey, B. G., and Hokin, L. E. (1958). Phospholipids and adrenaline secretion in guinea pig adrenal medulla. *J. Biol. Chem.* **233**, 814–817.

Holmsen, H., Dangelmaier, C. A., and Holmsen, H.-K. (1981). Thrombin-induced platelet responses differ in requirement for receptor occupancy. *J. Biol. Chem.* **256**, 9393–9396.

Homma, Y., Onozaki, K., Hashimoto, T., Nagai, Y, and Takenawa, T. (1982). Differential activation of phospholipids metabolism by formylated peptide and ionophore A23187 in guinea pig peritoneal macrophages. *J. Immunol.* **129**, 1619–1626.

Horrocks, L. A., Ansell, G. B., and Porcellati, G. (1982). "Phospholipids in the Nervous System," Vol. 1: Metabolism. Raven, New York.

Hunyady, L., Balla, T., Nagy, K., and Spat, A. (1982). Control of phosphatidylinositol turnover in adrenal glomerulosa cells. *Biochim. Biophys. Acta* **713**, 352–357.

Ieyasu, H., Takai, Y., Kaibuchi, K., Sawamura, M., and Nishizuka, Y. (1982). A role of calcium-activated, phospholipid-dependent protein kinase in platelet-activating factor-induced serotonin release from rabbit platelets. *Biochem. Biophys. Res. Commun.* **108**, 1701–1708.

Imai, A., Ishizuka, Y., Kawai, K., and Nozawa, Y. (1982). Evidence for coupling of phosphatidic acid formation and calcium influx in thrombin-activated human platelets. *Biochem. Biophys. Res. Commun.* **108**, 752–759.

Imai, A., Makashima, S., and Nozawa, Y. (1983). The rapid polyphosphoinositide metabolism may be a triggering event for thrombin-mediated stimulation of human platelets. *Biochem. Biophys. Res. Commun.* **110**, 108–115.

Irvine, R. F., Dawson, R. M. C., and Freinkel, N. (1982). Stimulated phosphatidylinositol turnover, a brief appraisal. *In* "Contemporary Metabolism" (N. Freinkel, ed.), Vol. 2, pp. 301–343. Plenum, New York.

Joseph, S. K., Thomas, A. P. Williams, R. J., Irvine, R. F., and Williamson, J. R. (1984). A second messenger for the hormonal mobilization of intracellular Ca^{2+} in liver. *J. Biol. Chem.* **259**, 3077–3081.

Jungalwala, F. B., Freinkel, N., and Dawson, R. M. C. (1971). The metabolism of phosphatidylinositol in the thyroid gland of the pig. *Biochem. J.* **123**, 19–33.

Kaibuchi, K., Takai, Y., Sawamura, M., Hoshijima, M., Fujikura, T., and Nishizuka, Y. (1983). Synergistic functions of protein phosphorylation and calcium mobilization in platelet activation. *J. Biol. Chem.* **258**, 6701–6704.

Kawahara, K., Takai, Y., Minakuchi, R., Sano, K., and Nishizuka, Y. (1980). Phospholipid turnover as a possible transmembrane signal for protein phosphorylation during human platelet activation by thrombin. *Biochem. Biophys. Res. Commun.* **97**, 309–317.

Kirk, C. J. (1982). Ligand-stimulated inositol lipid metabolism in the liver: Relationship to receptor function. *Cell Calcium* **3**, 399–412.

Kirk, C. J., Verrinder, T. R., and Hems, D. A. (1978). The influence of extracellular calcium concentration on the vasopressin-stimulated incorporation of inorganic phosphate into phosphatidylinositol in hepatocyte suspensions. *Biochem. Soc. Trans.* **6**, 1031–1033.

Kirk, C. J., Michell, R. H., and Hems, D. A. (1981a). Phosphatidylinositol metabolism in rat hepatocytes stimulated by vasopressin. *Biochem. J.* **184**, 155–165.

Kirk, C. J., Creba, J. A., Downs, C. P., and Michell, R. H. (1981b). Hormone-stimulated metabolism of inositol lipids and its relationship to hepatic receptor function. *Biochem. Soc. Trans.* **9**, 377–379.

Kishimoto, A., Mori, T., Kikkawa, U., and Nishizuka, Y. (1980). Activation of calcium and phospholipid-dependent protein kinase by diacylglycerol, its possible relation to phosphatidylinositol turnover. *J. Biol. Chem.* **266**, 2273–2276.

Lapetina, E. G. (1983). Metabolism of inositides and the activation of platelets. *Life Sci.* **32**, 2069–2082.

Lapetina, E. G., Schmitges, C. J., Chandrabose, K., and Cuatrecasas, P. (1977). Cyclic adenosine 3′,5′-monophosphate and prostacyclin inhibit membrane phospholipase activity in platelets. *Biochem. Biophys. Res. Commun.* **76**, 818–835.

Lefebvre, Y. A., White, D. A., and Hawthorne, J. N. (1976). Diphosphoinositide metabolism in bovine adrenal medulla. *Can. J. Biochem.* **54**, 746–753.

Lin, S. H., and Fain, J. N. (1981). Vasopressin and epinephrine stimulation of phosphatidylinositol breakdown in the plasma membrane of rat hepatocytes. *Life Sci.* **18**, 1905–1912.

Lin, S.-H., Wallace, M. A., and Fain, J. N. (1983). Regulation of $Ca^{2+}–Mg^{2+}$-ATPase activity in hepatocyte plasma membranes by vasopressin and phenylephrine. *Endocrinology* **113**, 2268–2275.

Litosch, I., Saito, Y., and Fain, J. N. (1982a). 5-HT-stimulated arachidonic acid release from labeled phosphatidylinositol in blowfly salivary glands. *Am. J. Physiol.* **243**, C222–C226.

Litosch, I., Fradin, M., Kasaian, M., Lee, H. S., and Fain, J. N. (1982b). Regulation of adenylate cyclase and cyclic AMP phosphodiesterase by 5-hydroxytryptamine and calcium ions in blowfly salivary-gland homogenates. *Biochem. J.* **204**, 153–159.

Litosch, I., Saito, Y., and Fain, J. N. (1982c). Forskolin as an activator of cyclic AMP accumulation and secretion in blowfly salivary glands. *Biochem. J.* **204**, 147–151.

Litosch, I., Lin, S.-H., and Fain, J. N. (1983). Rapid changes in hepatocyte phosphoinositides induced by vasopressin. *J. Biol. Chem.* **258**, 13727–13732.

Litosch, I., Lee, H. S., and Fain, J. N. (1984). Phosphoinositide breakdown in blowfly salivary glands. *Am. J. Physiol.* **246**, C141–147.

Lloyd, J. V., Nishizawa, E. E., Haldar, J., and Mustard, J. F. (1972). Changes in ^{32}P-labeling of rabbit platelet phospholipids in response to ADP. *Br. J. Haematol.* **23**, 571–585.

Lloyd, J. V., Nishizawa, E. E., Joist, J. H., and Mustard, J. F. (1973). Effect of ADP-induced aggregation on ^{32}PO$_4$ incorporation into phosphatidic acid and the phosphoinositides of rabbit platelets. *Br. J. Haematol.* **24**, 589–604.

Lunt, G. G., and Pickard, M. R. (1975). The subcellular localization of carbamylcholine-stimulated phosphatidylinositol turnover in rat cerebral cortex *in vivo*. *J. Neurochem.* **24**, 1203–1208.

Malbon, C. C., Gilman, H. R., and Fain, J. N. (1980). Hormonal stimulation of cyclic AMP accumulation and glycogen phosphorylase activity in calcium-depleted hepatocytes from euthyroid and hypothyroid rats. *Biochem. J.* **188**, 593–599.

Mastro, A. M., and Smith, M. C. (1983). Calcium-dependent activation of lymphocytes by ionophore, A23187, and a phorbol ester tumor promoter. *J. Cell. Physiol.* **116**, 51–56.

Michell, R. H. (1975). Inositol phospholipids and cell surface receptor function. *Biochem. Biophys. Acta* **415**, 81–147.

Michell, R. H. (1982). Is phosphatidylinositol really out of the calcium gate? *Nature (London)* **296**, 492–493.

Michell, R. H. (1983). Polyphosphoinositide breakdown as the initiating reaction in receptor-stimulated inositol phospholipid metabolism. *Life Sci.* **32**, 2083–2086.

Michell, R. H., and Kirk, C. J. (1982). The unknown meaning of receptor stimulated inositol lipid metabolism. *Trends Pharmacol. Sci.* **April**, 140–141.

Michell, R. H., Kirk, C. J., Jones, L. M., Downes, C. P., and Creba, J. A. (1981). The stimulation of inositol lipid metabolism that accompanies calcium mobilization in stimulated cells: Defined characteristics and unanswered questions. *Philos. Trans. R. Soc. London Ser. B* **296**, 123–137.

Peroutka, S. J., and Snyder, S. H. (1979). Multiple serotonin receptors: Differential binding of ^{3}H-hydroxytryptamine, ^{3}H-lysergic acid diethylamide and ^{3}H-spiroperidol. *Mol. Pharmacol.* **16**, 686–699.

Perret, B. P., Plantavid, M., Chap, H., and Douste-Blazy, L. (1983). Are polyphosphoinositides involved in platelet activation? *Biochem. Biophys. Res. Commun.* **110**, 660–667.

Phillips, J. H. (1973). Phosphatidylinositol kinase. A component of the chromaffin-granule membrane. *Biochem. J.* **136**, 579–587.

Prescott, S. M., and Majerus, P. W. (1983). Characterization of 1,2-diacylglycerol hydrolysis in human platelets. *J. Biol. Chem.* **258**, 764–769.

Prpic, V., Blackmore, P. F., and Exton, J. H. (1982). Phosphatidylinositol breakdown induced by vasopressin and epinephrine in hepatocytes is calcium-dependent. *J. Biol. Chem.* **257**, 11323–11331.

Putney, J. W., Jr., Weiss, S. J., Van de Walle, C., and Haddas, R. A. (1980). Is phosphatidic acid a calcium ionophore under neurohumoral control? *Nature (London)* **285**, 345–347.

Rhodes, D., Prpic, V., Exton, J. H., and Blackmore, P. F. (1983). Stimulation of phosphatidylinositol 4,5-bisphosphate hydrolysis in hepatocytes by vasopressin. *J. Biol. Chem.* **258**, 2770–2773.

Rittenhouse-Simmons, S. (1979). Production of diglyceride from phosphatidylinositol in activated human platelets. *J. Clin. Invest.* **63**, 580–587.

Rubin, R., Weiss, G., and Putney, J. (1984). *Proc. FASEB Calcium Symp., 1983.*

Sadler, K., Litosch, I., and Fain, J. N. (1984). Stimulation of phosphatidylinositol 4,5-bisphosphate formation by prior incubation of blowfly salivary glands with 5-HT. *Biochem. J.* **222** (in press).

Salmon, D. M., and Honeyman, T. W. (1980). Proposed mechanism of cholinergic action in smooth muscle. *Nature (London)* **284**, 344–345.

Shattil, S. J., McDonough, M., Turnbull, J., and Insel, P. A. (1981). Characterization of alpha-adrenergic receptors in human platelets using [³H]clonidine. *Mol. Pharmacol.* **19**, 179–183.

Sherman, W. R., Leavitt, A. L., Honchar, M. P., Hallcher, L. M., and Phillips, B. E. (1981). Evidence that lithium alters phosphoinositide metabolism: Chronic administration elevates primarily D-myo-1-phosphate in cerebral cortex of the rat. *J. Neurochem.* **36**, 1947–1951.

Shukla, S. D., and Hanahan, D. J. (1982). AGEPC (Platelet activating factor) induced stimulation of rabbit platelets: Effects on phosphatidylinositol, di- and tri-phosphoinositides and phosphatidic acid metabolism. *Biochem. Biophys. Res. Commun.* **106**, 697–703.

Soukup, J., and Schanberg, S. (1982). Involvement of alpha noradrenergic receptors in mediation of brain polyphosphoinositide metabolism *in vivo*. *J. Pharmacol. Exp. Ther.* **222**, 209–214.

Soukup, J. F., Friedel, R. O., and Schanberg, S. M. (1978). Cholinergic stimulation of polyphosphoinositide metabolism in brain *in vivo*. *Biochem. Pharmacol.* **27**, 1239–1243.

Streb, H., Irvine, R. F., Berridge, M. J., and Schulz, I. (1983). Release of Ca²⁺ from a nonmitochondrial intracellular store in pancreatic acinar cells by inositol-1,4,5-trisphosphate. *Nature (London)* **306**, 67–69.

Takai, Y., Kikkawa, U., Kaibuchi, K., and Nishizuka, Y. (1984). Membrane phospholipid metabolism and signal transduction for protein phosphorylation. *Adv. Cyclic Nucleotid Res.* (in press).

Takenawa, T., Saito, M., Nagai, Y., and Egawa, K. (1977). Solubilization of the enzyme catalyzing CDP-diglyceride-independent incorporation of myo-inositol into phosphatidylinositol and its comparison to CDP-diglyceride: Inositol transferase. *Arch. Biochem. Biophys.* **182**, 244–250.

Takenawa, T., Homma, Y., and Nagai, Y. (1982). Increased formation of phosphatidic acid induced with vasopressin or Ca²⁺ ionophore A23187 in rat hepatocytes. *Biochem. Pharmacol.* **31**, 2663–2667.

Takenawa, T., Homma, Y., and Nagai, Y. (1983). Role of Ca²⁺ in phosphatidylinositol response and arachidonic acid release in formylated tripeptide or Ca²⁺ ionophore A23187–stimulated guinea pig neutrophils *J. Immunol.* **130**, 2849–2855.

Thomas, A. P., Marks, J. S., Coll, K. E., and Williamson, J. R. (1983). Quantitation and early kinetics of inositol lipid changes induced by vasopressin in isolated and cultured hepatocytes. *J. Biol. Chem.* **258**, 5716–5725.

Tolbert, M. E. M., White, A. C., Aspry, K., Cutts, J., and Fain, J. N. (1980). Stimulation by vasopressin and α-catecholamines of phosphatidylinositol formation in isolated rat liver parenchymal cells. *J. Biol. Chem.* **255**, 1938–1944.

Trifaro, J. M., and Dworkind, J. (1975). Phosphorylation of the membrane components of chromaffin granules: Synthesis of diphosphatidylinositol and presence of phosphatidylinositol kinase in granule membranes. *Can. J. Physiol. Pharmacol.* **53**, 479–492.

Van Rooijen, L. A. A., Seguin, E. B., and Agranoff, B. W. (1983). Phosphodiesterase breakdown of endogenous polyphosphoinositides in nerve ending membranes. *Biochem. Biophys. Res. Commun.* **112**, 919–926.

Volpi, M., Yassin, R., Naccache, P. H., and Shaafi, R. I. (1983). Chemotactic factor causes rapid decreases in phosphatidylinositol 4,5-bisphosphate and phosphatidylinositol 4-monophosphate in rabbit neutrophils. *Biochem. Biophys. Res. Commun.* **112**, 957–964.

Wallace, M. A., and Fain, J. N. (1984). Analysis of hormone-induced changes of phosphoinositide metabolism in rat liver. *In* "Methods in Enzymology," Vol. 109. Academic Press, New York (in press).

Wallace, M. A., Agarwal, K. C., Garcia-Sainz, J. A., and Fain, J. N. (1982a). Alpha-adrenergic stimulation of phosphatidylinositol synthesis in human platelets as an alpha₂ effect secondary to platelet aggregation *J. Cell. Biochem.* **28**, 213–220.

Wallace, M. A., Randazzo, P., Li, S.-Y., and Fain, J. N. (1982b). Direct stimulation of phosphatidylinositol degradation by addition of vasopressin to purified rat liver plasma membranes. *Endocrinology* **111**, 341–343.

Wallace, M. A., Giraud, F., Poggioli, J., and Claret, M. 1983). Norepinephrine-induced loss of phosphatidylinositol from isolated rat liver plasma membrane. *FEBS Lett.* **156**, 239–243.

Warfield, A. S., and Segal, S. (1978). Myoinositol and phosphatidylinositol metabolism in synaptosomes from galactose-fed rats. *Proc. Natl. Acad. Sci. U.S.A.* **75**, 4568–4572.

Williamson, J. R., Cooper, R. H., and Hoek, J. B. (1981). Role of calcium in the hormonal regulation of liver metabolism. *Biochim. Biophys. Acta* **639**, 243–295.

Wooton, J. A., and Kinsella, J. E. (1977). Properties of cytidine diphosphodiacyl sn-glycerol: Myoinositol transferase of bovine mammary tissue. *Int. J. Biochem.* **8**, 449–456.

VITAMINS AND HORMONES, VOL. 41

The Chemistry and Physiology of Erythropoietin

JUDITH B. SHERWOOD

Department of Medicine,
Albert Einstein College of Medicine,
Bronx, New York

I. Introduction 161
II. Chemistry of Erythropoietin and Structure–Function Relationships 168
III. Purification of Erythropoietin 178
   A. Sheep Plasma Erythropoietin 179
   B. Human Urinary Erythropoietin 181
IV. Assays for Erythropoietin 186
V. Site of Erythropoietin Production 194
   A. Anephric Models 194
   B. Perfusion Studies 195
   C. Clinical Observations 196
   D. Production of Erythropoietin by Renal and Nonrenal Tumors 196
   E. Cell Origin of Erythropoietin 199
VI. Conclusions 202
   References 203

I. INTRODUCTION

Erythropoietin is the primary regulator of erythropoiesis in mammals. It is a glycoprotein hormone produced primarily in the kidney and secreted into the circulation, acting on the bone marrow to induce the differentiation of hematopoietic stem cells along erythroid lines.

The maintenance of a constant circulating red cell mass under normal physiological conditions had been recognized for some time, but the factors involved in this homeostatic regulation were unknown. The inverse correlation observed between red cell production and atmospheric oxygen supply led initially to the hypothesis that erythropoiesis is under the control of local marrow oxygen tension. A specific endocrine regulation of erythropoiesis was suggested by Carnot and Déflandre in 1906, based on observations that injection of serum from bled anemic rabbits produced an increased red cell count in normal rabbits. Definitive evidence, however, that erythropoiesis is controlled by a circulating factor acting directly on the marrow rather than on the level of marrow oxygenation was first provided by the observations of Reissmann (1950), Stohlman et al. (1954), and others in the 1950s.

161

Reissman (1950) observed, using parabiosed rats, that lowering the blood oxygen saturation to 63% in one of the rats was followed by increased erythropoiesis in both the hypoxic rat and the partner breathing room air and with a blood oxygen saturation of 97%. Stohlman and co-workers (1954) studied a patient with a patent ductus arteriosus and normal oxygen saturation above the diaphragm but with decreased oxygenation below the diaphragm. Erythroid hyperplasia was observed in the sternal marrow despite a normal marrow oxygen saturation, suggesting that a humoral factor produced below the diaphragm in response to hypoxia, rather than local marrow oxygen tension, regulates erythropoiesis.

Subsequent studies have confirmed these initial observations. Gordon and co-workers (Gordon, 1959; Gordon et al., 1954, 1964), Plzak and co-workers (1955), Erslev (1959), Borsook and co-workers (1959), and other investigators have shown that plasma from anemic or hypoxic animals produces a significant increase in reticulocyte count, hematocrit, marrow nucleated erythroid cells, and ^{59}Fe incorporation into red cells (Plzak et al., 1955), when injected into normal animals. This plasma factor that increased erythropoiesis was named "erythropoietin" (Gordon, 1959) in recognition of its role as the hormone involved exclusively with red cell production.

In the ensuing decades, an erythropoiesis-stimulating factor, produced in response to hypoxia and capable of stimulating erythropoiesis in vivo, has been identified in widely diverse animal species. It has been found in rats (Erslev and Lavietes, 1954; Fried et al., 1956; Plzak et al., 1955), mice (Jacobson et al., 1959), rabbits (Erslev, 1953; Gordon et al., 1955), monkeys (Mirand et al., 1964), cows (Jatkar and Kreier, 1967), swine (McClellan, 1963), dogs (Naets, 1959), llamas, chinchillas, and vicunas (Scaro and Aggio, 1966), goats (Borsook, 1959), and guinea pigs (Scaro et al., 1963). Erythropoiesis in birds similarly appears to be under hormonal control, increased in response to hypoxia, phlebotomy, and hemolysis and decreased in response to fasting. Plasma from anemic birds, however, appears to show species specificity, stimulating erythropoiesis only in polycythemic birds and not in polycythemic mice; likewise, anemic human serum is erythropoietically inactive in polycythemic birds (Rosse and Waldmann, 1966). Erythropoietin has also been identified in the plasma of the Blue Gourami fish (Trichogaster trichopterus) (Zanjani et al., 1969).

Mammalian erythropoietins appear to show relatively little species specificity with regard to biologic activity. Anemic plasma and serum can stimulate erythropoiesis in polycythemic hosts of either the same or unrelated mammalian species, thereby allowing the use of a standardized assay animal, the polycythemic mouse or the fasted rat. Likewise, tissue and circulating erythropoietins from several mammalian species react with an antibody to the human urinary hormone and inhibit binding of the pure human urinary erythropoietin tracer in the radioimmunoassay (Sherwood and Goldwasser, 1979; Garcia *et al.,* 1979). Dose–response curves parallel to those generated with human urinary standard erythropoietin have been obtained with sera and plasma from baboons and monkeys (Garcia *et al.,* 1979), cats, dogs, horses, mice, and rats (Sherwood, unpublished observations), and with extracts of rabbit and dog kidneys and fetal calf livers (Sherwood and Goldwasser, 1979; Sherwood, unpublished observations).

Species differences have been observed, both in biologic and immunologic activity. For example, in a series of studies, preparations of sheep erythropoietin did not give dose–response curves parallel to those for human material assayed in the polycythemic mouse system (Annable *et al.,* 1972). Significant differences between human and nonhuman hormone with regard to reactivity with the antihuman antibody have been found, as suggested by the discrepancy between the amounts of bovine erythropoietin found by bioassay and radioimmunoassay (Sherwood and Goldwasser, 1979), and the inability of the antihuman antibody to completely neutralize sheep erythropoietin (Schooley and Mahlmann, 1972).

The reactivity of erythropoietin from either human or nonhuman sources with an antiserum against human hormone and the erythropoietic activity in a variety of assay animals suggest that these erythropoietins share certain structural similarities.

The chemical and structural relationships, however, between erythropoietins from diverse animal sources are unknown. At present, erythropoietin has been purified from only two sources, sheep plasma (Goldwasser and Kung, 1971; Goldwasser *et al.,* 1962a,b) and human urine (Miyake *et al.,* 1977; Lee-Huang, 1980). The recent isolation and purification of human urinary erythropoietin have provided the stimulus for the current studies on erythropoietin structure and physiology and have permitted the development of a radioimmunoassay for erythropoietin (Sherwood and Goldwasser, 1979; Garcia *et al.,* 1979; Cotes, 1982; Zaroulis *et al.,* 1981) to help in approaching these problems.

Prior to development of the radioimmunoassay, biologic assays have been used to measure the hormone. The biologic assays all rely on the specific response induced by erythropoietin—namely, the differentiation of hematopoietic precursor cells along erythroid lines (Fig. 1). Hemoglobin synthesis is the marker in the most commonly utilized

ERYTHROPOIESIS (SCHEMATIC)

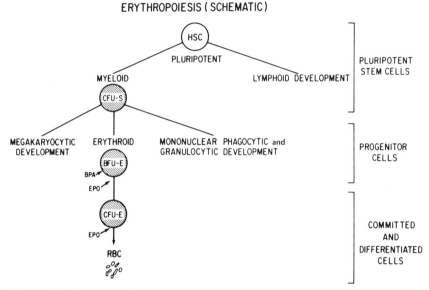

FIG. 1. The formation of red blood cells. Pluripotent hematopoietic stem cells in the bone marrow (HSC) differentiate along both myeloid and lymphoid lines. Myeloid stem cells (CFU-S) develop into erythroid progenitor cells (BFU-E) as well as along monocytic, granulocytic, and megakaryocytic lines. The BFU-E, under the influence of burst-promoting activity (BPA) and erythropoietin (EPO), differentiate along erythroid lines, to the colony-forming cells (CFU-E) and ending with the mature hemoglobinized red cells (RBC). Courtesy of Dr. E. Richard Stanley.

bioassays, for example, the *in vivo* cultured rat bone marrow (Goldwasser *et al.*, 1975) and fetal liver cell (Dunn *et al.*, 1975) assays, and the *in vivo* polycythemic mouse (Jacobson *et al.*, 1957), and fasted rat (Fried *et al.*, 1957) assays. The ^{59}Fe uptake into newly synthesized hemoglobin is directly related to the amount of erythropoietin added to the system, and a log dose–response curve is obtained.

   The standardization of erythropoietin is based upon the erythropoietic activity of cobalt chloride ($CoCl_2$). It had been observed that increasing amounts of a crude preparation of anemic sheep erythropoietin and of cobalt chloride at a concentration range between 5 and 10 μM generated parallel dose–response curves in the fasted rat assay. One unit of erythropoietin was therefore defined as the amount of erythropoietin creating a response equivalent to 5 μmol of $CoCl_2$ in the fasted rat assay (White *et al.*, 1960). Currently, there are international reference preparations of erythropoietin, consisting of lyophilized crude extracts of urine from anemic human beings (Annable *et al.*, 1972; Cotes and Bangham, 1966).

A considerable number of observations, both clinical and experimental, suggest that the erythropoietin content of plasma and urine is regulated by oxygen supply at the site of erythropoietin production, with an inverse correlation between these parameters. Thus, anemic hypoxia (bleeding, hemolytic anemia), hypobaric hypoxia (reduced barometric pressure, etc.), and histotoxic hypoxia (cobalt-induced, etc.) serve as stimuli for increased erythropoietin production. In contrast, erythropoietin titers are decreased with hyperoxia (Linman and Pierre, 1968) or a plethora of red cells (Adamson and Finch, 1966).

The inverse relationship between a red cell mass and hemoglobin concentration and circulating erythropoietin titer has been amply demonstrated and extensively reviewed. For example, in a child with thalassemia major, Gordon *et al.* (1964) found high urine and plasma levels of erythropoietin when the hemoglobin concentration was 5 g%; however, when the hemoglobin concentration was brought to 12 g% by transfusion, the erythropoietin titer fell to undetectable levels. Sherwood *et al.* (1981) found that, in either sickle cell or non-hemoglobinopathy-associated anemia, plasma immunoreactive erythropoietin was inversely correlated with plasma hemoglobin. In a study using the radioimmunoassay for erythropoietin, a normal subject was bled over a 3-day period; the serum erythropoietin content and hematocrit were inversely correlated, with the erythropoietin rising from a baseline of

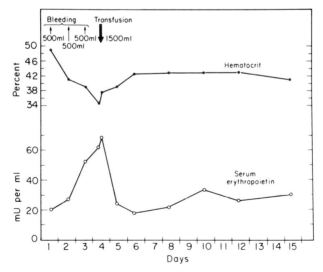

FIG. 2. Serum erythropoietin concentrations in a normal human being undergoing bleeding and transfusion. Erythropoietin was measured in the radioimmunoassay. From Garcia *et al.* (1979).

20 mU/ml to a peak of 68 mU/ml as the hematocrit fell from 49 to 34 (Garcia et al., 1979) (Fig. 2).

Moreover, at normal oxygen tension, conditions such as hypophysectomy, starvation, and hypothyroidism which reduce oxygen consumption lead to decreased erythropoiesis; increased rates of oxygen consumption with hyperthyroidism are often associated with increased erythropoiesis (Jacobson et al., 1959). Thus, the data indicate that erythropoietin production is regulated by the relationship of oxygen supply in the tissues to the demand for oxygen.

Although a considerable body of information exists on the correlation between erythropoietin production and such parameters involved in oxygen supply as hemoglobin concentration, red cell mass, and ambient p_{O_2}, little attention has been paid to a significant factor in the control of tissue oxygenation, namely the hemoglobin oxygen dissociation curve. Erythrocytosis has been observed in patients with hemoglobins of high oxygen affinity, for example, hemoglobin H Cape Town (Botha et al., 1966), hemoglobin Ypsilanti (Glynn et al., 1968), Hb Yakima (Novy et al., 1967), and Hb Kempsey (Reed et al., 1968). Other hemodynamic factors such as arterial oxygen pressure, oxygen consumption, and resting cardiac output were normal in these patients.

Modulation of the oxygen equilibrium curve by intrinsic changes in the hemoglobin molecule such as are found in sickle cell disease and the above-mentioned hemoglobinopathies and by such red cell parameters as 2,3-DPG levels, intracellular pH, etc. has a significant impact on oxygen delivery. A rightward shift of the curve—represented by an elevated p_{50}—leads to increased oxygenation of the tissues, while a leftward shift has the opposite effect (Jepson, 1979) (Fig. 3).

The shift to the right in the oxygen equilibrium curve found in renal insufficiency, sickle cell disease, and other disorders, by allowing for better oxygen delivery to the tissues, may eliminate the ability to respond to the anemia by increased production of erythropoietin. Indeed, Sherwood et al. (1981) observed that in patients with sickle cell anemia, the erythropoietin response was significantly correlated with anemia only below 9 g/dl. The mean erythropoietin level of the sickle cell anemic patients was significantly lower than that of patients with non-hemoglobinopathy-associated anemias, in spite of the greater degree of anemia in the sickle cell patients. Red cells taken from patients with sickle cell anemia in this study displayed the characteristic reduced oxygen affinity (expressed as higher p_{50}), an anomaly caused by the lower oxygen affinity of the hemoglobin S polymer (Bromberg and Jensen, 1967), and the increased intracellular 2,3-DPG levels (Charache et al., 1970).

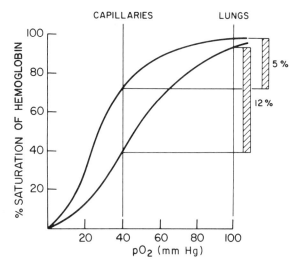

FIG. 3. Two hemoglobin oxygen binding curves illustrating the influence of hemo-globin oxygen affinity on the quantity of oxygen (in Vol%) released at a tissue (capillary) p_{O_2} of 40 mm Hg. At a given tissue p_{O_2}, the hemoglobin with the right-shifted curve (decreased affinity for oxygen) will release a greater total quantity of oxygen than a hemoglobin with a left-shifted curve (increased oxygen affinity). The position of the oxygen dissociation curve can be characterized by that partial pressure of oxygen (p_{O_2}) at which 50% of the hemoglobin is saturated, i.e., the p_{50}. Courtesy of Dr. Ronald L. Nagel.

Studies *in vitro* on regulation of erythropoietin production have uti-lized the isolated perfused kidney preparation. Kuratowska *et al.* (1961) showed that erythropoietin could be produced during perfusion with hypoxemic media; Fisher and Birdwell (1961) found increased titers after perfusion with blood containing cobalt. Perfusion of the kidney with prostaglandin E_1 (Paulo *et al.*, 1973) and E_2 (Gross *et al.*, 1976) or with arachidonic acid (Foley *et al.*, 1978), a precursor for prostaglandins, produced a significant increase in the erythropoietin titers in the perfusates which was blocked by pretreatment with the prostaglandin synthetase inhibitor indomethacin. Recent observations by Jelkmann *et al.* (1979) that albuterol can stimulate erythropoietin production by the perfused kidney suggest a β-adrenergic mechanism for erythropoietin regulation. Interpretation of these studies on per-fused kidney preparations is difficult, however, due to effects of agents in the perfusate on renal vasculature, effects on cells other than erythropoietin-producing cells, incomplete oxygenation of the prepara-tion, cell death due to high perfusion pressures, etc.

The present body of data suggests that *in vivo* erythropoietin produc-tion may be regulated by hemoglobin–oxygen affinity in addition to parameters such as hemoglobin concentration, red cell mass, and ambient p_{O_2}. There is, however, little information available from *in vitro* systems.

In this article we attempt to present the most interesting and potentially most important information currently being obtained on erythropoietin. Topics that have been extensively reviewed elsewhere will be discussed only in passing, if at all.

II. Chemistry of Erythropoietin and Structure–Function Relationships

The development of purification procedures for significant quantities of pure erythropoietin has made it possible to initiate studies on the structure of this hormone. Erythropoietin is an acidic glycoprotein with carbohydrate comprising approximately 25–30% of the molecule (Goldwasser, 1981b). The acidic properties are due to the high content of sialic acid which constitutes a large percentage of the terminal carbohydrate residues in the molecule.

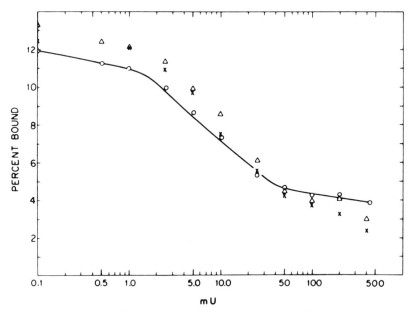

Fig. 4. Comparison of three forms of human erythropoietin. The pure α fraction (○) was compared with the pure β form (×) and with asialoerythropoietin (△). From Sherwood and Goldwasser (1979).

TABLE I
CARBOHYDRATE COMPOSITION OF HUMAN URINARY
ERYTHROPOIETIN[a]

Carbohydrate	Moles per mole of erythropoietin	
	α	β
Fucose	4.9 ± 0.9	4.4 ± 0.1
Galactose	13.4 ± 1.6	11.6 ± 0.2
Mannose	9.8 ± 1.5	8.2 ± 1
N-Acetylglucosamine	13.5 ± 0.2	9.3 ± 0.6[b]
N-Acetylneuraminic acid	18.1 ± 2.5	13.2 ± 1[b]

[a]Carbohydrate composition was determined by gas–liquid chromatography of the trifluoroacetate derivatives of methyl glycosides. α-Erythropoietin is eluted from hydroxylapatite with 1 mM phosphate and β with 2 mM phosphate. Calculations are based upon the apparent molecular weight of 39,000.

[b]The differences between α and β are statistically significant. Data from Dordal and Goldwasser (1982).

Two fractions, α and β, have been isolated by hydroxylapatite fractionation. These forms appear identical on sodium dodecyl sulfate gels but show different mobilities on gel electrophoresis at pH 9; biological activities are similar (Miyake et al., 1977). Dose–response curves for the α and β forms are identical in the radioimmunoassay (Fig. 4) (Sherwood and Goldwasser, 1979). The presence of two forms of similar molecular size and antigenic reactivity suggests a degree of carbohydrate microheterogeneity characteristic of many glycoproteins. Analysis of the carbohydrate composition by gas–liquid chromatography suggests that the heterogeneity might be accounted for by the small but significant difference in the number of N-acetylglucosamine and N-acetylneuraminic acid residues (Table I) (Dordal and Goldwasser, 1982).

Erythropoietin contains approximately 130 amino acid residues with a high proportion of hydrophobic residues (Goldwasser, 1981a). Although the amino acid composition has been determined (Table II), a complete amino acid sequence has not as yet been elucidated. Goldwasser (1981b) described the 26 amino acid NH_2-terminal peptide with the sequence

H_2N-Ala-Pro-Pro-Arg-Leu-Ile-Asn-Asp-Ser-Arg-Val-Leu-Glu-Arg-Tyr-Leu-Leu-Glu-Ala-Lys-Glu-Ala-Glu-Lys-Ile-Thr

TABLE II
AMINO ACID COMPOSITION OF
HUMAN URINARY
ERYTHROPOIETIN[a]

Amino acid	Residues per mole
Asp	11
Thr	9
Ser	9
Glu	17
Pro	8
Gly	9
Ala	16
Val	9
Met	2
Ile	7
Leu	21
Tyr	4
Phe	4
His	2
Lys	6
Arg	10
CysSH	3
Trp	2

[a] According to Goldwasser (1981a).

In recent studies by Sue and Sytkowski (1983), antibodies made against this peptide immunoprecipitated pure ^{125}I-labeled erythropoietin and biologically active unlabeled erythropoietin. Peptide and unlabeled erythropoietin inhibited the antibody–[125]I-labeled erythropoietin interaction with identical inhibition constants. These results indicate that the amino acid sequence is at least partially correct. The inability of antipeptide antibodies to neutralize erythropoietin suggests that the active site is located in a different region of the molecule.

The apparent molecular weight of native human erythropoietin is 39,000 and of the asialo form is 34,000 by sodium dodecyl sulfate gel electrophoresis (Miyake et al., 1977), as compared with 46,000 for the native and 41,000 for the asialo sheep plasma hormone (Goldwasser and Kung, 1972a,b) determined by the same method. Determination of molecular weight by this method, however, may be inaccurate for heavily sialylated glycoproteins possibly due to unblocked charges on sialic acid residues (Goldwasser and Kung, 1972a,b). The protein moiety of human urinary erythropoietin, prepared by deglycosylating the native form with protease-free mixed glycosidases, shows an apparent molecular weight of 28,500 by SDS–polyacrylamide gel electrophoresis (Dordal and Goldwasser, 1982). It has been suggested that erythropoietin is an elongated molecule (Rosse et al., 1963), in which case molecular weight determination may be distorted by the Stokes' radius, since the mobility of nonglobular proteins is better correlated with molecular (Stokes') radius than with molecular weight (Siegel and Monty, 1966). Electrophoresis of erythropoietin in sodium dodecyl sulfate and dithiothreitol at pH 7 does not produce a change in mobility, suggesting that both the α and β forms are monomeric (Miyake et al., 1977).

Although the primary structure of erythropoietin has not as yet been determined, studies of the functional importance of known structural features are currently underway. The involvement of tyrosine and free amino groups in biological activity has been suggested because of the loss of activity on production of iodotyrosine by standard iodination methods and on acylation of amino groups with ^{125}I-labeled p-hydroxyphenylpropionic acid (Miyake et al., 1977; Sherwood and Goldwasser, 1979).

The role of the carbohydrate moiety is not as yet known. Sialic acid comprises approximately 30% of the carbohydrate, and evidence concerning its functional importance is accumulating. Erythropoietin devoid of sialic acid is biologically inactive in vivo (Lowy et al., 1960), but is fully active in vitro, inducing erythropoietic differentiation in bone marrow cells in culture (Goldwasser et al., 1968). In vivo activity of asialoerythropoietin can be restored by modification of its terminal galactose residues. For example, oxidation of asialoerythropoietin with galactose oxidase allowed 40–50% restoration of in vivo activity (Table III) (Goldwasser et al., 1974). Pretreatment of animals with other glycoproteins having terminal galactose residues likewise restores some in vivo activity, possibly by competitive inhibition of galactose-recognition sites. Asialoerythropoietin showed 25–30% of its original activity in rats pretreated with asialoorosomucoid or stachyose (Table IV) (Goldwasser et al., 1974). Perfusion of rat livers with blood containing either native or disialylated erythropoietin causes rapid loss of desialylated but not of native erythropoietin activity. The loss of erythropoietic activity was prevented by addition of desialylated but not native orosomucoid (Briggs et al., 1974). All of the above data suggest that erythropoietin is rapidly cleared by the liver after desialylation.

Sialic acid, an acidic monosaccharide found only at the terminal position of glycoprotein carbohydrate side chains, appears to be impor-

TABLE III

EFFECT OF OXIDATION OF GALACTOSE RESIDUES ON ASIALOERYTHROPOIETIN
ACTIVITY in Vivo[a]

Preparation	Units of erythropoietin recovered	Activity restored (%)
Erythropoietin	9.0	100
Asialoerythropoietin (soluble sialidase)[b]	0.0	0
Asialoerythropoietin after galactose oxidase treatment[b]	3.7	41[c]
Erythropoietin	8.3	100
Asialoerythropoietin (acid hydrolyzed)[b]	0.7	8
Asialoerythropoietin after galactose oxidase treatment[b]	4.1	49[c]

[a]From Goldwasser et al. (1974).
[b]Nine units of desialated erythropoietin injected per rat.
[c]Significantly different from the "no erythropoietin" control group, at $p < 0.02$ (41%) + $p < 0.001$ (49%) levels.

tant in determining the half life of glycoproteins in the circulation. Removal of terminal sialic groups exposes the penultimate galactose residues; such desialylated glycoproteins are rapidly cleared from the circulation by catabolism in hepatic parenchymal cells (Morell et al., 1971). Hepatic cell plasma membranes contain specific saturable binding sites for the desialylated glycoproteins (Morell and Scheinberg, 1972; Pricer and Ashwell, 1971; Van Lenten and Ashwell, 1972).

TABLE IV

EFFECTS OF GALACTOSE-TERMINAL GLYCOPROTEINS INJECTED INTO TEST ANIMALS[a]

Preparation	Units of erythropoietin per rat	Activity recovered (%)
Erythropoietin	8.1	100
Asialoerythropoietin	0.0	0
Asialoerythropoietin + asialoorosomucoid[b]	2.0	25[c]
Asialoerythropoietin + stachyose[d]	2.6	32[c]
Asialoerythropoietin + lactose[d]	0.1	0

[a]From Goldwasser et al. (1974).
[b]Asialoorosomucoid given intravenously, 10 mg at $-1, 0$, and $+1$ hours with respect to erythropoietin injections.
[c]Significantly different from the "no erythropoietin" control group, at $p < 0.02$ (25%) and $p < 0.05$ (32%) levels.
[d]Stachyose given intravenously, 3 mg at $-2, 0$, and $+2$ hours with respect to erythropoietin injections. Lactose was administered in the same manner as stachyose.

Asialoerythropoietin is significantly more active than the native hormone *in vitro* in bone marrow cell cultures (a threefold difference seen at low doses) (Goldwasser *et al.*, 1974). This phenomenon has been noted for other glycoproteins such as human luteinizing hormone and chorionic gonadotropin (Dufau *et al.*, 1971). Native erythropoietin bears a significant negative charge due to sialic acid moieties, and the target cells in the marrow may likewise have a large number of anionic groups on the cell surface. Removal of the sialic acid residues would reduce charge repulsion and thus may facilitate interaction between the cell and the erythropoietin molecule (Goldwasser *et al.*, 1974), perhaps accounting for the increased activity of the asialo form.

Asialoerythropoietin is significantly more labile toward heat and tryptic hydrolysis than is the native hormone. The half-life of the native erythropoietin exposed to trypsin or to 100°C was 2.3-fold greater than that of the asialo form (Goldwasser *et al.*, 1974). These differences suggest that sialic acid may help maintain the conformational integrity of the erythropoietin molecule. In the radioimmunoassay, however, dose–response curves for native erythropoietin (both α and β forms) and for asialoerythropoietin were parallel, indicating immunological similarity (Fig. 4) (Sherwood and Goldwasser, 1979).

Erythropoietin stripped of its carbohydrate by use of protease-free mixed glycosidases from *Streptococcus pneumoniae* retained up to 66% of control activity in the *in vitro* bone marrow assay, but lost a significant amount of immunoreactivity (Dordal and Goldwasser, 1982), suggesting that the carbohydrate moiety is involved in the antigenic sites and, to a lesser extent, in the active site. It can therefore be suggested that glycosylation of erythropoietin confers specific conformational properties.

Glycoslyation of proteins could be an important feature in protecting the molecule from proteolysis. Tunicamycin inhibition of glycoslyation of the *Xenopus laevis* adrenocorticotropin–β-lipotropin precursor led to rapid degradation with formation and secretion of atypical peptides by the neurointermediate lobe. Secretion of the processed peptides appeared to be unaltered (Loh and Gainer, 1978). It is possible that the carbohydrate moieties at specific regions of the protein molecule protect the molecule from nonspecific proteolysis and confer a specific conformation that could direct a programmed limited proteolysis that provides for correct processing (Loh and Gainer, 1978). It has been postulated that glycosylation is a requirement for secretion of proteins such as thyroglobulin (Monaco *et al.*, 1975), although it does not appear to be necessary for secretion of the adrenocorticotropin–β-lipotropin precursor (Loh and Gainer, 1978).

Many polypeptide hormones are synthesized as longer prohormones which are processed to the final active hormone by limited proteolysis. A "proerythropoietin" has not as yet been identified, although it had been suggested that biologically active erythropoietin is released from a liver-derived precursor after cleavage by a renal enzyme (Gordon et al., 1967). Recent studies have not supported this concept. This proposed mechanism of erythropoietin formation bears examination because of the emphasis it has received in the hematological literature.

Despite evidence that the kidney is the site of erythropoietin production, previous attempts to extract large amounts of active erythropoietin from renal tissue had been unsuccessful (Contrera and Gordon, 1966; Demopoulos et al., 1965; Naets, 1960). To explain these failures, Gordon et al.(1967) proposed that erythropoietin is synthesized in a manner analogous to the renin–angiotensin system; that the kidney synthesizes an enzyme which is capable of generating the active hormone from an inactive circulating plasma precursor. Contrera and Gordon (1966, 1968; Contrera et al., 1966; Wong et al., 1968) observed that the light mitochondrial fraction of renal tissue from hypoxic rats contained no detectable erythropoietic activity when assayed alone in the polycythemic mouse but, after incubation in vitro with normal rat serum, showed detectable activity. This enzyme was called "erythrogenin" by Gordon et al. Erythrogenin and plasma substrate production are presumably affected by the same factors that regulate erythropoietin production. Renal erythrogenin levels were increased by hypobaric hypoxia, bleeding, and cobalt (Gordon, 1973; Rodgers et al., 1975; Kaplan et al., 1977) and depressed by red cell plethora (Gordon et al., 1968) and hyperoxia (Kaplan et al., 1977).

Kuratowska et al. (1964; Kuratowska and Lewartowski, 1962) localized a factor in the nuclear fraction of hypoxic kidney tissue that similarly required prior incubation with plasma or serum in order to show detectable erythropoietic activity in the polycythemic mouse assay. These workers, however, suggested that their factor was an erythropoietin precursor processed by or complexed to a plasma globulin to generate activity. This proposed mechanism for the biogenesis of erythropoietin is shown in Scheme 1.

Although Gordon and co-workers have presented much evidence in support of the erythrogenin concept of erythropoietin synthesis, recent studies do not support this hypothesis. Erslev and Kazal (1969) did not detect erythrogenin in extracts from hypoxic renal tissue and, in subsequent studies, Erslev found biologically active erythropoietin after perfusion of hypoxic kidneys with serum-free tissue culture medium and without incubation with serum (Erslev, 1974).

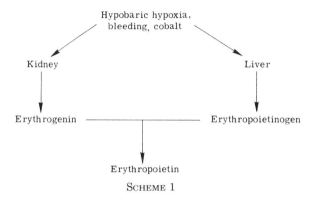

SCHEME 1

Sherwood and Goldwasser (1978) extracted significant amounts of active erythropoietin from the kidneys of normal rats, cattle, dogs, and rabbits by homogenization of the organs in 0.1 M phosphate buffer; these extracts were completely active without incubation with serum. The mean erythropoietin activity of the extracts, as determined in the starved-rat bioassay, was 0.26 units/g of beef kidney, 0.41 units/g of dog kidney, and 0.11 units/g of rat kidney. The dog kidney extracts showed a mean activity of 0.35 units/g in the *in vitro* cultured rat bone marrow assay, and produced a dose-dependent stimulation of ^{59}Fe incorporation into circulating red cells when assayed in the polycythemic mouse assay. The mean activity of five rabbit kidney cortical preparations was 2.12 units/g, as measured by stimulation of hemoglobin synthesis in the cultured rat bone marrow cells. The individual values are presented in Table V. Tests of erythropoietin from rabbit kidney cortex in either the radioimmunoassay or the marrow cell culture assay gave good agreement between biologically active (2.7 units/ml) and immunoreactive erythropoietin (2.9 units). Dog kidney homogenates yielded erythropoietin activity adsorbable to DEAE-cellulose from 0.01 M acetate buffer, pH 4.5, and elutable by 0.1 M Na$_2$HPO$_4$–0.5 M NaCl, pH 8 (Sherwood and Goldwasser, 1978), chromatographic behavior identical to that of sheep plasma erythropoietin (Goldwasser *et al.*, 1962a,b). An antibody made against human urinary erythropoietin completely inactivated the erythropoietic factor in the dog kidney extract (Table VI) (Sherwood and Goldwasser, 1978).

The erythropoietic activity of the extracts was not due to active plasma trapped in the renal vasculature, as serum from the dogs as well as from normal animals of other species did not contain amounts of erythropoietin detectable in *in vivo* assays. Based on the observations of Contrera *et al.* (1965) that there is 0.17 ml of residual plasma/g

TABLE V

STIMULATION OF HEMOGLOBIN SYNTHESIS BY EXTRACTS OF RABBIT
KIDNEY CORTEX[a,b]

Sample	^{59}Fe (cpm)	Units of erythropoietin/g tissue
Control	162 ± 14	
Experiment		
1	233 ± 23	1.24
2	226 ± 26	1.16
3	246 ± 38	2.22
4	286 ± 32	4.72
5	228 ± 30	1.24

[a]From Sherwood and Goldwasser (1978).

[b]Assays were done by the *in vitro* method. The 1_n dose–1_n response curve for simultaneously run erythropoietin standards gave a slope of 0.54, an intercept of 3.89, and a correlation coefficient of 0.98. All activities were significantly different from control values. For each experiment, the cortex from the kidneys of one rabbit was used.

of unwashed normal kidneys, Sherwood and Goldwasser (1978) calculated that the sera from the normal donor animals would have to contain 0.6–3 units of erythropoietin/ml of plasma for rat, dog, and beef kidneys and 6.8–27.8 units for rabbit kidney to attribute activity in kidney extracts to contaminating plasma. These observations have been confirmed by the work of Fried *et al.* (1980, 1981, 1982), in which active erythropoietin was extracted from the kidneys of rats.

The studies of Sherwood and Goldwasser (1978) provide evidence that the kidney contains erythropoietin similar in structure to that

TABLE VI

EFFECT OF ANTIERYTHROPOIETIN ON ACTIVITY OF DOG KIDNEY EXTRACT[a,b]

Sample	^{59}Fe (cpm)	Activity lost (%)
Control	48 ± 8	
Erythropoietin (3 mU)	89 ± 2	
Erythropoietin and antibody	49 ± 7[c]	100
Dog kidney extract	69 ± 6	
Dog kidney extract and antibody	45 ± 4[c]	100

[a]From Sherwood and Goldwasser (1978).

[b]All assays were done by the *in vitro* method. The values for antibody-treated samples were not significantly different from control values. The other values were significantly different at the $p < 0.02$ level.

[c]Antibody-treated samples.

found in plasma as shown by cross-reactivity with antibodies against human urinary erythropoietin (i.e., in the radioimmunoassay) or sheep plasma hormone (i.e., neutralization of activity) and by chromatographic behavior on DEAE-cellulose. These data do not support the hypothesis that the kidney synthesizes and secretes an enzyme erythrogenin that interacts with a plasma substrate. Our observations, however, do not negate the possibility that erythropoietin is synthesized as a prohormone and processed within the kidney.

Several explanations other than a renal erythropoietic factor–substrate interaction are possible to explain the previous observations that incubation of erythropoietically inactive kidney extract and normal serum produces an erythropoietically active incubation mixture. Since these studies have relied upon the relatively insensitive polycythemic mouse assay, it is possible that the kidney and the serum each contains active erythropoietin, but at concentrations below the sensitivity of this assay, approximately 0.05 units. When these components are combined in an incubation mixture, the combined erythropoietin level may be high enough to be detected in the bioassay. Indeed, the activity generated by incubating the renal factor and normal rat serum has been reported to be in the range of 0.02–0.10 units of erythropoietin/2 ml of incubation mixture (Gordon and Zanjani, 1970), and Contrera et al. (1966) reported that some of their kidney extracts contained low levels of activity. This possibility may explain the observations of Sherwood et al. (1972), that the supernatant fluids of organ cultures prepared from kidneys of hypoxic rats did not contain erythropoietic activity until after incubation with normal rat serum, a level of activity in the range of 0.04–0.09 units/ml of culture medium. Utilizing the more sensitive cultured bone marrow cell assay, Sherwood and Goldwasser (1976) found that human renal carcinoma cells in culture produced erythropoietin that was completely active without incubation with serum but was completely neutralized by antibody to human urinary erythropoietin.

It is also possible that erythropoietin forms a complex which slowly dissociates in solution, releasing the active hormone. Sytkowski (1980) showed that erythropoietin isolated from human urine exhibited a time-dependent increase in biological activity in solution independent of protease activity. Chromatography on BioGel of this erythropoietin incubated for varying periods suggested that the erythropoietin was in two forms—the native form and an erythropoietin–protein complex (Sytkowski, 1980). The nature of this proposed complex is unknown but might consist of erythropoietin bound to a protein molecule or of aggregates of erythropoietin molecules, perhaps reflecting interaction of glycoproteins through carbohydrate residues. Indeed, Miyake *et al.* (1977) found that either pure native or asialo erythropoietin shows considerable tendency to aggregate at pH 6. [After initial homogenization procedures, renal tissue extracts are often at low pH (Sherwood and Goldwasser, unpublished observations).]

The results presented in this article as well as by others indicate that active erythropoietin is produced within the kidney. Whether erythropoietin is synthesized in prohormone form and subsequently glycosylated and processed prior to secretion is as yet unknown.

Recent cloning studies by Lee-Huang (1984) suggest that the kidney contains the erythropoietin message. In the studies performed by Lee-Huang, poly(A)$^+$ RNA was prepared from a human renal carcinoma; cDNA was then synthesized and inserted into *Escherichia coli*. Recombinant colonies containing protein that reacted with monoclonal antibodies to human erythropoietin were found.

III. PURIFICATION OF ERYTHROPOIETIN

The major impediment to investigation of erythropoietin chemistry and physiology has been the scarcity of pure erythropoietin. Purification of this acidic glycoprotein has proved to be a formidable task, because it exists in extremely small quantities in plasma and urine, is contaminated with plasma and urinary proteins of similar physicochemical properties, and uniform sources of high content are difficult to obtain. In anemia and hypoxic stress, high concentrations of erythropoietin are found in plasma and excreted in urine. Therefore, patients and animals with severe anemia have been considered as possible sources of this hormone. Sheep made anemic by phenylhydrazine injection (White *et al.*, 1960; White and Josh, 1959) have become a major source of commercially available erythropoietin preparations. Plasma from these sheep contains an average of 4–6 units/ml (Painter *et al.*, 1968), representing approximately 0.0001% of the plasma proteins. Human urine is an increasingly important source of erythropoietin for studies of structural, chemical, and biological properties, for development of radioimmunoassays, and potentially for clinical trials. The major sources of this human material are patients with hemoglobin concentrations below 6 g/dl, e.g., erythropoietin has been obtained from the urine of patients with aplastic anemia (Miyake *et al.*, 1977), and the anemia associated with hookworm infection (Espada *et al.*, 1972, 1973).

A. Sheep Plasma Erythropoietin

Most studies on purification of plasma erythropoietin have utilized sheep made anemic with phenylhydrazine (Goldwasser et al., 1962a,b; Goldwasser and Kung, 1968; Painter et al., 1968; White et al., 1960; White and Josh, 1959). Erythropoietin concentrations are inversely correlated with the severity of the anemia; White et al. (1960) demonstrated that the erythropoietin concentration in blood rises significantly at a hematocrit below 15%. Therefore, in order to obtain hightiter plasma, sheep are subjected to whole body irradiation (800 rads ^{60}Co γ rays) which inhibits erythropoietic differentiation, in addition to injections of phenylhydrazine. By means of this method, levels as high as 10,000 units have been reached (Painter et al., 1968).

Initial attempts to purify erythropoietin from plasma involved the removal of contaminating plasma proteins by precipitation methods such as acidification of the plasma (Borsook, 1959; Linman and Bethell, 1956), perchloric acid percipitation (Goldwasser et al., 1962a,b), alcohol precipitation (Kuratowska et al., 1962), precipitation by ammonium sulfate (Borsook, 1959; White et al., 1960), or a combination of these methods (Lowy and Keighley, 1966). These procedures, however, led to considerable losses of activity and yielded preparations containing at least 33 distinct components when chromatographed on calcium phosphate gel; erythropoietic activity was associated with a minor component (Goldwasser et al., 1962a,b). Subsequent methods for purifying erythropoietin have involved a combination of ion-exchange, precipitation, and adsorption techniques.

Goldwasser and co-workers have described a procedure for obtaining pure preparations of sheep erythropoietin with approximately 8000 units/mg of protein, as follows. Erythropoietin in the anemic sheep plasma was absorbed on DEAE-cellulose at low pH and low salt concentration and was then eluted from the DEAE at high pH and high salt concentration. This fraction is Step I erythropoietin and contains 1 unit/mg protein. The Step I fraction was chromatographed on IRC-50 (Amberlite XE-97), a cation-exchange resin, at pH 6; contaminating proteins were absorbed and the activity was recovered in the effluent as Step II erythropoietin. The Step II fraction was chromatographed on IRC-50 at pH 6 and is called Step III erythropoietin. Step III was precipitated with 0.67 saturated ammonium sulfate to yield a Step IV fraction (Goldwasser et al., 1962a,b). The Step IV erythropoietin was dissolved in 3 M LiCl and precipitated with ethanol, with the activity precipitating between alcohol concentrations of 65 and 90%. This material was desalted and chromatographed on sulfoethyl-Sephadex. Elu-

TABLE VII

PURIFICATION OF SHEEP PLASMA ERYTHROPOIETIN[a]

Fraction	Units/mg protein[b]	Yield (%)	Purification factor
Anemic plasma	0.007	—	—
Step IV (ammonium sulfate fraction)	26	100	3,700
P7 (precipitated between alcohol concentrations of 65 and 90%)	250	76	35,700
SE 4,5,6 (pooled fractions eluted with 0.015, 0.0175, and 0.20 M acetate buffers)	570	20	81,300
Calcium phosphate gel eluate (eluted with 0.01 M phosphate)	1,670	6.6	238,000
Methylated albumin–Kieselguhr eluate (eluted with 0.01 M phosphate)[c]	7,450	2	1,050,000
	8,250	—	1,180,000

[a]Data from Goldwasser and Kung (1971).
[b]In vivo assays with the fasted rat and polycythemic mouse methods.
[c]This fraction was derived from a different experiment, utilizing more starting material.

tion was stepwise with acetate buffers of increasing molarity and pH. The activity eluted with the following acetate buffers—0.015 M, pH 5.0; 0.0175 M, pH 5.28; and 0.20 M, pH 5.6—and these fractions were pooled, desalted, and absorbed onto calcium phosphate gel. The major portion of the activity was eluted with 5×10^{-4} M phosphate buffer, pH 7.3, and this fraction was chromatographed on a methylated albumin–Kieselguhr column. The fraction eluted with 0.01 M phosphate buffer, pH 7.2, was of high potency—7450 and 8250 units/mg of protein (data derived from two separate purification procedures) (Goldwasser and Kung, 1971). This fractionation procedure is summarized in Table VII.

Enough material was obtained in these studies to perform preliminary analysis of biologic activity and homogeneity. Measurements of biologic activity were performed in the polycythemic mouse and starved rat assays, and a linear log dose–log response curve was obtained in the rat bone marrow culture assay. Analysis of ^{125}I-labeled material by microgel electrophoresis indicated a single peak, with a small shoulder on the slower side that contained 7.5% of the total label. Desialation of this material, using *Cholera vibrio* neuraminidase, caused loss of the shoulder and shift in the relative mobility of the single peak, suggesting that the shoulder represented partially or completely desialated erythropoietin (Goldwasser and Kung, 1971).

Although this sheep plasma erythropoietin preparation appears to be homogeneous or nearly so by polyacrylamide gel electrophoresis, the human erythropoietin recently purified by the same group (Miyake *et al.*, 1977) showed a potency 7–10 times greater than the sheep material when assayed by the same methods. This suggests either the presence of undetected contaminants in the sheep material or an artifact in the assay systems used, a possibility suggested by differences in dose–response slopes between sheep and human erythropoietin in the polycythemic mouse assay (Annable *et al.*, 1972), and in immunoreactivity with antibody against human erythropoietin (Schooley and Mahlmann, 1972).

B. HUMAN URINARY ERYTHROPOIETIN

Under conditions of anemic and hypoxic stress, large quantities of erythropoietin are excreted into the urine, thereby making this a potentially valuable source of the hormone. Efforts in several laboratories have been directed toward purification of erythropoietin from the urine of patients with the anemia of hookworm infection (Espada *et al.*, 1972, 1973), aplastic anemia (Miyake *et al.*, 1977), and other anemias associated with hemoglobin levels of 6 g/dl or less (Dukes, 1980). Urine from these patients usually contains at least 0.4 units/ml (Dukes, 1980), a concentration which makes this source usable as starting material for purification.

Purification of erythropoietin from urine presents problems, because of contamination with proteases and sialidases which inactivate erythropoietin (Chiba *et al.*, 1972), and with endotoxin (Spivak and Levin, 1977) and certain proteins such as colony-stimulating factor (Metcalf and Stanley, 1969), which can interact with hematopoietic stem cells (Metcalf and Stanley, 1969; Zuckerman *et al.*, 1979).

Erythropoietin is inactivated by a number of proteases, including trypsin, pepsin, chymotrypsin A, elastase, papain, ficin, and bromelain (Espada *et al.*, 1973; Winkert and Gordon, 1960), as well as by sialidase (Lowy *et al.*, 1960; Rosse and Waldmann, 1964; Winkert and Gordon, 1960). Crude preparations of human urinary erythropoietin contain protease activity sufficient to inactivate up to 60% of the hormone during storage at −20°C over a 20-week period (Chiba *et al.*, 1972). Although urine normally contains proteases such as uropepsin and urokinase, the enzymes responsible for inactivating urinary erythropoietin preparations have not been identified. Proteolytic activity in several crude preparations from human urine were not inhibited by protease inhibitors including phenylmethylsulfonyl fluoride, aprotinin, benzamidine, pepstatin, sodium tetrathionate, TLCK, and TPCK, nor by EDTA, EGTA, 2-mercaptoethanol, or guanidine. Heating at 50°C for 5 minutes inactivated the proteolytic activity but not erythropoietin (Mok and Spivak, 1982). Crude urinary erythropoietin loses biologic activity at pH 4.5 (Saidi and Gurney, 1970), suggesting activation of a protease such as uropepsin (Mok and Spivak, 1982), although mild acid hydrolysis, which removes terminal sialic acid residues, also inactivates the hormone (Rambach et al., 1958).

Treatment of the urine with 0.1% phenol (Dukes, 1980; Lowy and Keighley, 1961) and with phenol-p-aminosalicylate (Chiba et al., 1972; Miyake et al., 1977) effectively reduces the loss of erythropoietic activity and is now the method commonly employed during collection and concentration of erythropoietin-rich urine.

The need for large volumes of urine has been a major obstacle to purification, and several methods of concentrating erythropoietin have been utilized. The initial concentration steps most commonly employed are (1) hollow fiber dialysis-concentration, (2) membrane ultrafiltration, and (3) concentration by dialysis against Carbowax 20-M (polyethylene glycol), a drying agent (Dukes, 1980).

Current purification methods have employed (1) conventional chromatographic techniques based on molecular size and charge (Miyake et al., 1977), (2) affinity chromatography using lectin–agarose derivatives (Sieber, 1977; Spivak et al., 1977, 1978), based on the interaction between the lectin and specific carbohydrate moieties of erythropoietin, and (3) hydrophobic interaction chromatography (Lee-Huang, 1980). The recent development of monoclonal antibodies (Lee-Huang, 1982a,b; Weiss et al., 1982) has led to preliminary attempts to purify erythropoietin by immunoaffinity methods, which may prove to be a promising approach.

The first successful purification of erythropoietin from crude urinary material was accomplished by Goldwasser and co-workers in 1977 (Miyake et al., 1977), and involved a series of conventional chromatographic steps. The starting material was urine from patients with chronic aplastic anemia having 1–6 units/ml of erythropoietic activity. The urine was treated with phenol p-aminosalicylate (Chiba et al., 1972) to inactivate proteases and sialidases, desalted on Sephadex gel, and adsorbed on DEAE-cellulose at pH 5.5 and low ionic strength; the active fraction was eluted from the exchanger with 0.05 M Na$_2$HPO$_4$– 0.15 M NaCl, dialyzed free of salt and lyophilized. This material was dissolved in phosphate-buffered saline to which LiCl, which has been found to increase the solubility of proteins in ethanol (Lowy and Keighley, 1966), was added. Preliminary precipitation with ethanol re-

TABLE VIII
PURIFICATION OF HUMAN URINARY ERYTHROPOIETIN[a]

	Input		Product		Yield (%)	
Step	Units	Potency[b] (U/A)	Units	Potency[b] (U/A)	Each step	Overall
DEAE-cellulose			6,976,170	89	100	100
Phenol	7,059,670	91	5,115,110	110	72	72
Ethanol	5,186,690	88	4,750,740	660	92	66
DEAE-agarose	4,566,240	563	4,052,710	1,107	89	59
Sulfopropyl-Sephadex	2,480,400	1,750	1,352,810	11,170	55	32
Sephadex G-100	1,259,040	12,830	1,274,430	39,060	100	32
Hydroxylapatite	1,083,650	38,770	721,160	82,720[c]	67	21

[a]From Miyake et al. (1977).
[b]Potency (specific activity) is expressed as units of erythropoietic activity in the fasted rat bioassay per absorbance unit (A, 278 nm).
[c]The overall purification factor was 929, calculated from initial and final potencies.

moved contaminating proteins, and the active material was then precipitated when the supernatant was brought to 90% ethanol. The 90% ethanol precipitate was dissolved and chromatographed on DEAE-agarose; elution was accomplished with Tris–$CaCl_2$ buffers of increasing ionic strength, and approximately 90% of the activity was recovered in the 17 mM $CaCl_2$ eluate. This eluate was chromatographed on sulfopropyl-Sephadex and eluted with calcium acetate buffers of increasing ionic strength; 55% of the input activity was recovered in the 12.5 mM calcium acetate fraction. This material was gel filtered on Sephadex G-100, and 100% of the input activity was recovered in the fractions that eluted prior to the bovine serum albumin monomer marker. The active fractions were pooled, concentrated, and chromatographed on hydroxylapatite; elution was accomplished with phosphate buffers of increasing ionic strength. Most of the activity was contained in the fractions eluted with 1 mM phosphate (Fraction II, 32% of input activity) and 2 mM phosphate (Fraction IIIA, 21% of input activity). This purification scheme is summarized in Table VIII (Miyake et al., 1977).

The final pure material has a mean potency of 70,400 units/mg of protein. This material appears to be homogeneous in that it gave single peaks upon gel electrophoresis at pH 6, 9, and 7 in sodium dodecyl sulfate (Fig. 5). Recent evidence suggests that there is a single NH_2-terminal amino acid in this material (Goldwasser, 1982). Fractions II and IIIA (α and β) may represent microheterogeneity in the carbohy-

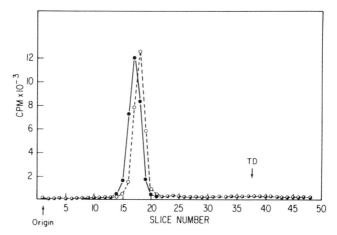

FIG. 5. Gel electrophoresis of ^{125}I-labeled erythropoietin at pH 6, in 0.05% Triton X-100. Native erythropoietin, hydroxylapatite Fraction II (alpha epo) (●); asialoerythropoietin (○); tracking dye (TD). From Miyake *et al.* (1977).

drate moiety, a characteristic of glycoproteins. These two fractions were discussed fully in Section II.

A preparative procedure for erythropoietin has been developed (Lee-Huang, 1980) based on the hydrophobicity of erythropoietin. The amino acid analysis of the human urinary material (Goldwasser, 1981a) indicates that a significant percentage of the amino acid residues is nonpolar (Table II). Therefore, hydrophobic interaction chromatography was utilized to separate erythropoietin from other urinary proteins of similar size and charge as well as carbohydrate structure. Unprocessed urine concentrates from anemic subjects were applied directly to phenyl-Sepharose columns, in a buffer with a high salt concentration (10 mM sodium phosphate containing 4 M NaCl), which facilitates the interaction of hydrophobic groups. Ninety percent of the contaminants were excluded and all of the erythropoietic activity was bound to the gel. The hormone was eluted with 20% ethylene glycol in 10 mM NaOH containing 4 M guanidine hydrochloride. Ethylene glycol decreases the strength of hydrophobic interactions and is essential in eluting erythropoietin from the phenyl-Sepharose. This single chromatography step produces 120-fold purification with a recovery of 85% of the activity.

The active fraction was subjected to affinity chromatography on concanavalin A-Sepharose (Lee-Huang, 1980), to which colony-stimulating factor (CSF) but not erythropoietin is bound (Spivak *et al.*, 1977, 1978; Lee-Huang, 1980). The excluded material from the Con A-

Sepharose column was chromatographed on phytohemagglutinin (E)-Sepharose, a lectin that binds oligosaccharides with a terminal sialic acid residue and a penultimate galactose (Kornfeld and Kornfeld, 1970), the carbohydrate structure found in erythropoietin (Dordal and Goldwasser, 1982). The active material from this step can be chromatographed on Sephadex G-100 to remove contaminants and the active fractions pooled and subjected to adsorption chromatography on hydroxylapatite. The majority of the erythropoietic activity elutes with 1 and 2 mM phosphate. This purification scheme (Lee-Huang, 1980; and personal communication) is summarized in Table IX.

The erythropoietin purified by this scheme shows a single major component in sodium dodecyl sulfate–polyacrylamide gel electrophoresis and disc gel electrofocusing, suggesting that this material is homogeneous. The molecular weight was determined by gel electrophoresis (SDS–PAGE) which gave a value of 38,000 (Lee-Huang, personal communication), which is in agreement with the value of 39,000 reported by Miyake et al. (1977) for sialoerythropoietin.

Lectin affinity chromatography has been utilized as a method for the partial purification of erythropoietin by Spivak et al. (1977, 1978; Rodman et al., 1981). Only wheat germ agglutinin and phytohemagglutinin show specific affinities for erythropoietin, whereas concana-

TABLE IX

PURIFICATION OF HUMAN URINARY ERYTHROPOIETIN BY HYDROPHOBIC INTERACTION CHROMATOGRAPHY[a]

Step	Potency[b] (U/mg)	Yield	Purification
Crude urine concentrate[c]	0.66	100	—
1. Phenyl-Sepharose CL-4B	79.20	85	120
2. Con A-Sepharose 4B			
3. PHA (E)-Sepharose 4B			
4. Sephadex G-100			
5. Hydroxylapatite			
Unconcentrated urine[c]	1.1	100	—
1. Phenyl-Sepharose CL-4B	116	84	105

[a]According to Lee-Huang (1980), and personal communication.

[b]Potency is expressed as units of erythropoietin/mg of protein. Erythropoietin was measured in the exhypoxic polycythemic mouse assay.

[c]From crude urine from anemic patients.

valin A binds colony-stimulating factor, a glycoprotein hemopoietin with properties similar to erythropoietin.

The development of monoclonal antibodies to erythropoietin (Lee-Huang, 1982a,b; Weiss *et al.*, 1982) now permits the use of immunoaffinity methods for the purification of erythropoietin. Yanagawa *et al.* (1984) recently described the isolation of human erythropoietin using an immunoadsorbent column of monoclonal antibodies against erythropoietin. The purified hormone had a specific activity of 81,600 U/mg of protein. The presence of a single NH_2-terminal alanine suggests that the preparation is homogeneous.

Purification of erythropoietin has been hampered by lack of a rich source of the hormone and by the lack of efficient purification schemes. Recent approaches to purification of erythropoietin have utilized fewer steps, with the aim of increasing yield. This objective has not yet been accomplished, however. The end point, based on the previously published purification of Miyake *et al.* (1977), is a potency of approximately 70,000 units/mg of protein.

IV. ASSAYS FOR ERYTHROPOIETIN

One of the major impediments to the study of erythropoietin physiology has been the lack of assays sensitive enough to detect normal amounts of the hormone in human plasma, as well as fluctuations of hormone levels. The three major categories of assays presently in use are the *in vivo* plethoric mouse and fasted rat bioassays, the *in vitro* bioassays utilizing cultured bone marrow or liver cells, and the immunoassays (Table X).

The bioassays are based on the specific biologic response induced by erythropoietin, namely, the differentiation of hematopoietic precursor cells along erythroid lines. Two major classes of erythroid progenitor cells have been recognized—erythroid burst-forming units (BFU-E) and erythroid colony-forming units (CFU-E), which are progeny of the BFU-E (Iscove and Guilbert, 1978; Iscove and Sieber, 1975). Erythropoietin regulates the growth of the CFU-E in particular, although it may regulate the BFU-E also, and induces the process of differentiation leading to hemoglobin synthesis (Iscove and Guilbert, 1978) (Fig. 1).

All of the bioassays currently in use measure one of the following three end points.

TABLE X
ASSAYS FOR ERYTHROPOIETIN

Assay	Parameter measured	Limit of sensitivity (units)
In vivo bioassays		
Exhypoxic polycythemic mouse	^{59}Fe uptake into peripheral red cells	0.05
Plethoric mouse		0.05
Fasted rat		1.00
In vitro bioassays		
Bone marrow (rat, mouse, rabbit, etc.)	^{59}Fe uptake into hemoglobin Erythroid colony formation	0.002
Fetal liver (mouse, etc.)	[^{3}H]Uridine incorporation into RNA Erythroid colony formation ^{59}Fe uptake into hemoglobin	0.002
Immunoassays		
Radioimmunoassays	Displacement of labeled tracer (^{125}I-labeled erythropoietin)	0.001

1. Colony formation. Both BFU-E and CFU-E are found in populations of bone marrow cells and grow in agar and plasma clot cultures as colonies of cells which can be distinguished on the basis of colony growth pattern and the length of time required for colony formation. The number of colonies per culture dish can be correlated with the amount of erythropoietin added to the dish (Iscove and Guilbert, 1978; Iscove and Sieber, 1975).

2. Increase in RNA synthesis. Stimulation of RNA synthesis is the earliest detectable event after exposure of erythrocyte precursors to erythropoietin (Goldwasser, 1975). Bessler *et al.* (1980) obtained a dose–response relationship between erythropoietin concentration and [^{3}H]uridine incorporation in cultured 12-day-old fetal mouse liver proerythroblasts.

3. Increased hemoglobin synthesis. This is the marker most relied upon in erythropoietin bioassays, both in *in vivo* and *in vitro* systems. ^{59}Fe uptake into newly synthesized hemoglobin is directly related to the amount of erythropoietin added to the assay system, and a log dose–response curve is obtained.

The most widely used assays, and the first to be developed, are the *in vivo* bioassays. These assays utilize a test animal in which endogenous erythropoietin production has been suppressed by fasting (Fried *et al.*, 1957) or by induction of polycythemia with transfusion of packed red cells or exposure to atmospheric hypoxia with subsequent mainte- nance at normal oxygen tension (Cotes and Bangham, 1961; Jacobson *et al.*, 1957). These animals are sensitive to erythropoietic stimuli; the percentage of ^{59}Fe incorporated into peripheral red blood cells is di- rectly related to the amount of erythropoietin injected. A minimum dose of 1 unit of erythropoietin in the starved rat and of 0.02–0.05 units in the exhypoxic and polycythemic mouse is necessary to induce a statistically significant increase in the percentage of ^{59}Fe incorporat- ed into the red cells. Therefore, this assay does not detect normal or subnormal amounts of erythropoietin in human serum.

The tissue culture assays utilizing bone marrow (Goldwasser *et al.*, 1975) or fetal liver (Dunn *et al.*, 1975) cells which are rich in erythroid precursors are significantly more sensitive than the *in vivo* bioassays, detecting from 1 to 5 mU of erythropoietin. Figure 6 shows a typical dose–response curve obtained with the mouse bone marrow cell culture assay (Goldwasser *et al.*, 1975). In addition to erythropoietin,

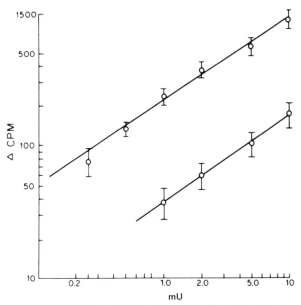

Fig. 6. Dose–response curve: ^{59}Fe uptake versus milliunits of erythropoietin standard in the cultured rat bone marrow cell assay. Upper curve, total ^{59}Fe uptake; lower curve, ^{59}Fe uptake into hematin; vertical bars ± 1 SD. From Goldwasser *et al.* (1975).

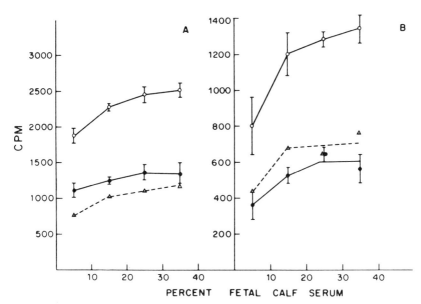

FIG. 7. Effect of fetal calf serum concentration on the total ^{59}Fe uptake (A) and on hematin synthesis (^{59}Fe uptake into hematin) (B). Controls (○), cells treated with 5 mU erythropoietin (●), change in cpm due to erythropoietin (△); vertical bars ± 1 SD. From Goldwasser *et al.* (1975).

these assay systems are modulated by numerous factors such as the concentration of iron and transferrin, the type of fetal calf serum, prostaglandins, and other inducing factors, and by inhibitors in serum such as complement-dependent antibodies (Fig. 7).

The need for a reliable, precise, highly sensitive, and specific radioimmunoassay for erythropoietin has long been evident. However, until pure erythropoietin was available, development of a radioimmunoassay was not feasible. There have been reports of immunologic assays for erythropoietin using impure hormone preparations (Cotes, 1973; Garcia, 1972; Lange *et al.*, 1968; Lertora *et al.*, 1975); the data from these assays are unreliable. The purification of erythropoietin by Miyake *et al.* (1977) permitted the development of a radioimmunoassay for erythropoietin simultaneously in two laboratories, using the same erythropoietin preparation (Sherwood and Goldwasser, 1979; Garcia *et al.*, 1979).

The Sherwood and Goldwasser assay will be described in this review, as this (with the assay of Garcia) was the first to be described (Sherwood and Goldwasser, 1979) and the one with which this author is most familiar. This radioimmunoassay (RIA) is specific for human erythropoietin, and sensitive enough to detect 0.002–0.003 units. With this method, normal, reduced, and elevated concentrations of human serum erythropoietin can be measured directly and accurately for the first time (Sherwood and Goldwasser, 1979).

The preparation of Miyake *et al.* (1977) is used as the labeled tracer and as standard. Radioiodination has been routinely performed by the method of Fraker and Speck (1978) using the water-insoluble oxidizing agent 1,3,4,6-tetrachloro-3,6-diphenylglycoluril (iodogen, Pierce Chemical Co.); the chloramine-T method and Bolton–Hunter reagent (1973) which acylates amino groups of the protein with the ^{125}I-labeled *p*-hydroxyphenylpropionic residue are also utilized. Although all methods of iodination have so far resulted in loss of biological activity, immunoreactivity is not altered as suggested by the similar standard curves produced with the two iodinated preparations as tracers (Fig. 8).

Antibodies were raised in rabbits, using a preparation of crude human urinary erythropoietin as immunogen. The antiserum we have been using at a dilution of 1:10,000 consistently gives a standard curve with the linear portion located between 1 mU (approximately 12 pg of

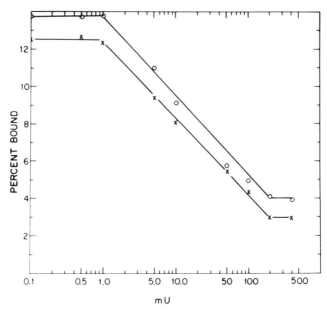

FIG. 8. Effect of iodination on immunoreactivity of erythropoietin. Iodogen method (○), Bolton–Hunter method (×). From Sherwood and Goldwasser (1979).

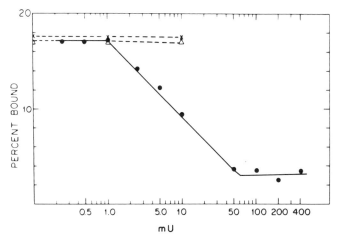

Fig. 9. Lack of reactivity of other glycoproteins with antibody to erythropoietin. Erythropoietin, human urinary standard (●) was compared with mouse lung cell colony-stimulating factor (×) at 10, 100, and 1000 pg and with human orosomucoid (△) at 0.1, 1.0, and 10 μg. From Sherwood and Goldwasser (1979).

protein) and 100–200 mU of erythropoietin, with a 50% inhibition of binding of ligand at 10–15 mU of erythropoietin (Fig. 8). This sensitivity is sufficient to detect normal or depressed concentrations of human serum erythropoietin.

Neither human serum orosomucoid nor pure mouse lung cell colony-stimulating factor, both glycoproteins with terminal sialic acid residues, compete with binding of ^{125}I-labeled erythropoietin to the antiserum (Fig. 9). Erythropoietin from nonhuman sources can be measured in this radioimmunoassay, although there appears to be a difference between human and some animal material with regard to reactivity with the antihuman erythropoietin antibody as suggested by the discrepancy between the bioassay and radioimmunoassay titers (Table XI). This confirms a report of Schooley and Mahlmann (1972) who showed that neutralization of sheep erythropoietin was not as effective as neutralization of human erythropoietin when an antiserum to the human hormone was used. Removal of sialic acid does not alter the immunoreactivity of erythropoietin, confirming the results of Garcia (1972), although *in vivo* biologic activity is lost, as shown by Goldwasser *et al.* (1974).

The competitive inhibition curves obtained with human serum samples are parallel to that produced by pure human erythropoietin stan-

TABLE XI

COMPARISON OF RADIOIMMUNOASSAY, MARROW CELL CULTURE ASSAY, AND *in Vivo*
ASSAY FOR ERYTHROPOIETIN FROM NONHUMAN SOURCES[a,b]

| | Erythropoietin (units/ml) found by | | |
Sample	Radioimmunoassay	Marrow cell culture	*In vivo* assay
Beef fetal liver extract	0.11	—	0.25
Dog kidney extract	0.09	—	0.95
Dog kidney extract	0.08	—	0.75
Sheep plasma erythropoietin	0.01	—	0.001
Rabbit kidney cortex extract			
1	0.56	1.16	—
2	6.00	4.70	—
3	1.95	1.24	—

[a]From Sherwood and Goldwasser (1979).

[b]The *in vivo* assays were done by the fasted rat method. For the radioimmunoassay, pure human urinary erythropoietin was used as the labeled tracer; the antibody was made against human urinary erythropoietin.

dard (Fig. 10), suggesting that the material in serum behaves immunologically like human erythropoietin. This evidence supports the interpretation that the substance detected in human serum by the radioimmunoassay is indeed erythropoietin.

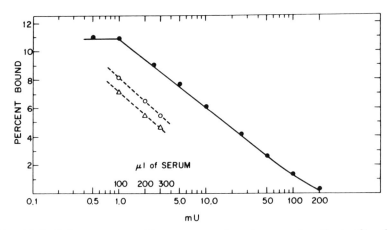

FIG. 10. Radioimmunoassay of human serum from two anemic patients (○ and △), compared with the human urinary erythropoietin standard (●). From Sherwood and Goldwasser (1979).

None of the assays used previously had been sensitive or specific enough to detect erythropoietin in normal human serum. The RIA now makes it possible to determine normal values. Sera from 66 normal healthy volunteers were assayed. The mean result was 21 ± 6 (SD) mU/ml with no significant difference between males and females and no correlation with hematocrit (hematocrit range: 37–49). Analysis of sera from patients showed the expected correlations between hypoxia, erythrocytosis, and elevated titers of erythropoietin found by RIA. For example (1) a patient with obstructive lung disease and hypoxia showed a titer of 122 mU/ml; (2) of six patients with erythrocytosis associated with heart or lung disease, five displayed titers above normal and one was normal; (3) two patients who received cadaver kidney transplants and subsequently developed increasingly high hematocrits (greater than 50%) with no evidence of secondary hypoxia or polycythemia vera showed erythropoietin titers of 49 and 350 mU/ml, re-

TABLE XII

ASSAY OF HUMAN SERUM SAMPLES[a]

Serum	Diagnosis	Units of erythropoietin/ml	
		RIA	Bioassay
Pool	Normal	0.020	—
J1	Normal	0.020	—
M1	Normal	0.036	—
J2	Polycythemia vera	0.025	—
M2	Anephric	0.010	0.02–0.005[b]
H1	Erythrocytosis secondary to hypoxia	0.086	0.054–0.015
J3	Chronic renal disease	0.240	0.085–0.02
B1	Chronic renal disease	0.160	0.02–0.008[b]
W1	Atypical myeloproliferative disease	2.18	2.46–0.5
W2	Atypical myeloproliferative disease	0.68	0.58–0.1
R	Hypoplastic anemia	0.16	0.16–0.02
J4	Iron-deficiency anemia	0.39	0.57–0.1

[a]From Sherwood and Goldwasser (1979).

[b]In this particular bioassay using the plethoric mouse method, the control ^{59}Fe uptake was 1.6%, 0.05 U yielded 8.8%, and 0.10 U, 13.4%. The sensitivity of the assay was sufficiently high to permit an appropriate estimate of the titers of the two 1-ml serum samples, using a log–log dose–response curve. Sample M2 showed 4.8% iron uptake and sample B1, 5.9%. If the curve is linear below the 0.05 U level, these estimates are reasonable; if the curve flattens at the low doses, these titers are overestimates.

spectively. Analyses by RIA and bioassay (plethoric mouse assay) showed reasonable agreement on serum taken from patients with diverse disorders (Table XII).

Discrepancies between bioassay and radioimmunoassay data (Table XII, sera J3 and B1) suggested that erythropoietin is found in native, biologically active form as well as in immunologically active but biologically inactive forms. Gel permeation chromatography of serum from normal individuals and from patients with chronic renal failure indicated that circulating erythropoietin appears as the native form, as high-molecular-weight material, and as fragments smaller than the native hormone (Goldwasser and Sherwood, 1981).

Other laboratories have recently reported on the development of radioimmunoassays, also using the Miyake and Goldwasser preparation of pure erythropoietin (Cotes, 1982; Zaroulis et al., 1981). Results for normal subjects with these radioimmunoassays agreed with those of Sherwood and Goldwasser (1979). As more pure hormone becomes available, it is expected that radioimmunoassays of greater sensitivity will be established.

V. SITE OF ERYTHROPOIETIN PRODUCTION

The primary role of the kidney in the formation of erythropoietin has been established by clinical observations such as the association between renal neoplasms and erythrocytosis and the presence of anemia in patients with chronic renal disease, and by the use of experimental systems employing anephric animals, perfused kidney preparations, extracts of kidney tissue, and renal tissue maintained in vitro. The initial studies were performed on nephrectomized or ureter-ligated animals and on isolated kidneys perfused with whole blood or experimental solutions. These studies have been extensively reviewed elsewhere and will not be discussed in depth in this article. Extraction of native erythropoietin from normal kidneys is a more recent development (Sherwood and Goldwasser, 1978) and has been described in the section on erythropoietin chemistry.

A. ANEPHRIC MODELS

Direct evidence that the kidney is the chief site of erythropoietin production was provided by the experiments of Jacobson and co-workers (Jacobson et al., 1957, 1959), showing that only bilateral nephrectomy and not removal of other organs abolished the capacity of rats and rabbits to produce increased amounts of erythropoietin in response to acute hemorrhage, administration of cobaltous chloride, or hypoxia. These results were not due to uremia, since bilateral ureteral ligation, producing a degree of uremia comparable to that of nephrectomy, did not inhibit erythropoietin production in response to the same types of stimuli (Jacobson *et al.*, 1957, 1959).

Of particular interest is the work of Naets (1960) which suggested that the kidney is the sole site of erythropoietin production in the dog. After nephrectomy, erythropoiesis ceased under control conditions and in response to bleeding. In contrast, dogs with bilateral ureteral ligation maintained erythropoietic function despite comparable uremia (Naets, 1960).

In species other than dogs, however, erythropoiesis and increased erythropoietin production are not completely inhibited by nephrectomy. This was found by Rosse and Waldmann (Rosse and Waldmann, 1962; Waldmann and Rosse, 1962) utilizing normal rats parabiosed to a normal, ureter-ligated, or nephrectomized partner. The highest percentage red blood cell radioiron incorporation was obtained with the normal or ureter-ligated partner exposed to hypoxia; exposure of the nephrectomized partner produced values that were low but significantly greater than in the controls (no exposure). Although it thus appears that the kidney is not fully required for rats to respond to hypoxic anoxia, Mirand *et al.* (1959) has suggested that it is required for increased erythropoietin production after challenge with anemic hypoxia or cobalt. Nephrectomized rabbits in the preuremic phase are capable of producing erythropoietin in response to challenge with acute anemic anoxia (Erslev, 1959).

These observations strongly suggest that, in some species, extrarenal tissues have the capacity to produce erythropoietin. The kidney, however, appears to be an important source of erythropoietin in all species studied so far.

B. Perfusion Studies

Direct evidence that the kidney is an important site of production or activation of erythropoietin has come from perfusion studies utilizing isolated organs. Isolated kidneys perfused with hypoxic blood (Fisher and Langston, 1967, 1968; Kuratowska *et al.*, 1961; Pavlovic-Kentera *et al.*, 1965; Reissmann and Nomura, 1962; Zangheri *et al.*, 1963) or with blood containing cobalt (Fisher and Langston, 1967, 1968; Fisher *et al.*, 1965) produced increased titers of erythropoietin in the perfusates. No significant increase was obtained with perfusates of blood at normal or increased oxygen tension, or from other organs. Histologic evaluation of the perfused kidneys indicates that the release of erythropoietin was not due to cell breakdown, i.e., histologic integrity was retained concomitant with significant elevations of erythropoietin content in the perfusates (Fisher and Langston, 1967, 1968). In addition, nephrotoxic substances such as organic and inorganic mercurials inhibited the response to erythropoietic stimuli (Gordon *et al.*, 1967).

C. Clinical Observations

The influence of the kidney on red blood cell formation was suggested by observations of anemia in chronic renal disease (Desforges and Dawson, 1958; Lange and Gallagher, 1962; Loge *et al.*, 1950; Naets *et al.*, 1968). Patients with renal insufficiency do not appear to show increased plasma levels of erythropoietin in response to the associated anemia (Sherwood *et al.*, 1981), while patients with normal renal function and a similar degree of anemia have elevated levels (Lange and Gallagher, 1962; Naets *et al.*, 1968; Sherwood *et al.*, 1981). The degree of anemia and renal excretory failure appears to be correlated, with the amount of erythropoietin produced by the kidney decreasing with increased excretory failure (Adamson *et al.*, 1968). In severe renal failure, the kidney can retain some capacity to produce erythropoietin (Caro *et al.*, 1979).

Denny *et al.* (1966) noted that in a series of patients undergoing renal homotransplantation, no plasma erythropoietin could be detected prior to bilateral nephrectomy and during the anephric state prior to transplantation. After transplantation, significant increases in erythropoietin titer were detected in the plasmas of certain patients, with no correlation noted between the usual parameters of renal function and the ability of the transplant to produce erythropoietin (Denny *et al.*, 1966; Naets *et al.*, 1968).

D. Production of Erythropoietin by Renal
and Nonrenal Tumors

Erythrocytosis is often observed in man in association with certain renal cysts (Rosse *et al.*, 1963; Waldmann *et al.*, 1968), and with renal tumors such as renal adenomas, hypernephromas, sarcomas, etc. (Donati *et al.*, 1963; Forssell, 1954; Waldmann *et al.*, 1968). In addition, erythrocytosis has been found in conjunction with nonrenal tumors, i.e., the ectopic hormone syndrome, such as cerebellar hemangioblastomas (Rosse *et al.*, 1963; Waldmann *et al.*, 1961), adrenal cortical carcinomas (Meineke, 1969), and hepatomas (Brownstein and Ballard, 1966; Gordon *et al.*, 1970). The clinical hematologic picture is characterized by high total red cell mass and, usually, by normal white blood cell count, platelet count, plasma volume, and erythroid hyperplasia in the bone marrow. Lack of the characteristics of polycythemia vera— elevated white cell count, platelet count, and splenomegaly—or secondary polycythemia—decreased arterial oxygen saturation—distinguishes between erythrocytosis observed with renal tumors as compared to ectopic tumors.

Erythrocytosis, however, is observed in only 5–10% of patients with renal cell carcinoma; anemia is found much more frequently in up to 25% of patients with localized tumors. Sufrin *et al.* (1977) determined erythropoietin in plasma from 57 patients with renal adenocarcinoma. Sixty-three percent of the patients showed erythropoietin levels that were detectable in the polycythemic mouse bioassay. The corresponding hematocrits of these patients showed no correlation with erythropoietin level, i.e., anemia in certain patients was not a stimulus for elevated erythropoietin production, and erythrocytosis did not necessarily accompany elevated erythropoietin levels. Bagley *et al.* (1982), using the radioimmunoassay of Sherwood and Goldwasser (1979), determined immunoreactive erythropoietin in 40 patients with renal adenocarcinoma, 7 with renal cysts, 1 with an echinococcal cyst, 1 with metastatic thryoid carcinoma to the kidney, and 3 with transitional cell carcinoma. Immunoreactive erythropoietin was elevated in 50% of all patients with adenocarcinoma of the kidney and in four out of five patients with stage-4 tumors, the most advanced neoplasms. High erythropoietin levels were not found in two of the patients with renal cysts nor in any of the patients with other types of carcinomas. In addition, higher erythropoietin concentrations were observed in the vein draining the tumor-containing kidney. Erythrocytosis did not occur in these patients.

High concentrations of erythropoietin have been detected in the plasma of patients with hepatic carcinoma (Gordon *et al.*, 1970) and pheochromocytoma (Waldmann and Bradley, 1961). Significant erythropoietic-stimulating activity has been found in fluids from renal cysts (Rosse *et al.*, 1963) and from cerebellar hemangioblastoma cysts (Waldmann *et al.*, 1961), as well as in saline extracts of hypernephroma tissue (Waldmann *et al.*, 1968), and of renal cyst wall (Nixon *et al.*, 1960).

The erythropoietic factor associated with these tumors and erythropoietin isolated from anemic and anoxic serum show identical phys-

TABLE XIII

ERYTHROPOIETIC ACTIVITY FROM CULTURES OF A HUMAN RENAL GRANULAR
CELL CARCINOMA[a]

Tumor cell culture medium	Age of culture[b] (days)	Units/ml[c]
Primary culture	66	0.44
Second passage	100	0.06
Third passage	115	0.08
Fourth passage	150	0.09
Normal monkey kidney (primary)	20	0.04

[a]From Sherwood and Goldwasser (1976).

[b]The age of the culture is the interval between the day on which the primary cultures are plated and the day of passage.

[c]Activities are expressed as units/ml of unconcentrated medium. All of the values were significantly different from those for control media (no cells) at the $p < 0.05$ level. Assays were done by the *in vitro* method. In this and other tables, data showing activities of unconcentrated media are calculated from the total ^{59}Fe uptake measurements made on the concentrated samples.

icochemical properties: both are inactivated by trypsin, sialidase, and an antibody to erythropoietin; both migrate as an α_2-globulin in zone electrophoresis, and show the same molecular weight (30,000 as determined by radiation inactivation) (Waldmann *et al.*, 1968). On the basis of these similarities, it appears that the erythropoietic factor isolated from these renal and ectopic lesions is erythropoietin.

These observations suggest the following possibilities: that the tumor produces erythropoietin, concentrates it from the plasma, or causes reduced metabolic clearance of circulating hormone. The *in vitro* studies of Sherwood and Goldwasser (1976) and Sherwood *et al.* (1983) showed that granular cell and clear cell carcinomas produce erythropoietin during maintenance in tissue culture for varying periods of time and for several passages (Table XIII). This material produced a dose-dependent increase in ^{59}Fe uptake into hemoglobin in the *in vitro* rat bone marrow cell assay and was completely neutralized by an antibody to human urinary erythropoietin (Sherwood and Goldwasser, 1976); it was detectable in the radioimmunoassay utilizing human urinary erythropoietin as tracer and an antibody developed against human urinary hormone (Sherwood *et al.*, 1983). The low activity of some of the tumor media in the *in vivo* bioassays and the chromatographic properties of the active material (i.e., activity was not adsorbed to DEAE at pH 4.5) suggested that the tumor-derived erythropoietin was largely asialoerythropoietin (Sherwood and Goldwasser, 1976). As asialoerythropoietin is biologically inactive *in vivo*, this finding could explain the observation that although plasma erythropoietin concentrations are elevated in patients with renal carcinoma, particularly by radioimmunoassay, erythrocytosis is infrequently present. These tissue culture studies, as well as a study by Toyama *et al.* (1979), indicate the renal adenocarcinoma is an erythropoietin-producing tumor.

E. Cell Origin of Erythropoietin

Although a considerable body of information exists implicating the kidney as the site of erythropoietin production, there is little information on the specific cell type involved. Diverse sites in the kidney have been suggested, based on extraction of renal tissue (Sherwood and Goldwasser, 1978), *in vitro* maintenance of kidney cells (Burlington *et al.*, 1972; Kurtz *et al.*, 1982; Sherwood *et al.*, 1972), immunofluorescence studies (Busuttil *et al.*, 1971, 1972; Gruber *et al.*, 1977), or the association between renal carcinoma and elevated erythropoietin concentrations (e.g., Bagley *et al.*, 1982; Sherwood and Goldwasser, 1976; Sufrin *et al.*, 1977).

Biologically active erythropoietin extracted from the renal cortices and medullas of normal rabbits is related immunologically to the native hormone in human serum (J. Sherwood and E. Goldwasser, 1978, 1979). These studies were discussed in Section II and are summarized in Table V. Equivalent amounts of erythropoietin have been extracted from the cortex and medulla, as measured in the radioimmunoassay and the *in vitro* rat bone marrow assay (J. Sherwood and E. Goldwasser, unpublished observations). These observations are in agreement with those of Zanjani *et al.* (1967) that a renal erythropoietic factor is found in all regions of the kidney.

The *in vitro* studies of Sherwood *et al.* (1972) likewise suggest that a cell type common to all segments of the kidney is involved in erythropoietin production. Explants of four anatomic regions of the rat kidney—inner and outer cortex, inner and outer medula—produced similar amounts of an erythropoietic factor during maintenance in organ culture (Table XIV). Associated with the production of erythropoietin was the existence of cells in the explants with histologic features characteristic of active protein synthesis, i.e., markedly hypertrophic Golgi, numerous polyribosomes, and extensive rough-surfaced endoplasmic reticulum (Sherwood *et al.*, 1972). These ultrastructural characteristics are reminiscent of the regenerating epithelial cells found in experimental tubular necrosis (Cuppage and Tate, 1969).

TABLE XIV

ERYTHROPOIETIC ACTIVITY IN CULTURE MEDIUM FROM ORGAN CULTURES OF RAT KIDNEY[a,b]

Region	Culture period[c]	Experiment 1		Experiment 2		Experiment 3	
		^{59}Fe incorporation (%)	ESF units (per ml medium)	^{59}Fe incorporation (%)	ESF units (per ml medium)	^{59}Fe incorporation (%)	ESF units (per ml medium)
Outer cortex	1	1.4 ± 0.5	—	1.3 ± 1.0	—	2.4 ± 0.4	—
	2	3.9 ± 0.2+[d]	0.06 ± 0.004	3.8 ± 1.5+[d]	0.05 ± 0.01	5.1 ± 1.0+[d]	0.09 ± 0.03
Inner cortex	1	4.7 ± 0.3+[d]	0.07 ± 0.01	2.0 ± 1.6	—	1.8 ± 0.1	—
	2	1.8 ± 0.6	—	5.1 ± 0.7	0.09 ± 0.02	4.9 ± 0.6+[d]	0.08 ± 0.02
Outer medulla	1	0.9 ± 0.04	—	2.8 ± 1.2	—	1.8 ± 0.5	—
	2	3.0 ± 0.8+[d]	0.04 ± 0.01	5.3 ± 2.4	0.10 ± 0.06	4.2 ± 1.2	0.06 ± 0.03
Inner medulla	1	1.7 ± 0.3	—			2.0 ± 0.2	—
	2	4.3 ± 0.3+[d]	0.06 ± 0.01			5.2 ± 0.4+[d]	0.09 ± 0.01
Control medium		1.2 ± 0.2		1.6 ± 0.5		1.6 ± 0.5	
Saline		1.0 ± 0.1		0.9 ± 0.2		0.9 ± 0.2	

[a]From Sherwood et al. (1972).

[b]Results shown are means ± SE. Media were tested in two assays: experiment 1 in the first and experiments 2 and 3 in the second. Each value refers to a total of 7–15 cultures, media from which were pooled, incubated with rat serum, and assayed in four to six assay mice. Each mouse was given the equivalent of 1 ml of original medium. Erythropoietin standards gave values of 3.61 ± 0.18% for 0.05 U and 7.24 ± 0.27% for 0.2 U and were similar in both assays.

[c]Culture period 1 represents the first 3.5 days in culture; period 2 the second 3.5 days.

[d]Significantly different from control medium ($p < 0.05$).

Erythropoietin production can be inhibited by agents such as $HgCl_2$ that produce renal tubular lesions. All of these observations implicate the renal tubule in erythropoietin production.

The juxtaglomerular apparatus has also been proposed as the site of synthesis, based on early observations that juxtaglomerular cell granularity is increased in certain anemic states (Hirashima and Takaku, 1962; Kaley and Demopoulos, 1963) and decreased in transfusion-induced polycythemia (Hirashima and Takaku, 1962). On the other hand, these changes in granularity may reflect alterations in renal vascular volume and perhaps renin secretion rather than fluctuations in erythropoietin production.

The glomerulus has been implicated as a site of production based on immunofluorescence studies (Busuttil *et al.*, 1971, 1972; Fisher *et al.*, 1965; Frenkel *et al.*, 1968; Gruber *et al.*, 1977) and tissue culture preparations of cells derived from the glomerular region (Burlington *et al.*, 1972; Kurtz *et al.*, 1982). In the immunofluorescence studies, antisera raised against impure preparations of erythropoietin bound preferentially to the glomerular tuft of the kidneys from anemic sheep (Fisher *et al.*, 1965; Frenkel *et al.*, 1968), anemic human beings (Busuttil *et al.*, 1971), hypoxic dogs (Busuttil *et al.*, 1972), or neonatal or adult hypoxic rats (Gruber *et al.*, 1977). Although these antisera were adsorbed with kidney tissue to remove the higher affinity antibodies, they still must be considered to be a mixture of antibodies against many kidney proteins as well as against erythropoietin. Therefore, data from these immunofluorescence studies are quite ambiguous and must be interpreted with caution.

Of potentially greater validity are the studies of erythropoietin production by glomerular cells maintained in tissue culture, although cells maintained *in vitro* for long periods of time may not retain the same characteristics as those *in vivo*. Burlington *et al.* (1972) demonstrated that goat kidney glomeruli, maintained in culture as confluent monolayers, produced an erythropoietin that was active in both the *in vitro* rat bone marrow cell assay and the exhypoxic polycythemic mouse assay; in the *in vivo* assay, activity appeared to be approximately 0.06 units/ml of culture medium for a 30-day interval between media changes. The activity was inhibited by anti-erythropoietin antibody (Table XV). Kurtz *et al.* (1982) cultured two types of cells derived from glomerular explant outgrowths: mesangial cells and glomerular epithelium. Erythropoietin was found in the medium of the cultures considered to be of mesangial cells (0.05 units/ml). However, as these investigators based the definition of cell type on the time interval between establishment of the primary culture and establishment of

TABLE XV

Erythropoietic Activity in Glomerular Culture Medium[a]

Sample[b]	^{59}Fe incorporation into erythrocytes (%) + SEM
Saline	0.24 ± 0.03
0.2 units of erythropoietin	3.61 ± 0.36
0.2 units of erythropoietin + antierythropoietin[c]	0.19 ± 0.03
Culture medium alone	2.03 ± 0.25
Culture medium + antierythropoietin	0.26 ± 0.25

[a]Data from Burlington et al. (1972).
[b]Samples assayed in transfused plethoric mice.
[c]Test substance and antierythropoietin incubated together. Antiserum to rabbit IgG was then added. The mixture was centrifuged and the supernatant was collected for assay.

the subcultures, one cannot conclude definitively that the mesangial cell is the erythropoietin-producing cell.

The kidney is a heterogeneous organ with each nephron containing many cell types with different functions. The specific cell type that synthesizes and/or secretes erythropoietin has yet to be found.

The ability of renal cell carcinomas to synthesize and secrete erythropoietin implicates the proximal convoluted tubule as a site of origin of this hormone, based on immunologic evidence suggesting that renal carcinomas are derived exclusively from cells of the proximal convoluted tubule. Renal carcinoma cells react with antibodies to brush border antigens (specific for cells of the proximal convoluted tubule) but not with antibodies to antigens of the distal convoluted tubule and loop of Henle (Tamm–Horsfall antigen) (Wallace and Nairn, 1972).

VI. Conclusions

In this review, we have presented some of the background studies of erythropoietin and discussed areas of research that we believe will be most applicable to future studies of the biochemistry and synthesis of the hormone. Progress with purification has permitted the establishment of sensitive and specific radioimmunoassays that can detect normal (or even less than normal) amounts of erythropoietin in human serum. The possibility has been raised that certain anemias, particularly the anemia of chronic renal disease, can be alleviated by administration of erythropoietin. With the radioimmunoassay, questions relevant to the regulation of erythropoietin physiology, its synthesis, secretion, and metabolic fate, can now be addressed. Problems of erythropoietin production in diverse hematologic and renal disorders such as inappropriate erythropoietin production, i.e., overproduction, underproduction, or secretion of biologically inactive hormone, and of inappropriate interaction between erythropoietin and the marrow target cells can now be analyzed.

REFERENCES

Adamson, J. W., and Finch, C. A. (1966). Mechanisms of erythroid marrow activation. *Trans. Assoc. Am. Phys.* **79**, 419.

Adamson, J. W., Eschbach, J., and Finch, C. A. (1968). The kidney and erythropoiesis. *Am. J. Med.* **44**, 725–733.

Adamson, J. W., Eschbach, J., and Finch., C. A. (1979). The kidney and erythropoiesis. *Am. J. Med.* **93**, 449–458.

Annable, L., Cotes, M., and Musset, M. V. (1972). The second international reference preparation of erythropoietin, human, urinary, for bioassay. *Bull. WHO* **47**, 99.

Bagley, D. H., Goldwasser, E., Sherwood, J., Albert, E., Appel, R., Banno, J. J., Javadpour, N., and Weiss, R. M. (1982). Erythropoietin in patients with renal cell carcinoma. *Trans. Am. Urol. Assoc.* (Abstr.).

Bessler, H., Notti, I., and Djaldetti, M. (1980). Quantitative determination of human plasma erythropoietin using embryonic mouse liver erythroblasts. *Acta Haematol.* **63**, 204–210.

Bolton, A. E., and Hunter, W. M. (1973). The labeling of proteins to high specific activities by conjugation to a 125 I containing acylating agent. *Biochem. J.* **133**, 529–539.

Borsook, H. A. (1959). A discussion of humoral erythropoietic factors. *Ann. N.Y. Acad. Sci.* **77**, 725.

Botha, M. C., Beale, D., Isaacs, W. A., and Lehmann, H. (1966). Haemoglobin. J. Cape Town-Alpha2 92 arginine → glutamine beta 2. *Nature (London)* **212**, 792.

Briggs, D. W., Fisher, J. W., and George W. J. (1974). Hepatic clearance of intact and desialylated erythropoietin. *Am. J. Physiol.* **227**, 1385–1388.

Bromberg, P. A., and Jensen, W. N. (1967). Blood oxygen dissociation curves in sickle cell disease. *J. Lab. Clin. Med.* **70**, 480–488.

Brownstein, M. H., and Ballard, H. S. (1966). Hepatoma associated with erythrocytosis. *Am. J. Med.* **40**, 204–210.

Burlington, H., Cronkite, E. P., Reincke, U., and Zanjani, E. D. (1972). Erythropoietin production in cultures of goat renal glomeruli. *Proc. Natl. Acad. Sci. U.S.A.* **69**, 3547–3550.

Busuttil, R. W., Roh, B. L., and Fisher, J. W. (1971). The cytological localization of erythropoietin in the human kidney using the fluorescent antibody technique. *Proc. Soc. Exp. Biol.* **137**, 327–330.

Busuttil, R. W., Roh, B. L., and Fisher, J. W. (1972). Localization of erythropoietin in the glomerulus of the hypoxic dog kidney using a fluorescent antibody technique. *Acta Haematol.* **47**, 238–242.

Caro, J., Brown, S., Miller, O. Murray, T., and Erslev, A. J. (1979). Erythropoietin levels in uremic nephric and anephric patients. *J. Lab. Clin. Med.* **93**, 449–458.

Charache, S., Grisolia, S., Fiedler, A. J., and Hellegers, A. (1970). Effect of 2,3-diphosphoglycerate on oxygen affinity of blood in sickle cell anemia. *J. Clin. Invest.* **49**, 806–812.

Chiba, S., Kung, C. K.-H., and Goldwasser, E. (1972). *Biochem. Biophys. Res. Commun.* **47**, 1372–1377.

Contrera, J. F., and Gordon, A. S. (1966). Erythropoietin: Production by a particulate fraction of rat kidney. *Science* **152**, 653–654.

Contrera, J. F., and Gordon, A. S. (1968). The renal erythropoietic factor. I. Studies on its purification and properties. *Ann. N.Y. Acad. Sci.* **149**, 114–119.

Contrera, J. F., Camiscoli, J. F., Weintraub, A. H., and Gordon, A. S. (1965). Extraction of erythropoietin from kidneys of hypoxic and phenylhydrazine-treated rats. *Blood* **25**, 809.

Contrera, J. F., Gordon, A. S., and Weintraub, A. H. (1966). Extraction of an erythropoietin-producing factor from a particulate fraction of rat kidney. *Blood* **28**, 330–342.

Cotes, P. M. (1973). Radioimmunoassay of erythropoietin. *Methods Invest. Diagn. Endocrinol.* pp. 1117–1123.

Cotes, P. M. (1982). Immunoreactive erythropoietin in serum. *Br. J. Haematol.* **50**, 427–438.

Cotes, P. M., and Bangham, D. R. (1961). Bio-assay of erythropoietin in mice made polycythemic by exposure to air at a reduced pressure. *Nature (London)* **191**, 1065–1067.

Cotes, P. M., and Bangham, D. R. (1966). The international reference preparation of erythropoietin. *Bull. WHO* **35**, 751.

Cuppage, F. E., and Tate, A. (1969). Repair of the nephron following injury with mercuric chloride. *Am. J. Pathol.* **51**, 405–429.

Demopoulos, H. B., Highman, B., Altland, P. D., Gerving, M. A., and Kaley, G. (1965). Effects of high altitude on granular juxtaglomerular cells and their possible role in erythropoietin production. *Am. J. Pathol.* **46**, 497.

Denny, W. F., Flanigan, W. J., and Zukoski, C. F. (1966). Serial erythropoietin studies in patients undergoing renal homotransplantation. *J. Lab. Clin. Med.* **67**, 386–397.

Desforges, J. F., and Dawson, J. P. (1958). The anemia of renal failure. *Am. Med. Assoc. Arch. Int. Med.* **101**, 326–332.

Donati, R. M., McCarthy, J. M., Lange, R. D., and Gallagher, N. I. (1963). Erythrocythemia and neoplastic tumors. *Ann. Intern. Med.* **58**, 47–55.

Dordal, M. S., and Goldwasser, E. (1982). Function and composition of the carbohydrate portion of human urinary erythropoietin. *Exp. Hematol.* **10** (Suppl. 11), 222.

Dufau, J. L., Catt, K. J., and Tsuruhara, T. (1971). *Biochem. Biophys. Res. Commun.* **44**, 1022.

Dukes, P. (1980). Preparation of Ep containing protein concentrates suitable for shipment to the collection center at the Hematopoiesis Research Laboratory-Childrens Hospital of Los Angeles. *Int. Conf. Exp. Hemato., 5th, 1980,* Suppl. 8, 41–51.

Dunn, C. D., Jarvis, J. H., and Greenman, J. M. (1975). A quantitative bioassay for erythropoietin using mouse fetal liver cells. *Exp. Haemotol.* **3**, 65–78.

Erslev, A. J. (1953). Humoral regulation of red cell production. *Blood* **8**, 349–357.

Erslev, A. J. (1959). Erythropoietic factor in the control of red cell production. *Ann. N.Y. Acad. Sci.* **77**, 627–637.

Erslev, A. (1974). In vitro production of erythropoietin by kidneys perfused with a serum-free solution. *Blood* **44**, 77–85.

Erslev, A., and Kazal, L. A. (1969). *Blood* **34**, 222–229.

Erslev, A. J., and Lavietes, P. H. (1954). Observations on the nature of the erythropoietic serum factor. *Blood* **9**, 1055.

Espada, J., Langton, A. A., and Dorado, M. (1972). Human erythropoietin: Studies on purity and partial characterization. *Biochim. Biophys. Acta* **285**, 427–35.

Espada, J., Brandan, N. C., and Dorado, M. (1973). Properties and characterization of human erythropoietin. *Acta Physiol. Lat. Am.* **23**, 540–2.

Fisher, J. W., and Birdwell, B. J. (1961). The production of an erythropoietic factor by the in situ perfused kidney. *Acta Haematol.* **26**, 244.

Fisher, J. W., and Langston, J. W. (1967). The influence of hypoxemia and cobalt on erythropoietin production in the isolated perfused dog kidney. *Blood* **29**, 114–125.

Fisher, J. W., and Langston, J. W. (1968). Effects of testosterone, cobalt and hypoxia on erythropoietin production in the isolated perfused dog kidney. *Ann. N.Y. Acad. Sci.* **149**, 75–87.

Fisher, J. W., Taylor, G., and Porteous, D. D. (1965). Localization of erythropoietin in glomeruli of sheep kidney by fluorescent antibody technique. *Nature (London)* **205**, 611–612.

Foley, J. W., Gross, D. M., Nelson, P. K., and Fisher, J. W. (1978). The effects of arachidonic acid on erythropoietin production in ex-hypoxic mice and the isolated perfused canine kidney. *J. Pharmacol. Exp. Ther.* **207**, 402–409.

Forsell, J. (1954). Polycythemia and hypernephroma. *Acta Med. Scand.* **150**, 155–161.

Fraker, P. J., and Speck, J. C., Jr. (1978). Protein and cell membrane iodination with a sparingly soluble chloroamide, 1,3,4,6-tetrachloride-3 alpha,6 alpha-diphenlglycoluril. *Biochem. Biophys. Res. Commun.* **80**, 849–857.

Frenkel, E. P., Suki, W., and Baum, J. (1968). Some observations on the localization of erythropoietin. *Ann. N.Y. Acad. Sci.* **149**, 292–293.

Fried, W., Plzak, L. F., Jacobson, L. O., and Goldwasser, E. (1956). Erythropoiesis. II. Assay of erythropoietin in hypophysectomized rats. *Proc. Soc. Exp. Biol. Med.* **92**, 203.

Fried, W., Plzak, L. F., Jacobson, L. O., and Goldwasser, E. (1957). Studies on erythropoiesis. III. Factors controlling erythropoietin production. *Proc. Soc. Exp. Biol. Med.* **94**, 237.

Fried, W., Barone-Varelas, J., and Berman, M. (1981). Detection of high erythropoietin titers in renal extracts of hypoxic rats. *J. Lab. Clin. Med.* **92**, 82–86.

Fried, W., Barone-Verelas, J., and Barone, T. (1982). The influence of age and sex on erythropoietin titers in the plasma and tissue homogenates of hypoxic rats. *Exp. Hematol.* **10**, 472–477.

Fried, W., Barone-Verelas, J., Barone, T., and Helfgott, M. (1980). Extraction of erythropoietin from kidneys. *Int. Conf. Exp. Hematol. 5th 1980:* Suppl. 8, 41–51.

Garcia, J. F. (1972). The radioimmunoassay of human plasma erythropoietin. In "Regulation of Erythropoiesis" (A. S. Gordon, M. Condorelli, and C. Peschle, eds.), pp. 132–153. Ponte, Milano.

Garcia, J. F., Sherwood, J., and Goldwasser, E. (1979). Radioimmunoassay of erythropoietin. *Blood Cells* **5**, 405–419.

Glynn, K. P., Penner, J. A., Smith, J. R., and Rucknagel, D. L. (1968). Familial erythrocytosis: Description of three families, one with hemoglobin Ypsilanti. *Ann. Intern. Med.* **69**, 769.

Goldwasser, E. (1975). Erythropoietin and the differentiation of red blood cells. *Fed. Proc., Fed. Am. Soc. Exp. Biol.* **34**, 2285–2292.

Goldwasser, E. (1981a). Erythropoietin and red cell differentiation. Control of cellular division and development: Part A: 487–494.

Goldwasser, E. (1981b). Erythropoietin: Progress report, 1981. *Blood* **58** (Suppl. 1), xlii.

Goldwasser, E., and Kung, K.-H. (1968). Progress in the purification of erythropoietin. *Ann. N.Y. Acad. Sci.* **149**, 49–53.

Goldwasser, E., and Kung, K.-H. (1971). Purification of erythropoietin. *Proc. Natl. Acad. Sci. U.S.A.* **68**, 697–698.

Goldwasser, E., and Kung, K.-H. (1972a). Purification and properties of erythropoietin. *In* "International Conference on Erythropoiesis. Regulation of Erythropoiesis" (A. S. Gordon, M. Condorelli, and C. Peschle, eds.), pp. 159–165. Ponte, Milano.

Goldwasser, E., and Kung, K.-H. (1972b). The molecular weight of sheep plasma erythropoietin. *J. BIol. Chem.* **247**, 5159–5160.

Goldwasser, E., and Sherwood, J. B. (1981). Annotation: Radioimmunoassay of erythropoietin. *Br. J. Haematol.* **48**, 359–363.

Goldwasser, E., White, W. F., and Taylor, K. B. (1962a). On the purification of sheep plasma erythropoietin. *In* "Erythropoiesis" (L. O. Jacobson and M. Doyle, eds.), pp. 43–49. Grune & Stratton, New York.

Goldwasser, E., White, W. F., and Taylor, K. B. (1962b). Further purification of sheep plasma erythropoietin. *Biochim. Biophys. Acta* **64**, 487.

Goldwasser, E., Kung, K.-H., and Eliason, J. (1968). Progress in the purification of erythropoietin. *Ann. N.Y. Acad. Sci.* **149**, 49–53.

Goldwasser, E., Kung, K.-H., and Eliason, J. (1974). On the mechanism of erythropoietin-induced differentiation. XIII. The role of sialic acid in erythropoietin action. *J. Biol. Chem.* **249**, 2402.

Goldwasser, E., Eliason, J. K., and Sikkema, D. (1975). An assay for erythropoietin in vitro at the milliunit level. *Endocrinology* **97**, 315–323.

Gordon, A. S. (1959). Hemopoietin. *Physiol. Rev.* **39**, 1–40.

Gordon, A. S. (1973). *Vitamin Horm.* **31**, 105–174.

Gordon, A. S., and Zanjani, E. D. (1970). *In* "Hemopoietic Cellular Proliferation" (F. Stohlman, ed.), p. 97. Grune & Stratton, New York.

Gordon, A. S., Piliero, S. J., Kleinberg, W. K., and Freedman, H. H. (1954). A plasma extract with erythropoietic activity. *Proc. Soc. Exp. Biol. Med.* **86**, 255–258.

Gordon, A. S., Piliero, S. J., and Tannenbaum, M. (1955). Erythropoietic activity of blood and tissues of anemic rabbits. *Am. J. Physiol.* **181**, 585.

Gordon, A. S., Weintraub. A. H., Camiscoli. J. F., and Contrera, J. F. (1964). Plasma and urinary levels of erythropoietin in Cooley's anemia. *Ann. N.Y. Acad. Sci.* **119**, 561–577.

Gordon, A. S., Cooper, G. W., and Zanjani, E. D. (1967). The kidney and erythropoiesis. *Semin. Hematol.* **4**, 337–358.

Gordon, A. S., Mirand, E. A., Wenig, J., Katz, R., and Zanjani, E. D. (1968). Androgen actions on erythropoiesis. *Ann. N.Y. Acad. Sci.* **149**, 318–335.

Gordon, A. S., Zanjani, E. D., and Zalusky, R. A. (1970). Possible mechanism for the erythrocytosis associated with hepatocellular carcinoma in man. *Blood* **35**, 151–157.

Gross, D. M., Brookins, J., Fink, G. D., and Fisher, J. W. (1976). Effects of prostaglandins A2, E2, and F2alpha on erythropoietin production. *J. Pharmacol. Exp. Ther.* **198**, 489.

Gruber, D. F., Zucali, J. R., Wleklinski, J., Larussa, V., and Mirand, E. A. (1977). Temporal transition in the site of rat erythropoietin production. *Exp. Hematol.* **5**, 399–407.

Hirashima, K., and Takaku, F. (1962). Experimental studies on erythropoietin. II. The relationship between juxtaglomerular cells and erythropoietin. *Blood* **20**, 1–8.

Iscove, N. N., and Guilbert, L. J. (1978). Erythropoietin-independence of early erythropoiesis and a two-regulator model of a proliferative control in the hematopoietic system. *In,* (M. J. Murphy, Jr., ed.), "In Vitro Aspects of Erythropoiesis" pp. 3–8. Springer-Verlag, Berlin and New York.

Iscove, N. N., and Sieber, F. (1975). Erythroid progenitors in mouse bone marrow detected by macroscopic colony formation in culture. *Exp. Hematol.* **3**, 32–43.

Jacobson, L. O., Goldwasser, E., Plzak, L. F., and Fried, W. (1957). Studies on erythropoiesis. IV. Reticulocyte response of hypophysectomized and polycythemic rodents to erythropoietin. *Proc. Soc. Exp. Biol. Med.* **94**, 243.

Jacobson, L. O., Goldwasser, E., Gurney, C. W., Fried, W., and Plzak, L. (1959). Studies on erythropoietin: The hormone regulating red cell production. *Ann. N.Y. Acad. Sci.* **77**, 551–573.

Jatkar, P. R., and Kreier, J. P. (1967). Relationship between severity of anemia and plasma erythropoietin titer in anaplasma-infected calves and sheep. *Am. J. Vet. Res.* **28**, 107.

Jelkmann, W., Brookins, J., and Fisher, J. W. (1979). Indomethacin blockade of albuterol-induced erythropoietin production in isolated perfused dog kidneys. *Proc. Soc. Exp. Biol. Med.* **162**, 65–70.

Jepson, J. H. (1979). "Hematologic Problems in Renal Disease," pp. 27–37. Addison-Wesley, Reading, Massachusetts.

Kaley, G., and Demopoulos, H. B. (1963). Effect of erythropoietic stimuli on renin content and juxtaglomerular cells. *Fed. Proc., Fed. Am. Soc. Exp. Biol.* **22**, 664.

Kaplan, S. M., Piliero, S. J., Gordon, A. S., and Meager, R. (1977). *Am. J. Med. Sci.* **273**, 71–77.

Kornfeld, R., and Kornfeld, S. (1970). The structure of a phytohemagglutinin receptor site from human erythrocytes. *J. Biol. Chem.* **245**, 2536–2545.

Kuratowska, Z., and Lewartowski, B. (1962). Studies on the active principle released by the hypoxic kidney into Tyrode's solution. *In* "Erythropoiesis" (L. O. Jacobson, and M. Doyle, eds.), p. 101. Grune & Stratton, New York.

Kuratowska, Z., Lewartowski, B., and Michalak, E. (1961). Studies on the production of erythropoietin by isolated perfused organs. *Blood* **18**, 527–534.

Kuratowska, Z., Kowalski, E., Lipinski, B., and Michalak, E. (1962). Preparation of the erythropoietic factor from human blood plasma. *Acta Biochim. Pol.* **9**, 189–197.

Kuratowska, Z., Lewartowski, B., and Lipinski, B. (1964). Chemical and biologic properties of an erythropoietin-generating substance obtained from perfusates of isolated anoxic kidneys. *J. Lab. Clin. Med.* **64**, 226–237.

Kurtz, A., Jelkmann, W., and Bauer, C. (1982). Mesangial cells derived from rat glomeruli produce an erythropoiesis stimulating factor in cell culture. *FEBS Lett.* **137**, 129–132.

Lange, R. D., and Gallagher, N. I. (1962). Clinical and experimental observations on the relationship of the kidney to erythropoietin production. *In* "Erythropoiesis" (L. O. Jacobson, and M. Doyle, eds.), pp. 361–373. Grune & Stratton, New York.

Lange, R. D., O'Grady, L. F., Lewis, J. P., and Trobaugh, F. E. (1968). Application of erythropoietin antisera to studies of erythropoiesis. *Ann. N.Y. Acad. Sci.* **149**, 281–291.

Lee-Huang, S. (1980). A new preparative method for isolation of human erythropoietin with hydrophobic interaction chromatography. *Blood* **56**, 620–624.

Lee-Huang, S. (1982a). Monoclonal antibodies to human erythropoietin. *Br. J. Haematol.* **50**, 427.

Lee-Huang, S. (1982b). Monoclonal antibodies to human erythropoietin. *Fed. Proc., Fed. Am. Soc. Exp. Biol.* **41**, 520.

Lee-Huang, S. (1984). Cloning of human erythropoietin gene. *Biophys. Soc. Meet.*

Lertora, J. J., Dargon, P. A., Rege, A. B., and Fisher, J. W. (1975). Studies on a radioimmunoassay for human erythropoietin. *J. Lab. Clin. Med.* **86**, 140–151.

Linman, J. W., and Bethell, F. H. (1956). Plasma erythropoietic stimulating factor: observations on circulating erythrocytes and bone marrow of rats receiving protein-free extracts of rabbit plasma. *Blood* **11**, 310–323.

Linman, J. W., and Pierre, R. V. (1968). Studies on the erythropoietic effects of hyperbaric hypoxia. *Ann. N.Y. Acad. Sci.* **149**, 25.

Linman, J. W., and Pierre, R. V. (1975). Studies on a radioimmunoassay for human erythropoietin. *J. Lab. Clin. Med.* **86**, 140–151.

Loge, J. P., Lange, R. D., and Moore, C. V. (1950). Characterization of the anemia associated with chronic renal insufficiency. *J. Clin. Invest.* **29**, 830.

Loh, Y. P., and Gainer, H. (1978). The role of glycosylation on the biosynthesis, degradation, and secretion of the ACTH-B-lipotropin common precursor and its peptide products. *FEBS Lett.* **96**, 269–272.

Lowy, P. H., and Keighley, G. (1961). Use of phenol in the isolation of erythropoietin glycoprotein. *Nature (London)* **192**, 75.

Lowy, P. H., and Keighley, G. L. (1966). Extraction of erythropoietin from human urine and rabbit plasma. *Clin. Chem. Acta* **13**, 491–497.

Lowy, P. H., Keighley, G., and Borsook, H. (1960). Inactivation of erythropoietin by neuraminidase and by mild substitution reactions. *Nature (London)* **185**, 102–103.

McClellan, R. O. (1963). Erythropoietin in miniature swine ingesting Sr-90. *USAEC Hanford Atomic Prod. Oper.* **HW-76000**, 93. 1963.

Maffezzoli, R. D., Kaplan, G. N., and Chrambach, A. (1972). Physical characterization by polyacrylamide gel electrophoresis of human follicle stimulating hormone from urinary extracts of children, men, and pre- and postmenopausal women. *J. Clin. Endocrinol.* **34**, 375–379.

Meineke, H. A. (1969). The origin of erythropoietin in rats with transplants of an adrenal cortical careinoma. *Proc. Soc. Exp. Biol. Med.* **132**, 651–655.

Metcalf, D., and Stanley, E. R. (1969). Quantitative studies on the stimulation of mouse bone marrow colony growth in vitro by normal human urine. *Aust. J. Exp. Biol. Med. Sci.* **47**, 453–466.

Mirand, E. A., Prentice, T. C., and Slaunwhite, W. R. (1959). Current studies on the role of erythropoietin on erythropoiesis. *Ann. N.Y. Acad. Sci.* **77**, 677–701.

Mirand, E. A., Prentice, T. C., and Grace, J. T., Jr. (1964). Ability of tamarins to produce and respond to erythropoietin. *Nature (London)* **204**, 1064.

Miyake, T., Kung, CK.-H., and Goldwasser, E. (1977). Purification of human erythropoietin. *J. Biol. Chem.* **252**, 5558–5564.

Mok, M., and Spivak, J. L. (1982). Protease activity in human urine erythropoietin preparations. *Exp. Hematol.* **10**, 300–306.

Monaco, F., Monaco, G., and Andreoli, M. (1975). *J. Endocrinol. Metab.* **41**, 253–259.

Morell, A. G., and Scheinberg, I. H. (1972). Solubilization of hepatic binding sites for asialo-glycoproteins. *Biochem. Biophys. Res. Commun.* **48**, 808–815.

Morell, A. G., Gregoriades, G., Scheinberg, I. H., Hickman, J., and Ashwell, G. (1971). The role of sialic acid in determining the survival of glycoproteins in the circulation. *J. Biol. Chem.* **246**, 1461–1467.

Naets, J. P. (1959). Erythropoietic activity in plasma and urine of dogs after bleeding. *Proc. Soc. Exp. Biol. Med.* **102**, 387.

Naets, J. P. (1960). Erythropoietic factor in kidney tissue of anemic dogs. *Proc. Soc. Exp. Biol. Med.* **103**, 129.

Naets, J. P., Wittek, M., Toussaint, C., and Van Geertruyden, J. (1968). Erythropoiesis in renal insufficiency and in anephric man. *Ann. N.Y. Acad. Sci.* **149**, 143–150.

Nixon, R. K., O'Rourke, W., Rupe, C. E., and Korst, D. R. (1960). Nephrogenic poly-cythemia. *Arch. Intern. Med.* **106,** 797–802.

Novy, M. J., Edwards, M. J., and Metcalf, J. (1967). Hemoglobin Yakima: II: High blood oxygen affinity associated with compensatory erythrocytosis and normal hemo-dynamics. *J. Clin. Invest.* **46,** 1848.

Painter, R. H., Bruce, W. R., and Goldwasser, E. (1968). The commercial production of erythropoietin from anemic sheep plasma. *Ann. N.Y. Acad. Sci.* **149,** 71–74.

Paulo, L. G., Wilkerson, R. D., Roh, B. L., George, W. I., and Fisher, J. W. (1973). The effects of prostaglandin E_1 on erythropoietin production. *Proc. Soc. Exp. Biol. Med.* **142,** 771–775.

Pavlovic-Kentera, V., Hall, D. P., Bragassa, C., and Lange, R. D. (1965). Unilateral renal hypoxia and production of erythropoietin. *J. Lab. Clin. Med.* **65,** 577–588.

Plzak, L. F., Fried, W., Jacobson, L. O., and Bethard, W. F. (1955). Demonstration of stimulation of erythropoiesis by plasma from anemic rats using Fe-59. *J. Lab. Clin. Med.* **46,** 671.

Pricer, W. E., Jr., and Ashwell, G. (1971). The binding of desialylated glycoproteins by plasma membranes of rat liver. *J. Biol. Chem.* **246,** 4825–4833.

Rambach, W. A., Shaw, R. A., Cooper, J. A. D., and Alt, H. L. (1958). Acid hydrolysis of erythropoietin. *Proc. Soc. Exp. Biol. Med.* **99,** 482.

Reed, C. S., Hampson, R., Gordon, S., Jones, R. T., Novy, M. J., Brimhall, B., Edwards, M. J., and Koler, R. D. (1968). Erythrocytosis secondary to increased oxygen affinity of a mutant hemoglobin, hemoglobin Kempsey. *Blood* **31,** 623.

Reissmann, K. R. (1950). Studies on the mechanism of erythropoietic stimulation in parabiotic rats during hypoxia. *Blood* **5,** 372–380.

Reissmann, K. R., and Nomura, T. (1962). Erythropoietin formation in isolated kidneys and liver. *In* "Erythropoiesis" (L. O. Jacobson and M. Doyle, eds.), pp. 71–77. Grune & Stratton, New York.

Rodgers, G. M., Fisher, J. W., and George, W. J. (1975). The role of adenosine 3′,5′-monophosphate in the control of erythropoietin production. *Am. J. Med.* **58,** 31–38.

Rodman, G. D., Spivak, J. L., and Zanjani, E. D. (1981). Stimulation of erythroid colony formation in vitro by erythropoietin immobilized on agarose-bound lectins. *J. Lab. Clin. Med.* **98,** 684–690.

Rosse, W. F., and Waldmann, T. A. (1962). The role of the kidney in the erythropoietic response to hypoxia in parabiotic rats. *Blood* **19,** 75–81.

Rosse, W. F., and Waldmann, T. A. (1964). A comparison of some physical and chemical properties of erythropoiesis-stimulating factors from different sources. *Blood* **24,** 739.

Rosse, W. F., and Waldmann, T. A. (1966). Factors controlling erythropoiesis in birds. *Blood* **27,** 654.

Rosse, W. F., Berry, R. J., and Waldmann, T. A. (1963). Some molecular characteristics of erythropoietin from different sources determined by inactivation by ionizing radi-ation. *J. Clin. Invest.* **42,** 124.

Ryan, R. J. (1969). A comparison of biologic and immunologic potency estimates of human luteinizing (lh) and follicle stimulating (fsh) hormones. *Karolins. Symp. Res. Methods Reprod. Endocrinol., 1st.* pp. 300–323.

Saidi, P., and Gurney, C. W. (1970). Attenuation of urinary erythropoietin activity under various conditions. *J. Lab. Clin. Med.* **76,** 659–667.

Scaro, J. L., and Aggio, M. C. (1966). Erythropoietin in high altitude resident animals. *Rev. Can. Biol.* **25,** 209.

Scaro, J. L., Keighley, G., and Lowy, P. H. (1963). Production and bioassay of erythropoi-etin in guinea pigs. *Acta Physiol. Lat.* **13,** 362.

Schooley, J. C., and Mahlmann, L. J. (1972). Studies with anti-erythropoietin serum. *In* "Regulation of Erythropoiesis" (A. S. Gordon, M. Condorelli, and C. Peschle, eds.), pp. 167–176. Ponte, Milano.

Sherwood, J. B., and Goldwasser, E. (1976). Erythropoietin production by human renal carcinoma cells in culture. *Endocrinology* **99**, 504–510.

Sherwood, J. B., and Goldwasser, E. (1978). Extraction of erythropoietin from normal kidneys. *Endocrinology* **103**, 866–870.

Sherwood, J. B., and Goldwasser, E. (1979). A radioimmunoassay for erythropoietin. *Blood* **54**, 885–893.

Sherwood, J. B., Robinson, S. H., Bassan, L. R., Rosen, S., and Gordon, A. S. (1972). Production of erythrogenin by organ cultures of rat kidney. *Blood* **40**, 189–197.

Sherwood, J. B., Chang, H., Mittman, N., Longnecker, R., Goldwasser, E., and Nagel, R. L. (1981). Erythropoietin titers in sickle cell disease and chronic renal failure. *Blood* **58**, (Abstr.).

Sherwood, J. B., Burns, E., and Shouval, D. (1983). Establishment of a human erythro-poietin-producing renal carcinoma cell line. *Am. Fed. Clin. Res.* **31**, 323A.

Sieber, F. (1977). Chromatography of human urinary erythropoietin and granulocyte colony-stimulating factor on insolubilized phytohaemagglutinin. *Biochim. Biophys. Acta* **496**, 146–154.

Siegel, L. M., and Monty, K. J. (1966). *Biochim. Biophys. Acta* **112**, 346.

Spivak, J. L., and Levin, J. (1977). Endotoxin contamination of some erythropoietin preparations. *Blood* **59**, 549.

Spivak, J. L., Small, D., and Hollenberg, M. D. (1977). Erythropoietin: Isolated by affinity chromatography with lectin-agarose derivatives. *Proc. Natl. Acad. Sci. U.S.A.* **74**, 4633–4635.

Spivak, J. L., Small, D., Shaper, J. H., and Hollenberg, M. D. (1978). Use of immobilized lectins and other ligands for the partial purification of erythropoietin. *Blood* **52**, 1178–1188.

Stohlman, F., Jr., Roth, C. E., and Rose, J. C. (1954). Evidence for a humoral regulation of erythropoiesis. *Blood* **9**, 721–733.

Sue, J. M., and Sytkowski, A. J. (1983). Site-specific antibodies to human erythropoietin directed toward the NH_2-terminal region. *Proc. Natl. Acad. Sci. U.S.A.* **80**, 3651–3655.

Sufrin, G., Mirand, E. A., Moore, R. H., Chu, T. M., and Murphy, G. P. (1977). Hormones in renal cancer. *J. Urol.* **117**, 433–438.

Sytkowski, A. (1980). Erythropoietin forms biologically inactive complexes in solution. *Biochem. Biophys. Res. Commun.* **93**, 354–359.

Toyama, K., Fujiyama, N., Suzuki, H., Chen, T. P., Tamaoki, N., & Ueyama, Y. (1979). Erythropoietin levels in the course of a patient with erythropoietin producing renal cell carcinoma and transplantation of this tumor in nude mice. *Blood* **54**, 245–253.

Van Lenten, L., & Ashwell, G. (1972). The binding of desialylated glycoproteins by plasma membranes of rat liver. Development of quantitative inhibition assay. *J. Biol. Chem.* **247**, 4633–4640.

Waldmann, T. A., and Bradley, J. E. (1961). Polycythemia secondary to a pheochromocy-toma with production of an erythropoiesis stimulating factor by the tumor. *Proc. Soc. Exp. Biol. Med.* **108**, 425–427.

Waldmann, T. A., and Rosse, W. F. (1962). Sites of formation of erythropoietin. *In* "Erythropoiesis" (L. D. Jacobson and M. Doyle, eds.), pp. 87–92. New York, Grune & Stratton, New York.

Waldmann, T. A., Levin, E. H., and Baldwin, M. (1961). The association of polycythemia with a cerebellar hemangioblastoma. The production of an erythropoiesis stimulating factor by the tumor. *Am. J. Med.* **31**, 318–324.

Waldmann, T. A., Rosse, W. F., and Swarm, R. L. (1968). The erythropoiesis-stimulating factors produced by tumors. *Ann. N.Y. Acad. Sci.* **149**, 509–515.

Wallace, A. C., and Nairn, R. C. (1972). Renal tubular antigens in kidney tumors. *Cancer* **29**, 977–981.

Weiss, T. L., Kavinsky, C. J., and Goldwasser, E. (1982). Characterization of a monoclonal antibody to human erythropoietin. *Proc. Natl. Acad. Sci. U.S.A.* **79**, 5465–5469.

White, W. F., and Josh, G. (1959). Studies on erythropoietin. II. Production of high-titer plasma in sheep. *Proc. Soc. Exp. Biol. Med.* **102**, 686.

White, W. F., Gurney, C. W., Goldwasser, E., and Jacobson, L. O. (1960). Studies on erythropoietin. *Recent Prog. Horm. Res.* **16**, 219.

Winkert, J., and Gordon, A. S. (1960). Enzymic actions on the human urinary erythropoietic-stimulating factor. *Biochim. Biophys. Acta* **42**, 170.

Wong, K. K., Zanjani, E. D., Cooper, G. W., and Gordon, A. S. (1968). The renal erythropoietic factor. V. Studies on its purification. *Proc. Soc. Exp. Biol. Med.* **128**, 67–70.

Yanagawa, S., Hirade, K., Ohnota, H., Sasaki, R., Chiba, H., Ueda, M., and Goto, M. (1984). Isolation of human erythropoietin with monoclonal antibodies. *J. Biol. Chem.* **259**, 2707–2710.

Zangheri, E. O., Campana, H., Ponce, F., Silva, J. C., Fernandez, F. O., and Suarez, J. R. (1963). Production of erythropoietin by anoxic perfusion of the isolated kidney. *Nature (London)* **199**, 572–573.

Zanjani, E. D., Cooper, G. W., Gordon, A. S., Wong, K. K., and Scribner, V. A. (1967). The renal erythropoietic factor (REF). IV. Distribution in mammalian kidneys. *Proc. Soc. Exp. Biol. Med.* **126**, 540–542.

Zanjani, E. D., Yu, M.-L. Perlmutter, A., and Gordon, A. S. (1969). Humoral factors influencing erythropoiesis in the fish (Blue Gourami-Trichogaster trichopterus). *Blood* **33**, 573.

Zaroulis, C. G., Hoffman, B. J., and Kourides, I. A. (1981). Serum concentrations of erythropoietin measured by radioimmunoassay in hematologic disorders and chronic renal failure. *Am. J. Hematol.* **11**, 85–92.

Zuckerman, K. S., Quesenberry, P. J., Levin, J., and Sullivan, R. (1979). Contamination of erythropoietin by endotoxin: In vivo and in vitro effects on murine erythropoiesis. *Blood* **54**, 146–158.

VITAMINS AND HORMONES, VOL. 41

Affinity Labeling of Receptors for Steroid and Thyroid Hormones

JOHN A. KATZENELLENBOGEN

Department of Chemistry, University of Illinois, Urbana, Illinois

BENITA S. KATZENELLENBOGEN

Department of Physiology and Biophysics, University of Illinois and University of Illinois College of Medicine, Urbana, Illinois

I. Introduction 213
II. Strategies in Covalent Attachment 215
  A. Critical Factors in Covalent Attachment 215
  B. An Overview of Covalent Attaching Functions 222
III. Affinity Labeling Studies on Receptor Properties
  and Mechanism of Action 225
  A. Types of Studies 225
  B. Affinity Labeling of Estrogen Receptors 229
  C. Affinity Labeling of Progestin Receptors 235
  D. Affinity Labeling of Glucocorticoid Receptors 241
  E. Affinity Labeling of Androgen Receptors 245
  F. Affinity Labeling of Thyroid Hormone Receptors 247
  G. Other Receptor Systems 252
IV. Affinity Labeling Studies on Enzymes
  and Extracellular Binding Proteins 253
  A. Electrophilic Affinity Labeling 254
  B. Photoaffinity Labeling 263
V. Conclusion 266
  References 267

I. Introduction

Affinity labeling is a technique for the selective, covalent labeling of binding sites in macromolecules. It involves initially the reversible binding of an affinity probe, which is a ligand modified so as to contain a reactive functional group (attaching function), within the binding site of the macromolecule, followed then by the covalent attachment of the affinity probe to the molecular constituents within or near the binding site. The selectivity of the labeling process derives from the selective interaction of the affinity probe with the binding site.

213

Methods of affinity labeling are generally classified according to the type of reaction involved in the covalent attachment. Thus, probes that embody electrophilic alkylating or acylating agents are conveniently termed electrophilic affinity labeling agents, while those whose reaction requires photochemical activation to generate a reactive species are termed photoactivated affinity labeling agents or more simply photoaffinity labeling agents. A more complete discussion of the differences between these types of agents will be given later.

Most of the early studies utilizing affinity probes were directed at elucidating the composition and topology of the binding sites in homogeneous protein preparations, particularly the active sites of enzymes. This early work has been reviewed extensively (Singer, 1967; Baker, 1967, 1970; Shaw, 1970a,b). But the real power of the affinity labeling technique, which is the selectivity that it derives from the sequestration of the affinity probe within the binding site prior to its covalent reaction, has enabled this method to be applied to systems of increased complexity, such as antibody binding sites, allosteric sites on enzymes and membrane transport systems, and multicomponent systems involving interactions between proteins and nucleotides such as ribosomes and tRNAs.

The application of concern to this article involves receptors for steroid and thyroid hormones, where the affinity labeling approach is being used to elucidate the physicochemical properties and the structure of receptors, to facilitate receptor purification and comparisons between receptors from different sources and to aid in elucidating the molecular basis of hormone action. In applications such as this, the requirement for high selectivity is particularly great, since in all but a few instances the receptor protein of interest constitutes only a very small fraction of the total proteins in the binding preparation being labeled. Since this is a field of great activity, a review indicating the fundamental bases of the labeling methods and outlining the scope and limitations of the method is timely.

The scope of this review will be restricted to recent work on the affinity labeling of receptors for steroids and thyroid hormones, and it will be divided into three sections. The first covers general considerations in the design and application of affinity probes—the nature of electrophilic and photoreactive attaching functions, considerations in affinity probe design, binding affinity, selectivity and efficiency in the labeling process, and methods for assaying covalent attachment. The second section deals with the receptors for the individual steroid hormones and for thyroid hormone, presenting strategies that have been utilized in achieving labeling with affinity probes and describing the types of studies that have been undertaken and the understanding that has resulted.

Studies involving the interaction of these same hormones with other proteins (enzymes and carrier proteins) will be referred to in the third section insofar as they relate to the applicability of the affinity labeling technique to receptors. There are, of course, many other systems in which affinity labeling is currently being used fruitfully. A description of these studies, as well as references to earlier studies, can be found in many recent review articles (Jakoby and Wilchek, 1977; Bayley and Knowles, 1977; Tometsko and Richard, 1980; Bayley, 1983; Chowdhary and Westheimer, 1979; Benisek et al., 1982; Simons and Thompson, 1982; Fedan, 1983).

A review on affinity labeling of hormone binding sites, written several years ago by one of the authors (Katzenellenbogen, 1977), concluded with the statement,

> the technique of affinity labeling is a general tool with great potential for specificity in studying binding sites. Its application to the field of hormone action is relatively new; consequently, present results are much more preliminary and tantalizing than definitive. . . . future successes will be limited only by the skill and imagination of future investigators.

The ways in which affinity labeling is currently being used in the study of steroid and thyroid hormone receptors are indeed a testament both to the power of the technique and the insightfulness of the investigators.

II. STRATEGIES IN COVALENT ATTACHMENT

A. CRITICAL FACTORS IN COVALENT ATTACHMENT

1. Labeling Efficiency and Labeling Selectivity

The labeling of receptors for hormones generally requires that a very small quantity of protein, generally present as a very minor component in a heterogeneous binding preparation, undergo covalent interaction with the affinity probe. In order for this to be done successfully, or at best optimally, the labeling process must be both efficient—that is, as much as possible (ideally all) of the receptor should become labeled—and selective—that is, as little as possible of the other nonreceptor proteins should become labeled. Thus, affinity probes that are efficient and selective can be used in situations where receptor concentrations are low and where receptors are not in a purified state, without interferences due to nonspecific labeling, i.e., the labeling of other proteins. The ultimate test of an affinity probe is its application in intact systems, whole cells in culture or tissues in organ culture or even *in vivo*.

Only a few of the affinity probes discussed in Section III approach this ideal behavior. Yet, even those with relatively low efficiency (such as the enone photoaffinity labeling agents) may be highly selective, so that when receptor levels are adequate, studies can be done in complex and intact systems, while others (such as the haloacetates), although efficient but relatively nonselective, have been used fruitfully in studies on purified or partially purified receptors or in conjunction with postlabeling separation methods such as electrophoresis.

In the development of affinity probes for receptors, it is important to evaluate the efficiency and selectivity of candidate agents. Often, these agents are obtained or prepared first in nonradiolabeled form; so, their interaction with the receptors can only be assayed indirectly by exchange assays. In such cases, only inactivation efficiencies, which would represent the upper limit of covalent attachment efficiencies, can be determined. Examples of such receptor inactivation assays are shown in Figs. 1 and 2.

Incubation of the electrophilic estrogen receptor affinity labeling agent, tamoxifen aziridine (**1**), with rat uterine cytosol causes a rapid consumption of binding sites (Fig. 1) (Robertson *et al.*, 1981). This consumption of binding sites is subject to protection by coincubation with an excess of estradiol sufficient to block access of the aziridine

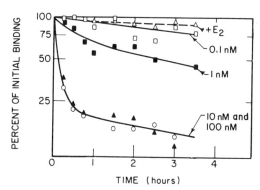

FIG. 1. Rate of inactivation of estrogen receptor from rat uterine cytosol by tamoxifen aziridine. Data are expressed as a percentage of initial estrogen-specific binding site concentration (2.1 nM), and are corrected for nonsaturable binding determined in the presence of a 100-fold excess of radioinert estradiol. The line labeled +E_2 demonstrates the protective effect of 30 nM estradiol in experiments utilizing 10 nM aziridine. (Modified from Robertson *et al.*, 1981, with permission.)

Tamoxifen Aziridine (I)   6-Oxoestradiol (2)

reagent to the receptor. Thus, the inactivation appears to be mediated through specific interaction with the estrogen-binding site of the receptor. Also, since the inactivation process is rapid and nearly complete, the azirdine would appear to be an efficient affinity labeling agent.

The results with the photoactivatable estrogen 6-oxoestradiol (2) appear similar (Katzenellenbogen et al., 1974). With this reagent (Fig. 2), the receptor is inactivated only upon ultraviolet irradiation of the receptor–photosensitive estrogen complex. The estrogen-protectable inactivation is >60%, indicating that this agent may be capable of covalent labeling of the receptor with considerable efficiency.

While receptor inactivation assays are a convenient way to estimate the covalent attachment efficiency of candidate affinity probes, they have their limitations. Inactivation efficiency does not necessarily correspond to labeling efficiency, especially with photoactivatable agents,[1] and the assay is not highly sensitive, so that inactivation efficiencies below 10–15% are difficult to determine. In addition, inactivation assays often do not reveal whether the labeling process is going to be selective.[2]

[1]It is possible that the interaction of an affinity probe with a receptor could cause destruction of the binding activity without covalent attachment of the ligand. This is more likely with photoaffinity reagents where the electronically excited ligand and the receptor could undergo a redox process that alters receptor but does not involve covalent attachment. The results with 6-oxoestradiol were of this nature—efficient, estrogen-specific receptor inactivation is produced, but with minimal covalent attachment (Katzenellenbogen, 1977; Katzenellenbogen et al., 1980). While it would appear that inactivation without covalent attachment is less likely with electrophilic labeling agents, it is conceivable that a cysteine residue on the receptor could attack a halocarbonyl compound on the halogen; this would generate a sulfenyl halide that could cross-link the receptor and destroy ligand binding activity, but would not effect covalent attachment of the halocarbonyl unit.

[2]Inactivation assays can provide information on the selectivity of labeling if substantial inactivation can be obtained using only a fewfold excess of the candidate inactivating agent. In this instance, the labeling process could not be too nonselective or no inactivation would be observed. With tamoxifen aziridine (cf. Fig. 1), ~ 0.8 nM of binding activity is inactivated by 1 nM of agent. Thus, labeling selectivity must be at least on the order of 80% in this receptor preparation.

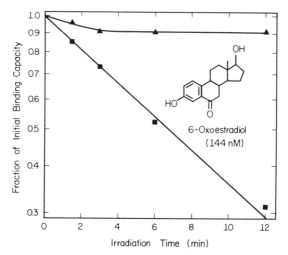

FIG. 2. Time course of irradiation of 6-oxoestradiol at 315 nm. This compound at 144 nM was irradiated in the presence of rat uterine cytosol, either with estradiol (30 nM) preincubation (▲) or without estradiol preincubation (■). Binding capacity was determined by exchange with [^{3}H]estradiol and is corrected for nonspecific binding. (From Katzenellenbogen *et al.*, 1974, with permission.)

Measurement of the attachment efficiency and selectivity of affinity probes available in radiolabeled form is straightforward: A receptor preparation is incubated with increasing concentrations of the agent, with or without an excess of unlabeled ligand for the receptor (to determine total and nonspecific attachment, respectively). Periodically, aliquots are removed and the extent of covalent attachment determined. With efficient, selective agents, the latter can be effected simply by precipitation of the receptor preparation with a denaturant, such as trichloroacetic acid or a hot organic solvent; this will suffice to release and extract unattached agent, the covalently attached probe remaining with the precipitated protein fraction. An example of such an attachment efficiency and selectivity determination is shown in Figs. 3 and 4.

The covalent attachment of tamoxifen aziridine (1) to the rat uterine estrogen receptor proceeds quite rapidly at 25°C (Fig. 3), reaching a maximum at 1 hour (B. S. Katzenellenbogen *et al.*, 1983). Nearly all of the receptor in this cytosol preparation (3.0 nM) is covalently labeled after a 1-hour exposure to 16 nM of [^{3}H]tamoxifen aziridine. The high efficiency of labeling can be appreciated by nothing that 3 nM of [^{3}H]tamoxifen aziridine, which represents only 1 equivalent relative to

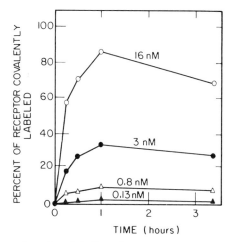

FIG. 3. Time course of covalent labeling of estrogen receptor in rat uterine cytosol. A rat uterine cytosol preparation containing 3.0 nM estrogen receptor was treated with the indicated concentrations of [^{3}H]tamoxifen aziridine in the absence or presence of 3000 nM of unlabeled estradiol. The extent of covalent labeling was determined by ethanol extraction of aliquots spotted on filter disks. The data plotted represent estrogen-specific covalent labeling (the difference between labeling in the absence and presence of unlabeled estradiol). (Modified from B. S. Katzenellenbogen *et al.*, 1983, with permission.)

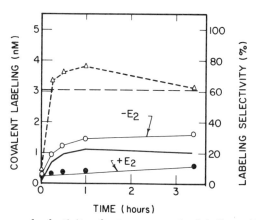

FIG. 4. Efficiency and selectivity of estrogen receptor labeling with [^{3}H]tamoxifen aziridine. Total ($-E_2$) and nonspecific ($+E_2$) labeling obtained with 6 nM [^{3}H]tamoxifen aziridine (TA), as described in Fig. 3, are plotted. The estrogen-specific binding is indicated by the boldface line, and the labeling selectivity (specific labeling as a percentage of total labeling) is indicated by the dashed line. The receptor concentration of this cytosol (3.0 nM) is indicated by the horizontal dashed line. (Modified from J. A. Katzenellenbogen *et al.*, 1983, with permission).

the receptor, labels nearly 40% of the sites, indicating that nearly half of the reagent is reacting with the receptor.

The selectivity of the covalent labeling can be appreciated by an analysis of the data presented in Fig. 4. Here is shown the complete time course of the covalent labeling in the absence of unlabeled estradiol (total labeling) and in the presence of estradiol (nonspecific labeling). The difference, shown in boldface, corresponds to the 3 nM curve plotted in Fig. 3. Estrogen-specific labeling as a percentage of total labeling is shown as the dotted curve and represents the selectivity of the labeling process for the receptor. The labeling selectivity during the first hour ranges between 65 and 75%.

In cases where the attachment efficiency and selectivity are lower or the receptor concentration or purity is lower, it may be necessary to employ a separation method such as polyacrylamide gel electrophoresis in order for the labeled receptor species to be observable over the background of nonspecific labeling (discussed further in Section III).

2. *Ligand Affinity and Exchange*

The binding affinity of an affinity labeling reagent to the receptor is related, though not in a simple manner, to the efficiency and selectivity of the labeling process. In general, however, high-affinity probes should be expected to have higher efficiencies and selectivities. It should be noted that measurement of the binding affinity of an affinity probe to the receptor is not straightforward: Electrophilic reagents may be undergoing covalent attachment during the time of the binding measurement; with photoactivated agents, one is not measuring the affinity of the reactive species, but that of its photochemical precursor. Thus, at best, one obtains a measure of "apparent" binding affinity.

There is one significant operational difference between earlier studies on enzyme affinity labeling and the receptor labeling studies discussed here. Ligand exchange with the enzyme active sites is generally rapid. Therefore, if a reagent (particularly an electrophilic agent) in the binding site underwent hydrolysis prior to covalent attachment, it could undergo exchange with fresh reagent, the exchange process providing multiple chances at binding site labeling. Generally, however, with receptors for steroid and thyroid hormones, the process of ligand exchange is very slow with respect to the times of labeling; so, the overall labeling efficiency of the process is the same as the inherent labeling efficiency of the reagent. It might be possible with inefficient agents to deliberately remove expended reagent and readd fresh reagent, thereby cycling the system, but this approach has not been tried.

3. Electrophilic vs Photoactivated Affinity Labeling: Comparison with Respect to Efficiency, Selectivity, and Applicability to Intact Systems

The most significant difference between electrophilic and photoaffinity labeling agents is that while the former undergo covalent attachment from the moment they are incubated with the receptor, the latter are inert until irradiated. Therefore, in principle, while electrophilic affinity labeling is a dynamic, "uncontrollable" process, one imagines that one can exert control over a photoaffinity labeling agent so as to obtain optimum labeling efficiency and selectivity. For example, with a photoreactive agent one could allow reversible binding to reach equilibrium in the dark, and then remove excess ligand by some rapid chromatographic separation or adsorption process, leaving the agent bound "only" in the desired high-affinity receptor binding site at the time of photoactivation, and thereby improving labeling selectivity. Furthermore, in principle, one should be able to increase the efficiency of labeling by cooling the receptor-photoaffinity label complex to low temperatures, thereby slowing the dissociation of the reactive intermediate generated by photolysis and increasing its chances of undergoing covalent attachment within the binding site (cf. Marver *et al.*, 1976).

Such arguments have been advanced to suggest an inherent superiority of the photoaffinity labeling approach for labeling binding sites in heterogeneous preparations, as is usually the case with receptors (Knowles, 1972). However, experience has not proven this to be true. Photoaffinity labeling agents, while they may be quite selective if their affinity is high, are often very inefficient. Furthermore, electrophilic affinity labeling agents can be both highly efficient and highly selective, showing great preference for reaction within the receptor site as compared to sites on nonreceptor proteins. Many examples will be given in Section III.

It is the characteristics of labeling efficiency and selectivity that determine the degree to which an affinity probe can be used in preparations of increasing heterogeneity or "intactness." The utility of agents with low efficiency and low selectivity will probably be restricted to cell-free preparations with partially purified receptors (or will need to be coupled with powerful separation processes after labeling). To achieve labeling in whole tissues or cells *in vitro* or *in vivo* will require agents with adequately high efficiency and selectivity. In such applications, operations, operational distinctions can again be made between the electrophilic and the photoaffinity labeling approaches.

With photolabeling, one can perform dynamic studies in which the actual time of covalent attachment is determined by the time of irradiation, which can be after any interval of time following the addition of the agent to the system under study. One does not have this flexibility with electrophilic affinity labeling agents, although one can do dynamic studies by the pulse–chase method. The consequences to the viability of the cell can also be different with the two types of reagents. If the conditions for photoactivation involve irradiation in the short wavelength UV region, cells may be killed; this would preclude the types of experiments that would involve studying the subsequent dynamics of covalently labeled receptors in viable cells. In addition, illumination can be provided only for relatively transparent, intact systems, such as cells in culture or thin segments of tissues (not whole animals!). On the other hand, electrophilic affinity labeling agents, if they are sufficiently selective for use in intact systems, which are generally rich in the highly nucleophilic sulfhydryl compounds (glutathione concentrations in cells are in the millimolar range), should have little effect on cell viability.

B. An Overview of Covalent Attaching Functions

1. *Electrophilic Attaching Functions*

Electrophilic covalent attaching functions used in affinity probes are generally the same as those utilized in simpler protein modifying reagents. A very brief summary of the reactivity characteristics of the commonly utilized attaching functions is provided below. The reactivity of these functions has been described in greater detail in some other reviews (Jakoby and Wilchek, 1977).

a. Halocarbonyl Groups. α-Halo ketones, esters, and amides, and the related sulfonate esters of α-hydroxycarbonyl compounds have long been known to be excellent alkylating agents, and numerous examples of their use in steroid receptor affinity labeling is documented (see Sections III and IV,A,1). In general, while such reagents may be highly efficient in their labeling of receptor in cell-free preparations, their high reactivity toward sulfhydryl compounds lowers the efficiency and selectivity of their reaction in intact systems. α-Halocarbonyl and related systems have been used as attaching functions in labeling the progesterone, androgens, glucocorticoid, and thyroid receptors as well as hormone-binding sites in enzymes and carrier proteins. While the α-carbonyl group is known to provide a large activation toward S_n2 displacement, such activation can also be provided by other adjacent centers of unsaturation (a double bond as in allylic halides and an aryl group as in benzylic halides).

b. Aziridines. Aziridines have not been widely used either in protein modification or in affinity labeling, but they are frequently utilized in DNA-directed cytotoxic compounds. Aziridines are relatively nonbasic, and since they are most reactive when protonated, (as the aziridinium ion), they may be particularly favorable agents to use in the selective labeling of binding sites containing an acidic function that might serve to protonate them selectively. This selective activation, coupled with a generally low inherent reactivity toward nucleophiles under physiological conditions, makes them appear promising in receptor labeling. Tamoxifen aziridine, a highly efficient and selective affinity label for the estrogen receptor, utilizes an aziridine attaching function (cf. Sections II,A,1 and III,B).

c. Oxiranes. Oxiranes or epoxides are similar to aziridines, being reactive on the basis of ring strain. Although their reactivity under neutral conditions is somewhat higher than that of the aziridines, they too are activated by acids. Although no receptor labeling has been done with oxirane derivatives, this function has been used in labeling studies on steroid isomerase enzymes (cf. Section IV,A,2).

d. Other Electrophilic Attaching Functions. Although they have not been yet successfully applied in electrophilic affinity labeling of receptors, there are many other organic functional groups with electrophilic activity. α,β-Unsaturated carbonyl compounds, provided the β-terminus is not sterically hindered, are known to be good electrophiles (Michael acceptors for thiols) and have been used to label hormone binding sites on enzymes (cf. Sections IV,A,3–5). A whole variety of acylating functions—active esters, imino esters—have been used in protein modification studies and in other affinity labeling studies. Mercurials, highly reactive toward sulfhydryl functions, have been utilized in some affinity labeling studies with the estrogen receptor (Muldoon, 1980).

2. Photoactivated Attaching Functions

a. Unsaturated Carbonyl Compounds. The photochemistry of unsaturated carbonyl compounds has been the subject of lively interest among photochemists. No actual photoadducts have been isolated and identified from receptor affinity labeling with ligands bearing unsaturated carbonyl chromophores; thus the detailed mechanism of photoattachment remains obscure. One may speculate that the $n\pi^*$ triplet excited state, having diradical character, might abstract a hydrogen atom from the protein, providing covalent attachment through coupling of the protein radical and the ligand radical (Turro, 1978, 1980).

Unsaturated ketone functional groups have been used with very considerable success in the labeling of progesterone, glucocorticoid, and androgen receptors and binding sites for ecdysone (cf. Section III). It has proven particularly convenient that this unsaturated ketone is present as an enone function in the natural ligands for these receptors. Dienone and trienone functions are part of several commercially prepared synthetic ligands. While usually highly selective, photoaffinity labeling mediated by unsaturated ketones is generally inefficient ($\sim$ 10%). Photochemical insertion reactions of aromatic ketones have been utilized successfully in photoaffinity labeling studies with peptide hormones (Galardy *et al.*, 1980), but not with the estrogen receptor (Katzenellenbogen *et al.*, 1974; Katzenellenbogen, 1977).

b. *Diazocarbonyl Compounds and Diazirines.* Diazocarbonyl compounds were among the first described photoactivatable protein labeling reagents. They have long been used in many systems, but thus far, not successfully in labeling steroid receptors, although the steroid-binding serum proteins α-fetoprotein and corticosteroid-binding globulin have been labeled with diazoketones (Section IV,B,2). Thyroid hormone-binding sites have been labeled by a diazoamide derivatives of the hormone (cf. Sections III,F and IV,B,2). The efficiency of labeling in these cases has been low ($\sim$ 10–15%), but labeling has been quite selective.

Although there is debate about the details of the mechanism, it is believed that α-diazocarbonyl compounds react by photochemical decomposition to α-ketocarbenes, which in the singlet state would undergo insertion into a variety of bonds found in amino acid residues (or in the triplet state, by hydrogen abstraction, radical coupling). The efficiency of photoattachment of diazocarbonyl compounds is believed to be compromised by two processes, Wolff rearrangement of the α-ketocarbene intermediate to an electrophilic, though less reactive ketene, and intramolecular transfer of a β-hydrogen. The former rearrangement is suppressed (and the inherent reactivity of the carbene thereby enhanced) by electron-withdrawing substituents on the α-carbon; hence the use of carbethoxy-substituted (diazomalonyl), or sulfonyl, and trifluoromethyl-substituted diazocarbonyl systems (Bayley, 1983). Problems with β-hydrogen transfer are avoided by designing systems that have no β-hydrogens.

Simple unsubstituted diazo compounds are too unstable for utilization with photoaffinity labeling agents, but the isomeric diaziridines are quite stable. Photolysis converts these functions, either directly or via the diazo form, into the carbene, with reactions and side reactions proceeding as with the ketocarbenes (Bayley, 1983). Despite the numerous cases in which diazocarbonyl and diaziridine functions have been utilized in photoaffinity labeling, it is not at all clear that optimally reactive structures for the ketocarbene intermediates have yet been defined.

c. *Azides*. While aliphatic azides are chemically stable, they do not have a chromophore that is readily accessible in the UV. Aromatic azides, on the other hand, have accessible chromophores, and upon irradiation decompose to species with capacity for covalent attachment to proteins. Electron-withdrawing auxochromes such as acyl or nitro groups probably increase chromophore accessibility and enhance covalent attachment efficiency (Knowles, 1972; Bayley, 1983). Again, the detailed photochemical processes by which this occurs are still not understood in detail; the scenario generally described is that photoinduced loss of nitrogen from the azide generates an aryl nitrene that undergoes either insertions as the singlet or hydrogen abstraction-radical center coupling as the triplet. It is quite likely that these courses of reaction are incorrect. Nevertheless, our lack of mechanistic understanding notwithstanding, aryl azides have been widely used in photoaffinity labeling studies (Bayley, 1983). With hormone receptors, however, only labeling of the estrogen receptor by an azide derivative has been described, and this proceeded in relatively low efficiency and selectivity (cf. Section III,B,1).

d. *Other*. Doubtless too there are many other functional groups that upon irradiation are transformed into a chemically reactive, electronically excited state or will undergo conversion into a reactive intermediate. Examples of some more unusual photoactive species of utility in receptor labeling are iodoaromatics and nitroanisoles. Thyroxine, itself an iodoaromatic, has the capacity of photolabeling of thyroid binding sites, although with very low efficiency (cf. Sections III,F and IV,B,3). *m*-Nitroanisoles, as well as many other aromatic systems, can be excited to electronically activated states where some of the substituents are readily subject to displacement by nucleophiles (Cornelisse and Havinga, 1975). This process has been utilized in protein labeling and cross-linking studies (Jelenc *et al.*, 1978) and may as well be applicable to receptor labeling (Katzenellenbogen *et al.*, 1980).

III. Affinity Labeling Studies on Receptor Properties and Mechanism of Action

A. Types of Studies

1. *Advantages and Limitations of Covalent Labeling: A Caveat*

Covalent labeling of a receptor with affinity labeling agent, if sufficiently selective and efficient, can be used to label receptor in heterogeneous preparations and even in intact systems. Covalently labeled receptors can be characterized in much greater detail by rigorous application of high-resolution biochemical separation methods under denaturing, disaggregating conditions, and in intact systems using dynamic and functional tests. In this section, we provide a comprehensive overview of studies utilizing affinity labeling in the steroid and thyroid hormone receptor systems. Appropriate reference will be given to subsequent sections in which these studies are discussed in greater detail. It is hoped that this section will be a presentation of worthy possibilities, many of which are still to be realized.

The action of hormones *in vivo* involves only reversible interaction between the hormonal agent and the receptor. Thus, receptors covalently labeled by an affinity method represent modified forms of receptor, possibly altered in structure as well as in its function. The covalently linked ligand–receptor complex may be "interpreted" differently by the cell than the reversibly associated hormone–receptor complex. The affinity labeling method is a powerful and convenient tool and a useful model system but a model nevertheless.[3]

2. Receptor Properties and Structure

Many receptors tend to aggregate, or as part of their action they may become associated with particulate fractions of the cell. These associations make them difficult to purify and characterize, as the methods for dissociation of these interactions may also disrupt their binding of reversible ligands. With a covalently labeled receptor, one can apply more rigorous methods for receptor purification and characterization, such as polyacrylamide gel electrophoresis in sodium dodecyl sulfate, isoelectric focusing in 8 M urea, and reversed phase high-performance liquid chromatography on denatured proteins. Since affinity labeling of receptors can often be performed on unpurified or only partially purified preparations, it enables comparisons of physicochemical properties of receptors from different species, different target tissues, or from target systems of varied responsiveness (mutant or variant cells in culture).

---

[3]In general, the "efficiency" of an affinity labeling experiment is considered to be the percentage of the total number of hormone-binding sites, determined in a binding experiment with a reversibly bound ligand, that become covalently labeled by the affinity probe. Ambiguities can develop when this efficiency is less than 100% and when there are multiple forms of the receptor, distinguishable after covalent labeling (but not before). In such a case, the relative concentration of the different receptor species labeled covalently may not be an accurate measure of their actual relative concentration, as the labeling efficiency of the different species may differ. Such ambiguities can complicate considerations of synthesis rates and analyses of precursor–product relationships between the different receptor species.

Many studies of receptor structure have utilized proteases to probe for domains of ligand binding and nucleotide interaction. When in the native state, most receptors seem to undergo proteolysis in clearly defined steps. With reversibly bound ligands, this selective proteolysis can be followed down to the level of the steroid-binding core, that has been termed in some systems the "mero" receptor. Such studies can be done very conveniently with covalently labeled receptor, especially since the size and charge of these species can be characterized at high resolution, under disaggregating conditions. But, in addition, these proteolytic degradation studies can be extended down beyond the point where the remaining receptor structure will no longer sustain the binding of a reversible ligand, and they can be performed on denatured receptor. Such studies have enabled important distinctions to be made between the structures of the progesterone A and B subunits, where it appears that evolutionary pressures have maintained nearly identical domains with respect to proteolytic cleavage of native receptor; differences in sequence, however, are revealed under denaturing conditions (Birnbaumer *et al.*, 1983a,b).

With covalently labeled receptor, degradation studies can be extended to the level of oligopeptides and even idividual amino acids bearing the covalently attached ligand. Thus, one can begin to investigate the composition and topology of the hormone binding site. While studies of this type are only beginning with the hormones in question (Holmes and Smith, 1983), this approach has been used extensively in characterizing active site residues in hormone-binding sites on enzymes and binding proteins (cf. Section IV).

One question concerning receptor proteolysis has to do with the true native form of the receptor and the degree to which receptor isolated after cell fractionation may have been acted upon by endogenous proteases or proteases activated during the preparation. This question can be addressed directly using affinity labels that are sufficiently selective to be used in intact systems: Receptor can be labeled in whole cells, and then the cells lysed directly under strongly denaturing conditions (such as hot sodium dodecyl sulfate–2-mercaptoethanol) that would inactivate degradative enzymes. Physicochemical comparison between receptor labeled *in situ* and receptor labeled after cell fractionation and purification allows studies on endogenous proteases (cf. Sections III,B,2 and III,C,2).

3. *Receptor Dynamics and Function*

Because covalently labeled receptor can be studied by high-resolution, disaggregating separation methods, such as two-dimensional gel electrophoresis, it is possible to investigate covalent modifications of receptors such as phosphorylation or acetylation that cause minor alterations in receptor charge. Such covalent modifications might represent different activity states of the receptor, altered by hormone exposure. Studies of this type have been done with the progesterone and glucocorticoid receptors (cf. Sections III,C and III,D).

Affinity labeling can also be used to study receptor turnover. The receptor in cells can be pulse labeled, either by photoaffinity labeling or by pulse-chase techniques. Then the subsequent fate of the receptor can be followed as to the rate of loss of native receptor and nature of processes degrading the receptor *in vivo*. Such studies have been performed on receptors for estrogens and thyroid hormone (cf. Sections III,B and III,F).

Receptors appear to act through association with other cellular macromolecules. These may be soluble "modifier" proteins or chromatin constituents. Regardless of the details of these ternary associations, such studies are assisted materially by affinity labeling coupled with cross-linking techniques. The covalent fixation of the ligand to the receptor converts the receptor itself into a stable probe for studying these ternary associations. These interactions can be studied under nondenaturing conditions by standard techniques, or after the application of bifunctional reagents to cross-link receptor to these macromolecules.[4] The physiochemical properties of the ternary complex, labeled by virtue of the covalent link of the affinity label to the receptor, can be studied in great detail under denaturing conditions. Both approaches should lead to more detailed information on the site of action of hormone receptors in the cell.

Autoradiography provides a direct approach to defining the subcellular localization of active hormonal agents. With diffusible substances such as steroid and thyroid hormones, sample processing must be done without exposure to fixatives, organic solvents, and embedding media (Roth *et al.*, 1977). This is not only awkward, but produces sections of poor quality. Covalent labeling of receptors provides a unique opportunity to perform autoradiographic studies on hormone subcellular localization. As autoradiography can be performed at the electron microscopic level, ultrastructural localization should also be possible. So far, however, studies of this type have not been reported.

Finally, irreversibly acting hormone analogs, analogous to affinity labels (particularly of the electrophilic type), might display unusual biological activity. While "prolonged" duration of action was once con-

---

[4]Prolonged photolysis at relatively low wavelength (e.g., 254 nm) has been proposed as a "zero spacer" cross-linker for protein–protein and protein–nucleic acid interactions (Kunkel *et al.*, 1981).

sidered to be an identifying characteristic of hormone analogs that react with receptor irreversibly, this has turned out to be only an idiosyncratic characteristic within the affinity labeling field: Altered pharmacokinetics of the hormone analog can give the impression of prolonged activity, and rapid turnover can limit duration of action of a covalently labeled receptor. Still, the *in vivo* activity of hormone analogs capable of covalent attachment to receptor sites is an interesting question.

B. AFFINITY LABELING OF ESTROGEN RECEPTORS

1. *Labeling Agents*

There are many reports that estrogen derivatives bearing alkylating groups may react covalently with estrogen receptors. This work was reviewed elsewhere (Katzenellenbogen, 1977), and much of it was done prior to the characterization of the estrogen receptor. Thus these reagents were not evaluated as receptor labels or inactivators. They were generally assayed in terms of the duration of their estrogenic activity, none of them appearing to have any unusual activity in this regard. It is unlikely that any of these reagents would be effective receptor affinity labels, but characterization at the biochemical level was insufficient to prove potential utility.

The potential of certain photoreactive estrogens as affinity labeling agents has been investigated by Katzenellenbogen (reviewed in Katzenellenbogen, 1977). The spectrum of compounds encompassed those bearing diazocarbonyl, azide, and unsaturated and aromatic carbonyl groups. These studies involved receptor binding and inactivation assays. Then on the basis of high receptor affinity and adequate receptor inactivation efficiency, two compounds, hexestrol azide (3) and 6-oxo-estradiol (2), were selected for further study and prepared in tritium-labeled from (Katzenellenbogen *et al.*, 1977).

Hexestrol azide (3) proved to have an attachment efficiency for receptor similar to its inactivation efficiency ($\sim$ 10–15%). In addition to being relatively inefficient, hexestrol azide also proved to be relatively nonselective in its photolabeling properties. Therefore, labeled recep-

Hexestrol Azide (**3**)　　　　　(**4**)

tor could be observed only in partially purified receptor preparations (Katzenellenbogen *et al.*, 1977).

The situation with 6-oxoestradiol (**2**) was very different: This compound has a good affinity for receptor and is efficient in the receptor photoinactivation assay (Katzenellenbogen *et al.*, 1974; cf. Section II,A,1, Fig. 2). However, it did *not* react covalently with receptor. Thus, it appears to be a representative of compounds that effect a site-specific inactivation of receptor (presumably through a photoactivated redox process), but do not themselves become attached to the protein.[1]

Although dienone systems were used successfully to photoattach affinity labeling agents to progestin, glucocorticoid, and androgen receptors, they have not proven effective as photoaffinity labeling agents for the estrogen receptor (R. J. Neeley, M. K. Mao, and J. A. Katzenellenbogen, unpublished). Examples of compounds that have been tried are shown in Scheme 1. It should be pointed out, however, that these reagents have been studied indirectly by receptor inactivation assays that might not detect low-efficiency labeling.

The aziridine analog of the nonsteroidal antiestrogen tamoxifen (**1**) is a very efficient and selective electrophilic affinity labeling agent for the estrogen receptor. This compound was chosen from several tamoxifen analogs having reactive functions in place of the side chain amino function, on the basis of potent receptor inactivating capacity in cell-free extracts and in whole uteri and cells *in vitro* (Robertson *et al.*, 1981). Once prepared in tritium-labeled form, it was found to label the receptor nearly quantitatively with high selectivity, in unfractionated cytosol preparations, in whole target tissues, in organ culture, and in estrogen-responsive cells in culture (B. S. Katzenellenbogen *et al.*, 1983). The utility of this compound in receptor studies is described in the next section.

Receptor affinity labeling studies have also been done with 4-mercuriestradiol (Muldoon and Warren, 1969; Muldoon, 1980). The non-

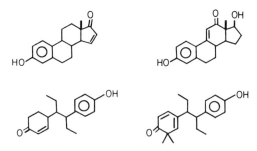

SCHEME 1. Estrogen enones that fail to inactivate receptor.

specific covalent reaction of this compound with free thiols limits its utility as a selective labeling agent, however. Studies with this compound have lead to interesting hypotheses about estrogen actions. Receptor labeling with a low-affinity estrogen disulfide derivative has also been reported (Ikeda, 1982).

11β-Chloromethylestradiol (Organon 4333, 4) has a very high apparent affinity for the estrogen receptor (230% that of estradiol), and appears to interact irreversibly with the estrogen receptor in whole cells and in cell extracts (Reiner and Katzenellenbogen, 1983; Reiner et al., 1984). Thus, it may be acting as a receptor affinity label. On the other hand, because of its high affinity, it may simply be bound reversibly, but so tightly that it fails to undergo exchange with [³H]estradiol under the usual conditions. The question of covalent attachment to receptor can be resolved only through studies with tritium-labeled material.

2. Studies on Estrogen Receptor Structure and Function

Tamoxifen aziridine (TA, 1), an electrophilic analog of the antiestrogen tamoxifen, was prepared by us (B. S. Katzenellenbogen et al., 1983) in tritium-labeled form (20 Ci/mmol) for direct studies on estrogen receptor structure. Initial studies with radioinert TA had suggested that this compound reacted irreversibly (covalently) with the estrogen receptor, in that there was a concentration and time-dependent loss of exchangeable binding activity as determined with tritiated estradiol (Fig. 1; Robertson et al., 1981). Subsequent studies with radiolabeled TA showed that the covalent labeling of receptor in cytosol preparations from rat uterus and breast cancer cells was very efficient, with essentially all of the receptors becoming labeled covalently (cf. Section II,A,1, Figs. 2 and 3). Labeling was rapid at room temperature, being complete within 1 hour, and it was highly selective for the estrogen receptor protein. Nearly complete labeling of receptor was achieved with only a few-fold excess of reagent, and there was minimal labeling of other, nonreceptor proteins. Labeling was estrogen specific in that it was blocked only by estrogens and antiestrogens, and it was not observed in nontarget cells and tissues lacking the estrogen receptor. The estrogen receptor in intact cells (MCF-7 human breast cancer cells) was similarly efficiently and selectively labeled by exposure of cells to tritiated-TA at 37°C (see below, Fig. 6). Receptor-negative MDA-MB-231 human breast cancer cells showed no estrogen-specific labeling.

SDS–polyacrylamide gel electrophoresis showed that the tamoxifen aziridine-labeled estrogen receptor appears to be ~ 63,000 Da (Fig. 5).

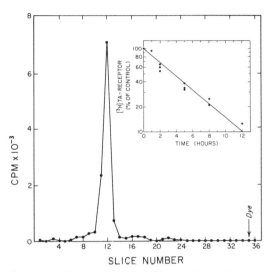

FIG. 5. Sodium dodecyl sulfate–polyacrylamide gel electrophoretic analysis of the MCF-7 nuclear receptor. Cells were labeled with 20 nM [³H]TA ± 2 μM estradiol for 1 hour at 37°C, and nuclear salt extracts were prepared and analyzed on SDS–polyacrylamide disc gels. Insert: Degradation of TA-labeled MCF-7 nuclear receptor. Nuclear receptor was labeled as described above, and the label was then chased with 10^{-6} M E_2 for various time periods ranging from 0 (no chase) to 12 hours.

This was found for receptor from rat or lamb uterus and from human MCF-7 breast cancer cells (Katzenellenbogen *et al.*, 1983b; B. S. Katzenellenbogen *et al.*, 1983; Monsma *et al.*, 1984). Both cytosolic estrogen receptor, labeled by treating cytosol with [³H]TA, and nuclear receptor, obtained from cells or tissues incubated with [³H]TA, show identical molecular weights. *In situ* labeling of nuclear receptor, as can be done with the MCF-7 cells, and lysis of cells in denaturing medium, showed that the molecular weight of receptor in intact cells was also 63,000 under conditions in which proteolytic degradation of receptor was not likely to occur.

Time-course studies with [³H]TA-labeled nuclear receptor indicate that the M_r 63,000 receptor form is stable for over 24 hours at 25°C in the nuclear salt extracts; cytosolic receptor from MCF-7 cells, however, is rapidly degraded to a 53,000 and then eventually to a 37,000 molecular weight species, this conversion being blocked completely by adding leupeptin or molybdate. Affinity-labeled receptor interacts with several monoclonal antibodies to MCF-7 estrogen receptor (prepared by Geoffrey L. Greene), and it can be purified extensively by immunoadsorbent chromatography on antireceptor antibody columns (Monsma *et al.*, 1984).

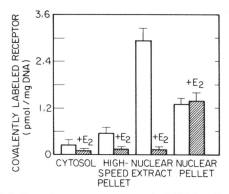

FIG. 6. Covalent labeling of estrogen receptors in MCF-7 cells with [³H]tamoxifen aziridine. Separate flasks of MCF-7 cells were exposed to 10 nM [³H]tamoxifen aziridine in the absence (open bars) or presence (shaded bars) of 1 μM estradiol for 1 hour at 37°C, and the indicated cell fractions were prepared. The extent of covalent binding was determined by the ethanol-filter disc assay. The error bars indicate the range of two experiments. (From B. S. Katzenellenbogen *et al.*, 1983, with permission.)

The labeling of whole cells with [³H]TA (Fig. 6) also indicates that there are at most only minor quantities of estrogen binding species in the particulate fractions (microsomal and membrane/nuclear pellet fractions) remaining after salt extraction. These findings, however, do not exclude the existence of estrogen receptors in subcellular fractions. These sites may simply not react covalently with TA or low levels of receptor could be masked by nonspecific background binding found in membrane fractions.

The TA-labeled estrogen receptors from R3 and R27 variants of MCF-7 cells resistant to the growth inhibitory effect of antiestrogens show molecular weights and isoelectric points indistinguishable from that of the wild-type cells (Miller and Katzenellenbogen, 1983b). These and other findings (Nawata *et al.*, 1981) suggest that the defect in antiestrogen responsiveness of these variant cells lies at steps beyond the initial binding of ligand.

It is difficult to determine the isoelectric point of estrogen receptor labeled with reversible ligands, because aggregation with other proteins prevents the receptor from entering the focusing gel and distorts the focusing pattern. Thus, with reversibly labeling ligands, it is not possible to determine accurately whether the cytosolic and the nuclear estrogen receptor show identical isoelectric points. With TA-labeled receptor, isoelectric focusing can be done in 8 M urea. Under these disaggregating conditions, both nuclear and cytosolic receptor are found to have pI values of ~ 5.7. In these experiments the protein bands on isoelectric focusing gels were relatively broad, suggesting charge heterogeneity possibly arising from varying degrees of receptor phosphorylation, acetylation, or other modification. Higher resolution assays with partially purified preparations are underway to determine the charge homogeneity/heterogeneity of estrogen receptors.

Finally, it is of note that although triphenylethylene antiestrogens such as tamoxifen interact with an additional class of antiestrogen specific binding sites that are distinct from the receptor (Sutherland *et al.*, 1980; Katzenellenbogen *et al.*, 1983a; Sudo *et al.*, 1983; Miller and Katzenellenbogen, 1983a,b), the interaction of TA with these sites is reversible and shows no evidence of covalent interaction (Monsma *et al.*, 1984).

3. *Studies on Estrogen Receptor Dynamics*

The high selectivity of TA permits its use to label estrogen receptors in MCF-7 cells in a pulse–chase manner. After the labeling period with [³H]TA, excess estradiol is added as a chase, and the fate of the covalently labeled receptor can be followed with time to determine the half-life of the receptor. As is seen in the inset to Fig. 5, it is evident that the 63,000 molecular weight receptor component is lost quite quickly with a half-time of 4 hours, consistent with the rate of receptor turnover in these cells determined by the technique of heavy amino acid-density shift (Eckert *et al.*, 1982, 1984). It is of note that smaller molecular weight fragments are not observed during the degradation of receptor in cells, either in the nuclear salt-extractable fraction or in the cytosol or the microsomal or salt-extracted nuclear pellet fractions (not shown). Thus, in MCF-7 cells the TA-labeled receptor must be broken down in such a manner that the portion retaining the label is quickly degraded to small-molecular-weight fragments that are no longer detectable by SDS–gel electrophoretic techniques (Katzenellenbogen *et al.*, 1983b; Monsma *et al.*, 1984).

TA behaves as an antiestrogen with bioactivity much like its reversibly binding parent compound, tamoxifen. It inhibits the growth of MCF-7 human breast cancer cells *in vitro*, suppresses estradiol-stimulated uterine growth in rats, and elicits the regression of hormone-dependent dimethylbenz[*a*]anthracene-induced mammary tumors in rats (Katzenellenbogen *et al.*, 1982). In all of these assays, TA is only slightly less potent than tamoxifen. It should be noted, however, that studies *in vivo* may be complicated by possible metabolism of TA, an aspect that has not yet been examined because the amounts of tritiated compound available are limited.

Muldoon and Warren (1969) and Muldoon (1980) have carefully

studied 4-mercuriestradiol, an interesting estradiol derivative which increases uterine cell proliferation and specific estrogen-stimulated enzyme activities in rat uterus. This compound has been shown to interact with uterine cytosol estrogen receptors in an affinity labeling manner. Although the apparent affinity of 4-mercuriestradiol for estrogen receptor is low, the compound interacted to form a nondissociable complex, and the stoichiometry of binding indicated that at least two to three times as many molecules of 4-mercuriestradiol as of estradiol became bound. Although the mercuriestradiol–receptor complex exhibited the same sedimentation properties as those of the estradiol–receptor complex on sucrose gradients, the mercuriestradiol–receptor complex showed very little binding to nuclei, DNA, or chromatin, and it did not stimulate RNA polymerase I activity in uterine nuclei. Hence, of particular interest was the observation that while warming of the estradiol- and the 4-mercuriestradiol–receptor complexes at 30°C elicits conversion of both complexes from the 4 S to a 5 S form, only the 5 S estradiol–receptor complex showed significant affinity for nuclear components. Subcellular distribution analysis following uterine intraluminal administration of 4-mercuri[³H]estradiol indicated very low levels of nuclear accumulation of receptor complexes but early accumulation of mercuriestradiol receptor complexes in the microsomal fraction, suggesting a possible extranuclear site of action of this affinity labeling estrogen (Muldoon, 1980).

Ikeda (1982) reported that rabbit uterine estrogen receptor is covalantly labeled with a 17-nitrophenyldithioestradiol derivative. This compound shows very low affinity for the receptor; nevertheless, the covalent labeling of an estrogen-specific binding component was demonstrated by polyacrylamide gel electrophoretic analysis. The validity of this labeling is uncertain, however, since the labeled receptor was not identified on sucrose gradients.

C. Affinity Labeling of Progestin Receptors

1. Labeling Agents

The progesterone receptor has been labeled with either photoaffinity or electrophilic affinity labeling agents. Most photolabeling studies have used the synthetic progestin R5020 (17α,21-dimethyl-19-norpregna-4,9-diene-3,20-dione (5); Roussel-Uclaf), which embodies a dienone system. Photoactivation of this compound by irradiation at 300 nm results in labeling of the receptor with a relatively modest efficiency; the labeling efficiency of receptor from human breast cancer cells

R 5020 (**5**)   RU 38486 (**6**)   ORG 2058(**7**)

(T47D cells), chick oviduct, or rabbit uterus was comparable (see Section III,C,2 below). Although the labeling is relatively inefficient, it is highly selective, so that in cytosol preparations essentially only receptor becomes labeled. In T47D cells, *in situ* labeling of receptor can also be performed selectively (Horwitz and Alexander, 1983). Another Roussel synthetic progestin RU 38,486 (**6**) may be a valid photoaffinity label for the progesterone receptor, but its labeling efficiency is very low (Horwitz *et al.*, 1983). A related synthetic progestin ^{3}H-labeled ORG 2058 (**7**) also was reported to photoaffinity label progesterone receptors in rabbit uterine cytosol (Westphal *et al.*, 1981), but this compound has received relatively little use thus far.

The progesterone receptor can be labeled using electrophilic bromoacetoxy derivatives (**8**). These compounds, prepared originally for affinity labeling studies on steroid dehydrogenases (cf. Section IV,A,1), label receptor efficiently, but with low selectivity, so that purified receptor must be used. Also, these derivatives are susceptible to hydrolysis, precluding use in prolonged incubations (Holmes *et al.*, 1981). They have the advantage that the covalently labeled residue in the proteins can be isolated as the carboxymethylated derivative, a form that permits ready identification.

Several other electrophilic progesterone derivatives were reported earlier as potential receptor affinity labeling agents. Again, their interaction with receptor was not investigated adequately. This work has been reviewed earlier (Katzenellenbogen, 1977).

2. Studies on Progesterone Receptor Structure

Dure *et al.* (1980) employed the synthetic progestin, tritiated R5020 (**5**), to photoaffinity label the chick oviduct progesterone receptor. This

	X	Y	Z
8a	$OCOCH_2Br$	——	——
8b	——	$OCOCH_2Br$	——
8c	——	——	$OCOCH_2Br$

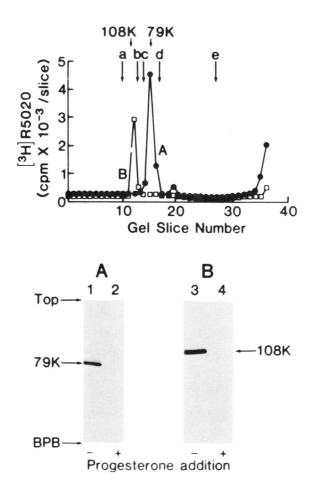

FIG. 7. Polyacrylamide gel electrophoretic analysis of covalently labeled proteins in receptor A-2 and B-2 preparation. Top, radioactive profiles of covalently labeled proteins in receptor A-2 (●) and B-2 (□) proteins; preparations separated by tube gel electrophoresis in 7.5% polyacrylamide containing SDS. Radioactivity in the last two to three slices is due to breakdown products of ³H-labeled R5020 formed during UV irradiation. Bottom, fluorography of covalently labeled proteins in partially purified receptor A-2 and B-2 preparations separated by slab gel electrophoresis in 7.5% polyacrylamide containing SDS. Lane 1, fluorography of receptor A-2 preparation labeled with ³H-labeled R5020 in the absence of unlabeled progesterone; Lane 3, fluorography of receptor B-2 preparation labeled with ³H-labeled R5020 in the absence of unlabeled progesterone; Lanes 2 and 4, fluorography of receptors A-2 and B-2 preparations obtained after carrying out incubations with ³H-labeled R5020 in the presence of 1 μM unlabeled progesterone. (From Birnbaumer et al., 1983a, with permission.)

ligand shows high affinity for the progesterone receptor (K_d approximately 2 nM) and a UV absorption maximum at 320 nm. Irradiation can be performed on crude cytosol extracts at wavelengths over 300 nm (through a Pyrex filter), so that damage to proteins is minimized. When the progesterone receptors in cytosol were complexed with tritiated R5020 and then irradiated with UV light, analysis of the protein mixture by SDS–polyacrylamide gels revealed two major components with molecular weights of 106,000 and 78,000, present in approximately equal amounts (Fig. 7). These proteins corresponded to receptor subunit proteins B and A. The time course of photoaffinity labeling of proteins A and B was similar, with maximal attachment being reached by 1–2 hours.

Use of a copper sulfate solution filter, which blocks all irradiation below ∼ 315 nm, raises the coupling efficiency to 5% and provides more selective labeling of the receptor (Birnbaumer *et al.,* 1983a). These studies, carried out in crude receptor preparations, showed highly selective covalent labeling of the receptor, but small amounts of other proteins were covalently labeled as well. They also provided further evidence for the existence of two dissimilar hormone-binding subunits as was found in earlier work on receptor protein purification. Results with the progesterone receptor in human breast cancer cells in culture (Lessey *et al.,* 1983) also reveal two hormone-binding components of dissimilar size, approximately 81,000 (A subunit) and 115,000 (B subunit), photoaffinity labeled in equal amounts, that differ also in affinity for DNA. Hence, in human cells there appear to be two progesterone receptor subunits analogous in many ways to those seen in the chicken oviduct.

The question of structural similarity in hormone binding domains in the chick oviduct progesterone receptor A and B subunits has been assessed by partial proteolysis of the photoaffinity labeled proteins under highly denaturing conditions (Birnbaumer *et al.,* 1983a). Partially purified and covalently labeled receptor A and B proteins were digested with *Staphylococcus aureus* V8 protease, an enzyme specific for glutamic acid residues. SDS-gel fluorographic analyses of the A and B protein products revealed similar patterns yielding a 9500 Da limit digest fragment that has the same isoelectric point (pI 5.9–6.0). Hence, the tritiated R5020 is bound to regions of receptor subunits A and B that show great similarity in charge and molecular weight. Since only a single radioactive spot was seen in two-dimensional gel analysis, it suggests that only a single locus of A and B is covalently labeled with R5020. In addition, since unlabeled progesterone prevents the covalent labeling with tritiated R5020, it appears that the site covalently labeled is at or near the progesterone binding site on the receptor subunits.

As found with *S. aureus* V8 protease, use of two other enzymes, trypsin and chymotrypsin, gave peptide patterns for covalently labeled A and B proteins characteristic for each protease but again indistinguishable for the A and B proteins (Fig. 8). This provided further evidence that the two proteins were similar if not identical in structural organization. Two-dimensional analysis, however, on iodinated A and B proteins, revealed both common as well as different peptides in the two proteins. Thus the A and B proteins do not bear a precursor–product relationship, are distinct from one another in amino acid se-

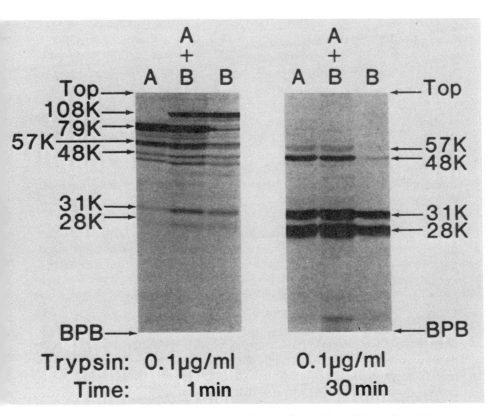

Fɪɢ. 8. Tryptic proteolysis. Tryptic proteolysis under mild conditions of partially purified A and B progesterone receptor proteins (not denatured) covalently labeled with ³H-labeled R5020 and comparison of fragment sizes obtained. The electrophoretic analysis was carried out in 12.5% polyacrylamide gel slabs. (From Birnbaumer *et al.*, 1983b, with permission.)

quences, but clearly share common structural features in the native state (Birnbaumer *et al.,* 1983b).

Progesterone receptors in rabbit uterine cytosol have been photoaffinity labeled with tritiated R5020 (Janne, 1982), or with tritiated ORG 2058 (**7**) (Westphal, *et al.,* 1981). Labeling of partially purified receptor preparations revealed species of 100,000, 80,000, and 65,000 molecular weight (Janne, 1982) or of 95,000 and 85,000 molecular weight (Westphal *et al.,* 1981); purified receptor migrated predominantly as a 70,000 molecular weight protein. The relationship of these several forms to the native receptor found *in vivo* remains under active consideration (Lamb *et al.,* 1982).

In recent experiments, Horwitz and Alexander (1983) have examined the nuclear progesterone receptor after *in situ* photolabeling of intact T47D breast cancer cells with tritiated R5020. Cells are exposed to tritiated R5020 to localize receptors in the nucleus, and then the intact cells are irradiated with ultraviolet light at 300 nm for 2 minutes. Approximately 15% of the receptors become covalently linked to R5020, and as was seen for cytosol receptors, two species of M_r 115,000 and 81,000 are observed. Hence, cytosol and nuclear progesterone receptors are of similar subunit size, suggesting that the acquisition of nuclear binding capacity does not involve major structural receptor modification. Similar size of the nuclear and cytosolic steroid hormone receptors was also found with affinity labeled estrogen receptors in human breast cancer MCF-7 cells (Katzenellenbogen *et al.,* 1983b; Monsma *et al.,* 1984).

In studies by Holmes *et al.* (1981), 11α-, 16α-, and 21-bromoacetoxyprogesterones (**8**) have been used to affinity label and characterize the progesterone receptor from human uterus. These reagents were used previously with success to label the progesterone binding site of the enzyme 20β-hydroxysteroid dehydrogenase (cf. Section IV,A,1). These alkylating progesterone derivatives are highly reactive and not very selective. Hence, the receptor must be purified extensively before reaction with the affinity label. Labeling with tritiated compounds reveals that these three derivatives bind to an $M_r = 45,000$ protein from human uterus, that is most likely a proteolytic fragment of the native intact receptor. Holmes and Smith (1983) have identified the particular amino acid residues that are alkylated by the 11α- and 16α-bromoacetates by employing hydrolysis of the steroid–receptor adducts followed by separation of the resulting carboxymethylated amino acids using high-performance liquid chromatography. The 11α-bromoacetate alkylates the 1 position of a histidine residue, and the 16α-bromoacetate alkylates the 3 position of a histidine residue, as well as a methionine residue. This report was the first instance wherein specific amino acid residues in the binding site of a steroid–hormone receptor were identified.

These studies reveal some interesting similarities between affinity labeling of the human progesterone receptor and human transcortin, also affinity labeled using progesterone analogs with bromoacetoxy groups on the C- and D-rings (cf. Section IV,A,1). With transcortin, a methionine residue was located near the 11β position, and histidine and methionine residues were located adjacent to the 16α and 17α positions. So, the data for the progesterone receptor concerning the binding site around the D-ring of progesterone are similar, in that histidine and methionine residues are present, but at the C-ring, the receptor differs from transcortin, in that histidine, not a methionine, was present near the 11α position.

D. Affinity Labeling of Glucocorticoid Receptors

1. *Labeling Agents*

The glucocorticoid receptor has been studied with both photoreactive and electrophilic affinity labeling agents. The synthetic progestin, R5020, which is useful as a photoaffinity labeling agent for the progesterone receptor, also binds to the glucocorticoid receptor and can be used as a photoaffinity label. The synthetic glucocorticoid triamcinolone acetonide (9), which contains a cross-conjugated dienone system, also has been used as a photoaffinity labeling agent. With either of these agents, labeling efficiency is low, but selectivity is high.

The 21-O-methanesulfonate (mesylate) derivatives of cortisol (10) and dexamethasone (11) have been used as electrophilic affinity labels for glucocorticoid receptors. The efficiency of receptor labeling with these agents is very good, but as with other α-keto alkylating agents, their selectivity is low, since they are generally reactive toward any strong nucleophile. So, most studies have been done in partially purified receptor preparations. It is possible, however, to conduct labeling studies in intact cells and observe receptor-specific labeling by analysis of the labeled proteins by polyacrylamide gel electrophoresis.

Triamcinolone Acetonide (9)   Cortisol Mesylate (10)   Dexamethasone Mesylate (11)

2. *Studies on Glucocorticoid Receptor Structure and Function*

Several groups have used photoactivation of triamcinolone acetonide (**9**) (Dellweg *et al.*, 1982; Gehring and Hotz, 1983) and R5020 (Nordeen *et al.*, 1981) to covalently label receptors in glucocorticoid-responsive wild-type and in nonresponsive mutant cells and to compare their physicochemical properties. Irradiation of crude cytosol–receptor complexes with triamcinolone acetonide yields only 2% covalent attachment of the ligand, but in partially purified receptor preparations, cross-linking is increased to 8–12% (Dellweg *et al.*, 1982). Tritiated R5020, which can covalently bind to the progesterone receptor, also displays low affinity for glucocorticoid receptors, and upon photoactivation, it also covalently labels the glucocorticoid receptor. The labeling efficiency of glucocorticoid receptor with R5020 is 2–5% (Nordeen *et al.*, 1981).

In wild-type mouse lymphoma (S49) cells, activated or nonactivated receptor complexes show the same molecular weight, approximately 94,000 by SDS gel electrophoresis of [^{3}H]triamcinolone acetonide-labeled material (Dellweg *et al.*, 1982; Gehring and Hotz, 1983). Examination of glucocorticoid receptors of wild-type lymphoid cells and of two classes of glucocorticoid-resistant variants of "nuclear transfer-deficient, nt$^-$" and "increased nuclear transfer, nt^i" phenotypes, revealed that wild-type and nt$^-$ variant receptors yielded radiolabeled receptor bands of M_r 94,000, while nt^i variant receptors gave a lower molecular weight of 40,000. Partial proteolysis of wild-type and nt$^-$ receptors with α-chymotrypsin yielded steroid-labeled receptor fragments of molecular weight 38,000, while nt^i variant receptors were unaffected by chymotrypsin treatment. The 39,000 Da chymotryptic fragment showed increased affinity for DNA that was indistinguishable from that of native nt^i variant receptors. Trypsin treatment of wild-type, nt$^-$, and nt^i receptors yielded in all cases steroid-labeled fragments of M_r approximately 29,000; these tryptic fragments were devoid of DNA binding ability regardless of the original receptor type.

These same 94,000 and 39,000 molecular weight species were found whether receptors were photolabeled with triamcinolone acetonide (**9**) (Gehring and Hotz, 1983) or with R5020 (**5**) (Nordeen *et al.*, 1981). In another steroid-resistant S49 mutant (S49r$^-$) that lacks hormone binding activity, no specific, covalently labeled species was detected (Nordeen *et al.*, 1981). In glucocorticoid-sensitive human lymphoblastic leukemia CEM-C7 cells (Gehring and Hotz, 1983) and in rat hepatoma HTC cells (Nordeen *et al.*, 1981), the same glucocorticoid receptor protein band with molecular weight estimated at 87,000–

94,000 was observed. Interestingly, in another mouse lymphoma with glucocorticoid-sensitive and resistant forms, the glucocorticoid receptor in the cortisol sensitive tumor was of M_r 94,000, while the glucocorticoid-resistant tumor CRP1798 showed the 39,000 receptor form and bound more tightly to DNA than did the receptor from the cortisol-sensitive lymphoma.

Hence, the binding form of the glucocorticoid receptor consists of a single polypeptide of M_r = ~ 90,000 in at least three different species, namely, rat, mouse, and human, and in wild-type cells of either lymphoid or hepatic origin. It is of interest that receptor from nuclear transfer-deficient cells, although reduced in affinity for DNA-cellulose compared to that of the wild-type receptor, showed a molecular weight identical to that of the wild-type receptor. In contrast, the nuclear transfer-increased S49 receptor and the CRP1798-resistant mouse lymphoma receptor bound more tightly to DNA cellulose and gave a molecular weight of 39,000. Mixing experiments and experiments with hybrids of nuclear transfer from wild-type and nuclear transfer-deficient cells (Yamamoto et al., 1976; Gehring, 1979) suggest that the 39,000 receptor species is not due to activity of an endogeneous protease. Rather, they suggest a possible mutation in the structural gene for the glucocorticoid receptor allowing synthesis of only "truncated" receptor, a species representing only a portion of the receptor (Nordeen et al., 1981; Gehring and Hotz, 1983), or a mutation causing premature protein chain termination.

Analyses provided by photoaffinity labeling of receptors in hormone-resistant cells, and other studies employing purified receptors (Wrange and Gustafsson, 1978) have provided evidence for three domains in the wild-type glucocorticoid receptor: a hormone-binding domain, a nuclear interaction domain, and a third domain that modulates nuclear interaction and DNA binding.

The covalent attachment of triamcinolone acetonide and R5020 to glucocorticoid receptor requires activation by light. In contrast, cortisol 21-mesylate (**10**) and dexamethasone mesylate (**11**) are electrophilic affinity labeling agents for the glucocorticoid receptor and thus do not require light activation for covalent binding to the receptor. Simons et al. (1980a,b) and Dunkerton et al. (1982) have prepared several chemically reactive derivatives of glucocorticoids as potential electrophilic affinity labels for the glucocorticoid receptor. Initial studies focused on cortisol 21-mesylate (**10**), an alkylating derivative of cortisol (Simons et al., 1980c). Studies with nonradiolabeled compound revealed that it had an apparent affinity 7% that of cortisol, and that it irreversibly inhibited tritiated dexamethasone binding to receptor in cell-free cytosol extracts of hepatoma tissue culture (HTC) cells. This compound behaved as an antiglucocorticoid. It did not induce tyrosine aminotransferase activity, and it inhibited induction of this enzyme by dexamethasone. In addition, it appeared to be a very long-acting compound, consistent with its presumed covalent interaction. However, with the nonradiolabeled compound there was no direct evidence for this (Simons et al., 1980c).

More recent studies have employed the 21-mesylate derivative of the more potent glucocorticoid dexamethasone (11) (Simons and Thompson, 1981, 1982). Dexamethasone mesylate has an apparent affinity for receptor 14% that of dexamethasone, but since dexamethasone has a higher affinity for receptor than does cortisol, dexamethasone mesylate displays an apparent affinity for glucocorticoid receptor that is approximately equal to that of cortisol (15-fold higher than that of cortisol mesylate). Dexamethasone mesylate behaves as a partial agonist as well as an antagonist of glucocorticoid action in HTC cells, and tritiated dexamethasone is unable to exchange into preformed dexamethasone mesylate–receptor complexes.

Labeling of cytosol with tritiated dexamethasone mesylate revealed a covalently labeled $M_r = 85,000$ species that appears to represent the glucocorticoid receptor, i.e., labeling was dexamethasone competable. Although the efficiency of labeling in this first report was only 13% (Simons and Thompson, 1981), labeling efficiency was increased to approximately 70–90% by raising the pH to 8–9, using concentrated receptor extracts, and optimizing the time and temperature of the incubation (Simons et al., 1983). Even with this enhanced efficiency of receptor labeling, however, there are many dexamethasone mesylate-labeled species in unfractionated cytosol extracts. DNA-cellulose affords substantial purification of the covalently labeled receptor and clearly reveals that this species is of molecular weight 90,000. The unactivated and activated rat liver and HTC cell receptors labeled by tritiated dexamethasone mesylate show identical molecular weights as determined by SDS-gel electrophoresis, and receptors labeled covalently with dexamethasone mesylate and receptors labeled reversibly with dexamethasone can be equally activated to a DNA binding form (i.e., approximately 30% of complexes become activated). The glucocorticoid receptor in rat thymocytes and human lymphoid cells can also be covalently labeled with dexamethasone mesylate, revealing a similar receptor size of M_r 95,000 (Foster et al., 1983).

Dexamethasone mesylate is very inefficient in labeling receptors in intact cells, and the extent of nonspecific covalent labeling is very high. However, it is possible to find low amounts of a specifically labeled 90,000 molecular weight species in both cytosol and nuclear salt extracts. Hence, dexamethasone mesylate shows only low nuclear transfer of receptor complexes in HTC cells (Simons *et al.*, 1983). This may be due to the fact that the internal intracellular pH is lower than optimal for covalent binding and/or that the high concentration of thiols in cells inactivates dexamethasone mesylate and blocks the covalent labeling reaction. In any event, these studies provide good evidence for the similarities in physicochemical properties of nuclear and cytosol glucocorticoid receptor species and for covalent and non-covalently labeled glucocorticoid receptors.

Weisz *et al.* (1983) have also used dexamethasone mesylate to label the glucocorticoid receptor in partially purified preparations from goat lactating mammary gland, and they report an apparent molecular weight of 75,000–80,000, slightly smaller than the 90,000 species reported for the nonproteolyzed receptor in other cells. In Syrian hamster melanoma cells, dexamethasone mesylate acted as a long-acting glucocorticoid agonist and showed little antiglucocorticoid activity (Weisz *et al.*, 1983). Hence, the biological character of dexamethasone mesylate appears to be different in HTC cells (Simons and Thompson, 1981), than in melanoma cells (Weisz, *et al.*, 1983), based upon the end points of bioactivity that have been examined.

Further studies by Housley and Pratt (1983a,b) reveal that the $M_r = 92,000$ glucocorticoid receptor in L cell cytosol is phosphorylated on serine residues and can be resolved into two species using isoelectric focusing. Charge heterogeneity of the glucocorticoid receptor has also been reported for the dexamethasone mesylate affinity labeled glucocorticoid receptor in human HeLa S3 cells. Treatment of receptors with human alkaline phosphatase generates a less heterogeneous receptor population with more basic isoelectric points, suggesting that the glucocorticoid receptor is a family of molecular species of varying isoelectric points that may reflect different states of phosphorylation (Cidlowski and Rishon, 1983).

E. Affinity Labeling of Androgen Receptors

1. *Labeling Agents*

Steroidal dienones were first used as photoaffinity labeling agents on androgen binding protein, an extracellular protein that is distinct from the androgen receptor (cf. Section IV,B,1). It was these studies that inspired the use of dienones as photoreactive labeling agents for progesterone and glucocorticoid receptors. Methyl trienolone (R1881) (**12**), a synthetic androgen embodying a trienone system, has been

Methyl Trienolone
R 1881 (**12**)   (**13**)

utilized for photoaffinity labeling of the androgen receptor. It has a binding affinity for receptor that is somewhat higher than that of testosterone. 5α-Dihydrotestosterone 17-bromoacetate (**13**) has been used as an electrophilic labeling agent.

2. Androgen Receptor Labeling Studies

There are only a few reports of affinity labeling of the androgen receptor. Chang *et al.* (1982) describe a 540,000-fold purification of the androgen receptor from steer seminal vesicles, using a simple procedure involving chromatography on two DNA-cellulose columns and a testosterone affinity column. By this process, they obtain in 48% yield, a homogeneous species that migrates on SDS-polyacrylamide gels with an apparent molecular weight of 60,000 and retains the binding specificity characteristic of the androgen receptor.

In order to verify the identity of this species as the androgen receptor, they have performed affinity labeling experiments on partially purified material. Upon electrophilic labeling with 5α-dihydrotestosterone 17-bromoacetate (**13**) or photolabeling with methyl trienolone (**12**), they observed radioactive incorporation into both a 60,000 and a 70,000 molecular weight species. This labeling is blocked by ligands for the androgen receptor, but is unaffected by steroids that do not bind. The partially purified preparation appears to contain two "receptor" species (60,000 and 70,000 molecular weight), with the larger being lost during the subsequent purification steps. Whether the smaller form arises by proteolytic degradation of the larger is not yet known.

A very similar procedure was used to purify the androgen receptor from rat ventral prostate (Chang *et al.*, 1983). Again, partially purified receptor was affinity labeled with methyl trienolone and 5α-dihydrotestosterone 17-bromoacetate, and both reagents labeled a species with an apparent molecular weight of 86,000 on SDS-polyacrylamide gels. Although there were many other protein components in the partially purified preparation, the photoreactive compound only labeled receptor. The bromoacetate, while giving predominantly receptor labeling, also labeled other, nonreceptor species. It is not certain at this point whether the different apparent molecular weights of the rat prostate androgen receptor (86,000) and the steer seminal vesicle receptor (60,000 and 70,000) represent species or organ differences or differential proteolysis.

F. AFFINITY LABELING OF THYROID HORMONE RECEPTORS

1. Labeling Agents

Receptors for thyroid hormones have been affinity labeled with photoreactive and electrophilic compounds. N-2-Diazo-3,3,3-trifluoropropionyl-3,5,3'-triiodo-L-thyronine (14a) has been used to photoaffinity label the thyroid receptor from GH1 cells. Labeling selectivity with this reagent is high, but efficiencies are only on the order of 10–15%. Aromatic iodo compounds are photolytically labile, and triiodothyronine (14b) and thyroxine (14c) themselves are capable of photolabeling the thyroid hormone receptor. The selectivity of this direct labeling is reasonably high, and the labeling efficiency depends upon the wavelength of irradiation and can be as high as 15–20%. N-Bromoacetyltriiodothyronine (14d) has also been used as an electrophilic affinity label; while labeling efficiency is high, selectivity is low.

2. Studies on Thyroid Hormone Receptor Structure and Function

Samuels and co-workers have synthesized a photoaffinity label derivative of 3,5,3'-triiodo-L-thyronine (L-T3), namely N-2-diazo-3,3,3-trifluoropropionyl-3,5,3'-triiodo-L-thyronine (L-T3-PAL) (14a), and have used it to photoaffinity label thyroid hormone nuclear receptors in intact pituitary tumor GH1 cells. In a series of careful experiments,

14a $\quad R = -\overset{O}{\underset{\underset{N_2}{\|}}{C}} - \underset{\|}{C} - CF_3 \quad X = H$

14b $\quad R = -H \quad\quad\quad X = H$

14c $\quad R = -H \quad\quad\quad X = I$

14d $\quad R = -\overset{O}{\overset{\|}{C}} - CH_2 Br \quad X = H$

Pascual *et al.* (1982) present good evidence that the photoaffinity label is indeed labeling the nuclear thyroid hormone receptor. The lines of evidence include mutually competitive binding to receptor, identical sedimentation coefficients (3.8 S) on sucrose gradients, identical Stokes' radii (3.4 nm) from high-performance liquid chromatography analysis of the L-T3 and L-T3-PAL-labeled nuclear-binding components (estimated molecular weight 54,000), and identical 6.5 S and 12.5 S forms excised by micrococcal nuclease digestion of nuclei.

After exposure of intact cells to the photoaffinity agent (**14a**) and irradiation of cells with UV light at 254 nm for 2 minutes (or for 1–30 minutes), salt extraction of nuclei and analysis on SDS gels revealed two covalently labeled species, a predominant species of $M_r = 47,000$ and a minor species of $M_r = 57,000$ representing approximately 25% of the total covalent radioactive species (Fig. 9). Both species are also observed upon photolabeling of nuclear extracts *in vitro*. Irradiation of cells at 310 nm, where damage to proteins should be less, allows labeling of the 47,000 species almost exclusively, although the UV coupling

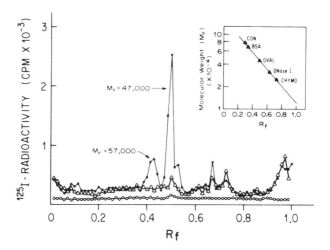

FIG. 9. SDS–polyacrylamide gel electrophoresis of nuclear protein covalently bound to L-[125I]T3-PAL (**14a**) after UV irradiation at 254 nm. GH1 cells were incubated with 3 nM L-[125I]T3-PAL (**14a**) without (●) or with (△) 5 μM L-T3 or with 0.5 nM L-[125I]T3 (○) for 1.5 hour. The cell monolayers were irradiated with UV light for 2 minutes at 4°C. Nuclear proteins extracted with 0.4 M KCl were adjusted to 1% SDS and precipitated in 80% ethanol at −20°C for 15 hours. The samples were centrifuged at 3000 *g* for 20 minutes and the derived pellet was washed an additional time with 70% ethanol. The precipitated material was dried and heated to 100°C with 1% 2-mercaptoethanol for 2 minutes and then was electrophoresed in SDS–10% polyacrylamide gels. (From Pascual *et al.*, 1982, with permission.)

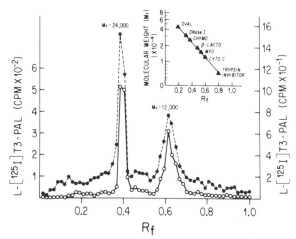

FIG. 10. Cleavage of the $M_r = 57,000$ and 47,000 binding components by *S. aureus* V8 protease. Three gel slices containing the ^{125}I-radioactive peaks were digested with 10 µg of enzyme during electrophoresis. Protein standards were electrophoresed in parallel gels. The cleavage fragments of the $M_r = 47,000$ (○) and the $M_r = 57,000$ (●) precursors are plotted as relative mobilities (R_f) to estimate the molecular weight of the derived fragments using the R_f of the protein standards (inset). (From Pascual *et al.*, 1982, with permission.)

at 310 nm is less efficient (only 40% that achieved at 254 nm). This latter finding implies that the 47,000 form is probably not due to UV-induced damage.

Pascual *et al.* (1982) have shown that the 47,000 species does not seem to be derived from the 57,000 species by the action of endogenous proteases. In addition, both forms seem to be closely related species. Nonradioactive T4 and T3 derivatives show similar affinities for the 57,000 and the 47,000 proteins, and the 47,000 and 57,000 species show identical size fragments upon incubation with *S. aureus* V8 protease and with trypsin (Fig. 10). These findings suggest that both forms are indeed related, being possibly prereceptor or postreceptor forms. It is also possible that a 10,000 molecular weight component, either a subunit of receptor or a chromatin-associated protein, may be associating tightly with receptor during protein cross-linking.

More recent studies (H. Samuels, unpublished) indicate that the sedimentation profiles of micrococcal nuclease-digested chromatin after photocross-linking of intact cells show that the 57,000 component is enriched in nucleosome particles compared to the 47,000 component. It is conceivable that the 57,000 component may be the primary translation product of the receptor mRNA and a precursor to the 47,000 component. The 57,000 component might be the biologically active receptor species which is then inactivated in the cell nucleus to the 47,000 component. A combination of photoaffinity labeling and dense amino acid labeling of receptor in these cells could be used to examine rates of synthesis and degradation of the 47,000 and 57,000 species; this should provide important information on the relationships between these two receptor species in hormone action. The relatively low efficiency of labeling of the two species, however, with the T3 photoaffinity label (and the possibility that the two species are labeled with different efficiencies) makes analysis of receptor synthesis and turnover rates difficult.[3]

David-Inouye et al. (1982) have used [^{125}I]T3 (**14b**) as a photoreactive probe for the thyroid hormone nuclear receptor from rat liver. The partially purified rat liver nuclear extracts were exposed to the probe for 100 seconds at 22°C with UV light at 254 nm. Although this labels many proteins, even in partially purified receptor preparations, the use of one- and two-dimensional polyacrylamide gels showed that labeling of one particular protein, with molecular weight of 47,000 and an isoelectric point of approximately 6.2, was inhibitable by the thyroid hormones T3 and T4. Hence, the rat liver receptor appears to have a molecular weight similar to that of the major receptor component identified in GH1 pituitary cells. Since a 57,000-Da species was not revealed in these studies, either this form does not exist in liver or it is not covalently labeled by photolysis of T3. It is also conceivable, however, that minor amounts of such a species might escape detection or be masked by other closely migrating proteins during gel analysis.

Both 57,000 and 47,000 receptor species exist in rat liver according to recent studies by H. J. Cahnmann (personal communication) and van der Walt et al. (1982). They have used un-derivatized thyroid hormones for photoaffinity labeling of serum thyroid hormone-binding proteins (cf. Section IV,A,3) and thyroid hormone receptors in nuclear extracts from rat liver. Irradiation of the thyroid hormones T4 (**14c**) and T3 (**14b**) with UV light at >300 nm causes homolytic fission of C–I bonds in both rings. In the presence of hormone-binding proteins, the phenyl radical thus produced and possibly also the iodine radical can form covalent bonds with certain amino acid residues in the binding site. Photoaffinity labeling of crude rat liver nuclear extracts was performed after preincubation with [^{125}I]T4 or [^{125}I]T3; SDS-gel analysis of the covalently labeled proteins revealed a predominant 45,000 molecular weight species and a minor 56,000 molecular weight species similar to that seen by Pascual et al. (1982) in GH1 cells. A portion of the photoaffinity labeling of these two species was reduced by exposure to unlabeled T4 or T3, suggesting that at least a portion of this labeling was due to interaction at a high affinity limited capacity binding site, and represented thyroid hormone receptors.

The photoattachment efficiency with T3 or T4 depends largely on the irradiation conditions. A photoattachment efficiency of 15–20% for [125I]T4 and 4–5% for [125I]T3 is obtained when long-wavelength UV light (below 300 nm) is used. Thiols drastically reduce photolabeling by T4 and T3 (Nikodem *et al.*, 1980). Irradiation of [125I]T3 at 254 nm (David-Inouye *et al.*, 1982) is much less favorable, giving very low coupling efficiencies of approximately 0.1%. Hence, the advantage of using unmodified hormones is that high affinity for nuclear receptors can be maintained, while introduction of modifications such as in the T3 photoaffinity label used by Pascual *et al.* (1982) reduces affinity for receptor to approximately 5% that of T3.

N-Bromoacetyl derivatives of T4 and T3 have been used to study thyroid hormone receptors (Nikodem *et al.*, 1980; Cheng, 1983; Horiuchi *et al.*, 1982). Although *N*-bromoacetyl-T3 has been reported to covalently modify a protein in nuclear extracts from rat liver and GH1 cell nuclei, estimated by SDS-gel analysis to have a molecular weight of 52,000 or 56,000, it is not clear whether this covalent attachment is inhibited by preincubation with excess T3 (Pascual *et al.*, 1982). Hence, the bromoacetyl-T3 may be covalently labeling a nonreceptor protein with a molecular weight similar to that of one of the thyroid hormone nuclear receptor species.

Horiuchi *et al.* (1982) and Cheng (1983) have used *N*-bromoacetyl-T3 to covalently label an M_r 55,000 T3-binding protein present in intact cells and in purified plasma membranes from GH3 rat pituitary tumor cells. The labeling of this membrane component is reduced 50% by unlabeled T3 and, hence, shows T3 specificity. A similar 55,000 molecular weight plasma membrane T3 binder has been identified by affinity labeling with *N*-bromoacetyl-T3 in a human and mouse cultured cell line. *S. aureus* and elastase digests of the 55,000 affinity labeled species from human epithelioid carcinoma A431 cells, Swiss 3T3-4 mouse fibroblasts, and rat GH3 pituitary tumor cells yield identical patterns indicating the structural similarity of this binder in the three species. It appears, however, from protease digest patterns that this protein is different from that of the nuclear thyroid hormone receptor. Its role in mediating thyroid hormone entry into cells and other possible functions of thyroid hormone remain aspects of considerable interest.

G. Other Receptor Systems

Xenopus oocytes contain a steroid-binding protein that appears to be involved in the steroid-induced stimulation of oocyte maturation. Photoaffinity labeling of oocyte membrane preparations with ³H-labeled R5020 provides highly selective labeling of a 110,000 molecular weight protein. Labeling is blocked by excess unlabeled R5020 and appears saturable with regard to time and R5020 concentration, although the labeling efficiency is not known (Sadler and Maller, 1982). Progesterone, which is active in inducing oocyte maturation, produces a curious effect on R5020 photolabeling. The rate of photolabeling increases fivefold as progesterone concentration increases from 0 to 4 μM, but then decreases somewhat at higher concentrations. The mechanism of this effect is not clear, but may involve allosteric or positive cooperative effects.

An interesting application of photoaffinity labeling has been in the characterization and *in vivo* distribution of binding proteins for the insect hormone ecdysone. Binding proteins for this hormone share some characteristics with the mammalian steroid hormone receptors, but show much lower affinities (reviewed by Bonner, 1982). Gronemeyer and Pongs (1980) localized ecdysterone (**15**)-binding sites in *Drosophila* salivary gland polytene chromosones using an indirect immunofluorescence approach. Endogenous (or exogenously supplied) hormone was irradiated at >300 nm, presumably affixing it covalently to its binding proteins through photoexcitation of the B-ring enone chromophore. The irradiated glands were then incubated with rabbit antibodies toward ecdysterone, and detected by fluorescein-labeled goat anti-rabbit immunoglobulin. Fluorescence appeared in bands that corresponded temporally with puff sites under hormonal regulation. In some instances fluorescence appeared as discrete spots within the bands, and as multiples of a basic fluorescence intensity (Gronemeyer

Ecdysterone (X = OH) (**15**)

Ponasterone (X = H) (**16**)

et al., 1981). In a subsequent study with either *Drosophila* salivary glands or *Drosophila* K_c tissue culture cells and tritium-labeled ponasterone A (**16**), an ecdysone analog bearing the same chromophore, Schaltmann and Pongs (1982) found specific photoaffinity labeling of a protein of molecular weight 130,000 and p*I* 5.8. Additional controls established that a photoreactive, but nonbinding analog, 2-acetylecdysterone, did not attach to this protein. The photolabeling technique was used to characterize the subcellular localization of the ecdysone-binding protein and its sedimentation properties under different states of hormone exposure.

IV. AFFINITY LABELING STUDIES ON ENZYMES AND EXTRACELLULAR BINDING PROTEINS

Steroid and thyroid hormones interact with macromolecular binding sites other than receptors, namely, with extracellular carrier proteins and with enzymes involved in biosynthesis and metabolism. The function and properties of these proteins are distinct from those of the intracellular receptors; nevertheless, the approaches taken in covalent labeling of the binding sites in these proteins are illustrative of methods and techniques that could be used in the labeling of receptors. For comparative purposes we discuss briefly relevant affinity labeling studies on these enzymes and binding proteins.

The presentation in this section is organized according to type of labeling process and reactive species, rather than the particular protein involved.

Many of the studies presented in this section deal with binding proteins or enzymes in a homogenous or highly purified state. Thus labeling specificity and applicability to more heterogeneous systems have not been stringently tested. Moreover, although affinity labeling of steroid metabolizing or biosynthetic enzymes can be approached with either electrophilic or photoreactive steroid derivatives, the catalytic activity of the enzymes provides an additional avenue for active site reaction: An appropriate substrate analog, with a potentially reactive functional group in a latent form, could be accepted as a substrate and acted upon by the enzyme. If this substrate analog were designed so that enzymatic activity revealed the reactive species, then the enzyme could become inactivated by the covalent interaction of the reactive product with active site residues. Such latently reactive substrate analogs have been termed, variously, suicide substrates, enzyme-activated irreversible inhibitors, or k_{cat} inhibitors (for a recent review see Walsch, 1982). Suicide substrates can be considered precursor forms of electrophilic affinity labeling agents.[5] Finally, in many of these studies, the only parameter monitored is loss of enzyme activity. Therefore, the covalent attachment of the reactive derivative with the protein can only be presumed.

A. ELECTROPHILIC AFFINITY LABELING

1. *Haloacetyl and Other Halo Compounds*

The popularity of haloacetyl compounds (haloacetates and haloacetamides) is well illustrated in these studies, emphasizing the advantage of these steroid derivatives as electrophilic affinity labels: The haloacetyl group alkylates nucleophilic amino acids, which, upon complete protein hydrolysis, can be isolated as carboxymethyl derivatives and thus readily identified by chromatographic comparisons with available standards.

Using a series of haloacetoxy and haloacetamido progesterone derivatives, Warren and co-workers have performed a very complete series of affinity labeling studies on the 20β-hydroxysteroid dehydrogenase of *Streptomyces hydrogenans*. This work has been reviewed extensively elsewhere (Benisek *et al.*, 1982; Katzenellenbogen, 1977; for more recent work, see Strickler *et al.*, 1981; Chin *et al.*, 1980, 1982a,b; Murdock and Warren, 1982), but a few additional comments are relevant. In each case, the electrophilic affinity labeling characteristics of these alkylating steroids toward the enzyme were documented very carefully through substrate protection, nucleophile competition, and comparative reactivity studies. In addition, in most instances, carboxymethylated amino acids were isolated and identified after complete hydrolysis of the affinity labeled protein. Because the active site of this enzyme has been studied with a multitudie of affinity labeling agents

---

[5]While not directly relevant to a discussion of affinity labeling, a conceptual distinction is made between "true" and "pseudo"suicide inactivation of an enzyme (Walsh, 1982). In true suicide inactivation, the enzyme is inactivated by the reactive species generated in the active site, prior to its dissociation from the site. This process, potentially, can be highly selective. Pseudosuicide inactivation, in contrast, derives from an enzyme-generated reactive species that is in equilibrium with the active site; that is, its reaction with the enzyme is slow relative to its dissociation from the active site. Such a process is, in effect, an enzyme-generated electrophilic affinity labeling process, and the overall result should be the same (that is, no more selective) as that produced by addition of the electrophilic enzyme-generated product. Careful kinetic analysis and studies on the effectiveness of nucleophilic scavengers can distinguish between the two processes.

bearing the labeling function at differing locations around the steroid structure, one can begin to construct a topological map of residues about the ligand in the active site from an analysis of the pattern of residue labeling. These studies illustrate nicely the type of structural information that can be obtained by multiple affinity labeling studies on one site.

Steroids bearing halogens attached directly to the steroid skeleton at positions 2, 6, and 16 have been studied as inactivators of other steroid dehydrogenases as well as the Δ^5-3-ketosteroid isomerase and estrogen synthetase (aromatase). These studies have also been reviewed elsewhere (Benisek *et al.*, 1982; Katzenellenbogen, 1977).

Corticosteroid binding globulin (CBG, transcortin) has been the target of affinity labeling in two studies with halo and haloacetyl steroids. Khan and Rosner (1977) found that 6β-bromoprogesterone reacted rapidly with human CBG with 1:1 stoichiometry, consuming a single accessible cysteine residue; progesterone-6-S-L-cysteine was obtained from complete acid hydrolysis of the labeled protein. Using a somewhat different preparation of human CBG (that did not have an accessible cysteine residue), LeGaillard and Dautrevaux (1977) found that 11α-bromoacetoxyprogesterone, 17β-O-bromoacetyltestosterone, and 16α-bromoacetoxyprogesterone acted as affinity labeling agents, with the last derivatives being the most efficient. Chromatographic analysis of acid hydrolyzates of CBG labeled with the three derivatives indicated the following residues as sites of alkylation: methionine, methionine and histidine at N-3, and histidine at N-1, respectively.

N-Bromoacetyl-L-thyroxine was used in a careful affinity labeling study of human thyroxine binding prealbumin (Cheng *et al.*, 1977). This derivative reacts covalently with glycine-1, and lysines-9 and -15 in a 29:63:8 ratio.

2. *Epoxides*

Epoxides have been utilized as attaching functions with enzymes involved in hydrolysis of glycosidic linkages (Thomas, 1977); here, the acidic functions that catalyze the hydrolysis reactions are presumed to protonate the epoxide and activate it toward reaction with nearby nucleophiles.

Epoxysteroids have been used to label the Δ^5-3-ketosteroid isomerase from *Pseudomonas testosteroni* (Pollack *et al.*, 1979; Bevins *et al.*, 1980; Kayser *et al.*, 1983). Catalysis of the isomerization process by this enzyme is thought to involve interaction of the oxygen of the 3-keto group with an acidic residue, and Pollack and coworkers found that steroid analogs with 3- and 17-substituted spiroepoxide groups

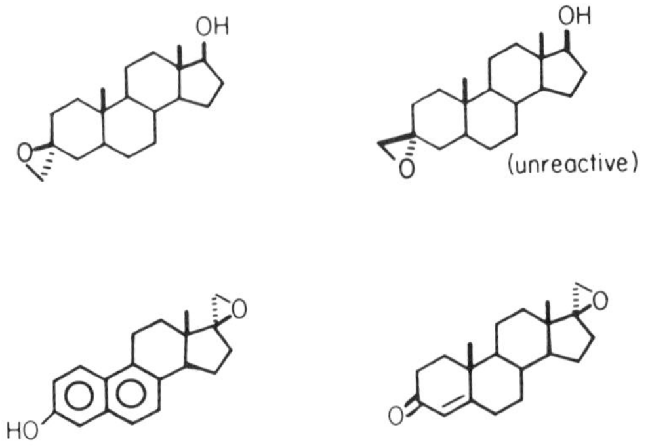

SCHEME 2. Steroid epoxides: Δ^5-3-ketosteroid isomerase inactivators.

(Scheme 2) were inactivators of the isomerase. The isomerase was inactivated only with epoxide oxygen β-oriented (presumed to be better situated for protonation of the epoxide oxygen by the enzyme; the α-epoxides are simple competitive inhibitors), but the effectiveness of both the 3- and 17-epoxysteroids suggests that the isomerase enzyme can accept steroids in either the normal or the "backward" orientation (A- and D-ring positions reversed). Further studies with two of the 17-spiroepoxides demonstrated a 1:1 inactivator–enzyme subunit labeling stoichiometry, and protein chemistry studies indicated that aspartate-38 was the residue affected by the alkylation (Kayser *et al.*, 1983). It is interesting that the epoxide appears to react with this residue by attack at both the methylene and the fully-substituted end.

3. Unsaturated Ketones: Enones (Scheme 3) and Dienones (Scheme 4)

16-Methylene estrone (**17**), a steroid derivative embodying a sterically accessible enone (Michael acceptor) system, is an irreversible inactivator of two human placental dehydrogenase activities (17β- and 20α-) (Thomas *et al.*, 1983). The enzyme(s) is also inactivated by the precursor allylic alcohol, 16-methylene-17β-estradiol, which is converted by the enzyme into the reactive enone, and thus acts as a suicide substrate.

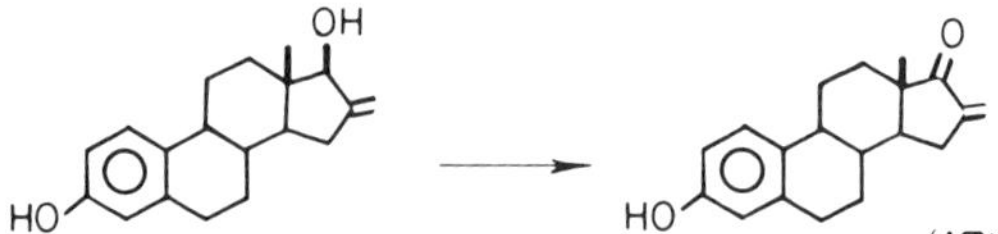

SCHEME 3. Steroid enone: 17β-hydroxysteroid dehydrogenase inactivator.

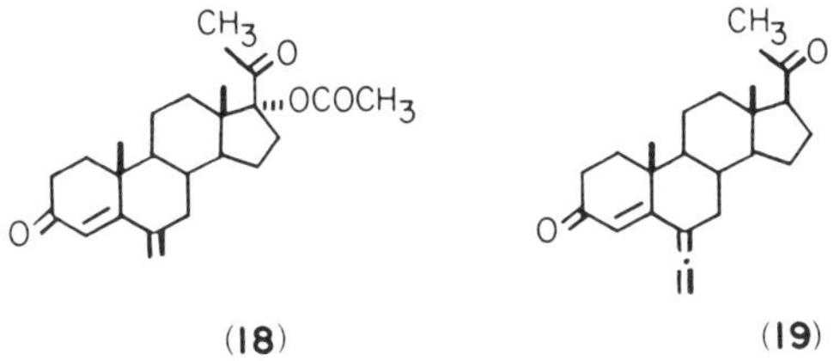

SCHEME 4. Steroid dienone: Δ^4-3-ketosteroid 5α-reductase inactivator.

Petrow and co-workers (Petrow *et al.*, 1981, 1983; Kadohama *et al.*, 1983), studying a series of unsaturated steroidal ketones as potential irreversible inactivators of the Δ^4-3-ketosteroid 5α-reductase, found the most active compound to be the 6-methylene-4-pregna-3,20-dione (18). This molecule embodies a sterically accessible dienone system, and is presumed to act as a Michael acceptor and thus to become covalently linked to the enzyme by addition of a nucleophilic residue to the 6 methylene group. As expected for this mechanism, the irreversible inactivating properties of the 6-methylene-Δ^4-3-ketosteroid system is reduced by substituents on the 6-methylene group and elsewhere on the steroid.

Petrow considers the 6-methylene compounds to be inactivators of the suicide type, because inactivation requires NADPH (Petrow *et al.*, 1981). It is difficult to imagine what reactive species might be generated by the addition of a hydride to the dienone system. Therefore, it would seem more likely that these agents act as classical electrophilic affinity labels, with the NADPH binding in some way being required to place the enzyme in a conformation better disposed for promoting interaction of the nucleophilic residue with the methylene terminus. In this regard, it is interesting that the 6-ethenylidine compound 19 is also an irreversible inactivator of the 5α-reductase, but does not require NADPH.

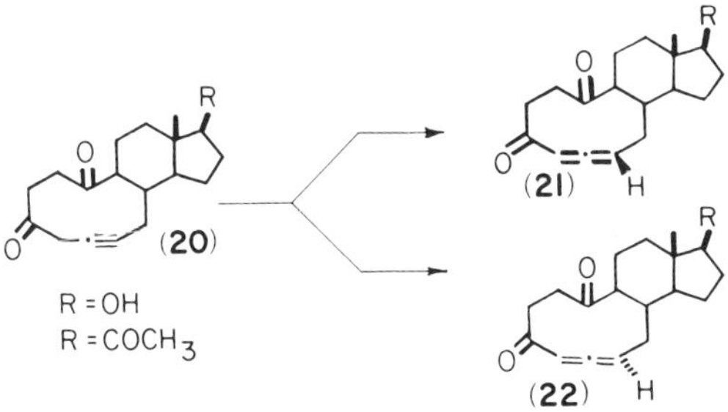

SCHEME 5. Allenic ketones: Δ^5-3-ketosteroid isomerase inactivators.

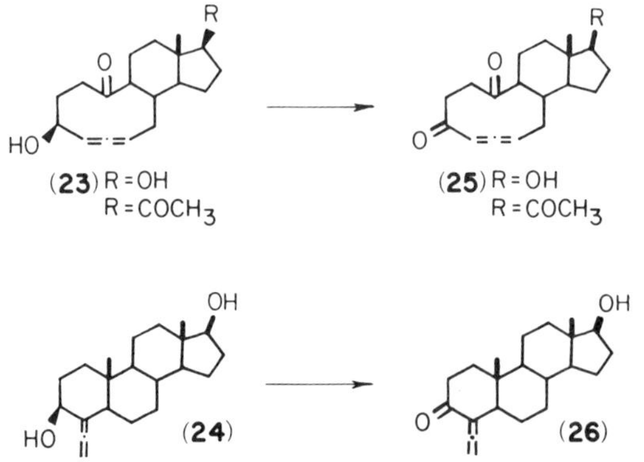

SCHEME 6. Allenic ketones and precursor allenic alcohols: Δ^5-3β-hydroxysteroid dehydrogenase inactivators.

4. *Unsaturated Ketones: Allenic Ketones (Schemes 5 and 6)*

Allenic ketones derived from secoandrogens and progestins are inactivators and active site alkylating agents for the bacterial Δ^5-3-ketosteroid isomerase enzyme from *P. testosteroni*. [This work has been reviewed by Benisek *et al.* (1982).] There are two diastereomeric allenic ketones (**21** and **22**), differing in allene stereochemistry. Both stereoisomers are generated from a single β-acetylenic ketosteroid **20**, either chemically by treatment with base or enzymatically by exposure to isomerase. The enzymatic conversion of acetylenic ketone into allenic ketone is rapid relative to reaction of the allenic ketones with the enzyme; thus, enzyme inactivation upon exposure to the acetylenic ketones would be considered pseudosuicide inactivation (Penning *et al.*, 1981).[5] Both allene stereoisomers react covalently with the enzyme, though at somewhat different rates, giving a 1:1 steroid:enzyme stoichiometry. The enzyme adduct, though covalently linked, is relatively labile. Nevertheless, careful enzymatic digestion and structural analysis suggested that attachment occurred at asparagine-57 (Penning *et al.*, 1982). It is believed that these same allenic ketones and their acetylenic ketone precursors inactivate the mammalian Δ^5-3-ketosteroid isomerase and the Δ^4-3-ketosteroid 5α-reductase enzymes (Robaire *et al.*, 1977; Batzold *et al.*, 1977; Voigt *et al.*, 1978).

The steroidal and secosteroidal allenic alcohols **23** and **24** act as suicide substrates for the Δ^5-3-hydroxysteroid dehydrogenase from mammalian sources (Balasubramanian and Robinson, 1981; Balasubramanian *et al.*, 1982). Inactivation was produced by oxidation of the allenic alcohols to allenic ketones **25** and **26,** which are potent

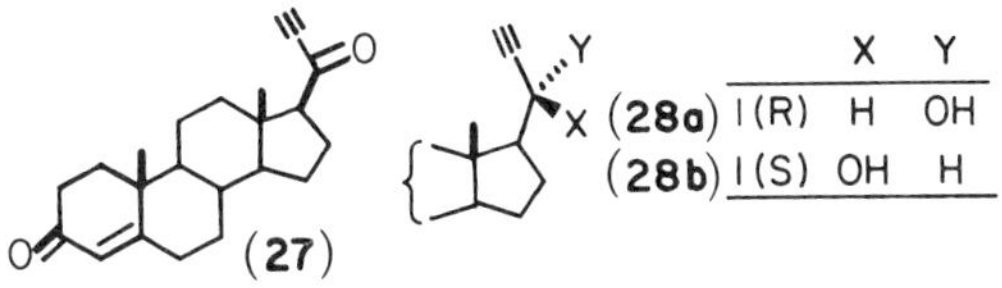

	X	Y
(28a)	1(R) H	OH
(28b)	1(S) OH	H

SCHEME 7. Acetylenic ketone and propargylic alcohol precursors: 17β- and 20α-hydroxysteroid dehydrogenase inactivators.

electrophiles and alkylate the active site of the enzyme by a pseudosuicide mechanism.[5] These allenic alcohols appeared to be oxidized only at C-17, by the 3β,17β-hydroxysteroid dehydrogenase activity from *P. testosteroni,* and thus, they failed to inactivate this enzyme; of the allenic ketones, only **26** inactivated the bacterial enzyme.

5. *Unsaturated Ketones: Acetylenic Ketones (Ynones) (Schemes 7–9)*

Acetylenic ketones have been utilized as inactivators of dehydrogenase and oxidase enzymes; generally, inactivation can be accomplished directly by incubation with the acetylenic ketone itself or indirectly by exposure to a propargyl or propargylic alcohol precursor form (suicide substrate) that is converted into the acetylenic ketone by the enzyme.

The placental enzyme with 17β- and 20α-hydroxysteroid dehydrogenase activity is inactivated by 17β-(1-oxo-2-propynyl)androst-4-en-3-one (**27**). The 1(R)-propargylic alcohol precursor **28a** acts as a suicide substrate for this enzyme, but the 1(S)-epimer **28b** does not (Tobias *et al.,* 1982). The same two acetylenic compounds also cause a parellel loss of the 3α- and 20β-hydroxysteroid dehydrogenase activities of the enzyme from *S. hydrogenans* (Strickler *et al.,* 1980).

Another instance of irreversible inactivation with acetylenic ketone was found with a different oxidative enzyme, the estrogen synthetase enzyme also known as aromatase. Aromatase is inactivated by exposure to the acetylenic ketone-substituted androstenedione **29** (Covey *et al.,* 1981; Marcotte and Robinson, 1982a). Because this enzyme can hydroxylate C-19, both the 19-propargyl (**29**) and the 19-hydroxypropargyl (**30**) substituted androstenediones act as suicide substrates. It is of note that only the 1(S)-hydroxypropargyl epimer (**30**) is reactive (Covey *et al.,* 1981).

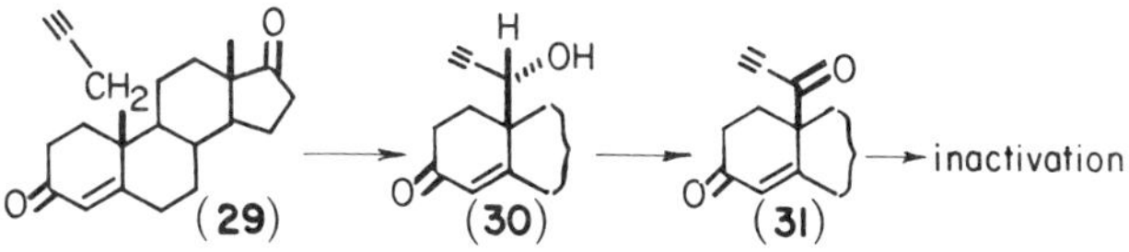

SCHEME 8. Acetylenic ketone and propargyl and propargylic alcohol precursors: aromatase inactivators.

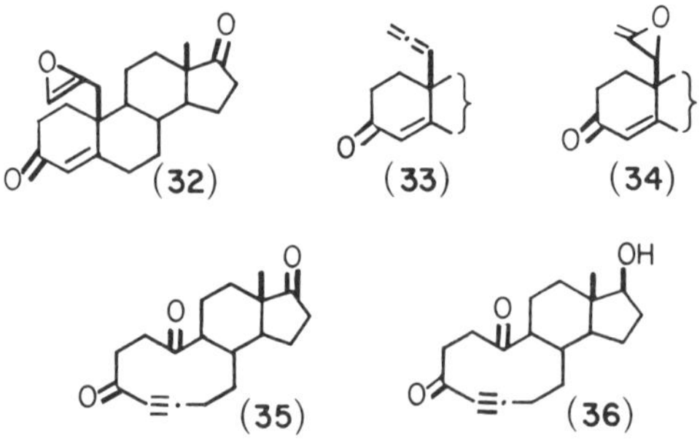

SCHEME 9. Acetylenic ketones: Δ^5-3-ketosteroid isomerase inactivators.

A somewhat contradictory report by Metcalf has appeared (Metcalf *et al.*, 1981). Based on kinetic isotope studies and his finding that the ethynyl ketone was not reactive he suggested that aromatase inactivation by the propargyl compound was due to reactive oxirine intermediate (**32**); the related allenic steroid **33** was proposed to inactivate via the related alkylidine oxirane **34**.

The same two acetylenic ketones (**27** and **31**) together with two acetylenic AB secosteroids (**35** and **36**) were studied as inactivators of Δ^5-3-ketosteroid isomerase activity; the bacterial isomerase from *P. testosteroni* was compared with two (C-19 and C-21) activities from beef adrenal (Penning and Covey, 1982). All four compounds act as irreversible inactivators, presumably through alkylation of active site residues. The kinetic specificity of these acetylenic ketones toward the activities from the two sources was markedly different, and differences in their activity toward the two isomerase activities from adrenal suggest that two separate enzymes may be involved.

It is uncertain at this time whether all four of these acetylenic ketones react with the same nucleophilic residues in the active site of each enzyme. The fact that four different compounds, bearing the reactive ynone function at three distinct regions about the steroid skeleton, are all active raises interesting questions as to whether substrates are bound in alternative orientations within the active site, as appeared to be the case in the reactions of steroidal epoxides with the *Pseudomonas* isomerase (Bevins *et al.*, 1980).

6. *Acylhalides and Sulfonyl Halides*

The 19-fluoro- and the 19,19-difluoro-substituted androstenediones **37** and **39** provide an interesting contrast as inactivators of estrogen synthetase (aromatase): The monofluoro compound is a substrate, the difluoro is a suicide inactivator (Marcotte and Robinson, 1982a,b). This is consistent with a process whereby hydroxylation at C-19 leads to loss of HF. From compound **37**, this process would generate an acyl fluoride **38**, a good candidate for active site acylation; compound **39**, on the other hand, would simply produce the 19-carboxaldehyde **40**, an intermediate in the normal aromatization sequence.

Dansyl chloride, a commonly used fluorescent derivatizing agent, contains a reactive sulfonyl chloride function that reacts with accessible nucleophilic residues. This reagent modifies selectively lysine-15 in the thyroxine-binding site of prealbumin (Cheng *et al.*, 1975). Although prealbumin is a tetramer composed of four identical subunits, only two thyroxine molecules are bound per tetramer; likewise, only two of the four identical lysine-15 residues are modified by dansyl chloride.

7. Subversion of a Covalently Bound Intermediate

The aromatase enzyme is inactivated in a time- and cofactor-dependent manner by several substrate analogs, e.g., 4-androstene-3,6,17-trione (**41**), 1,4,6-androstatrien-3,17-dione (**42**), and 4-hydroxy-4-androstene-3,17-dione (**43**) (Covey and Hood, 1981, 1982a). While the precise mode of reaction of these substrate analogs is not known, Covey has proposed an imaginative rationale based on a novel, mechanistic proposal for the aromatization process itself (Covey and Hood, 1982b). In brief, he proposes that aromatization, which is known to proceed via a series of hydroxylation steps, may actually involve a transient covalently bound intermediate. With normal substrates, this covalent link between enzyme and substrate is broken in a subsequent elimination step leading to the aromatized product. The inactivating substrate analogs, however, provide alternate pathways for this elimination reaction and lead to a stable covalently bound species, with the result that the enzyme is inactivated. Related mechanisms are proposed to account for the inactivating properties of all three substrate analogs.

8. Diazonium Compounds

An unusual intermediate appears to be involved in the inactivation of Δ^4-3-ketosteroid 5α-reductase by the 4-diazo-3-ketosteroid **44** (Blohm et al., 1980). This enzyme catalyzes the addition of a hydride ion (from NADPH) to C-5, and it is thought to provide a proton to neutralize the enolate intermediate. The diazo substituted substrate analog **44** already has the 5α-hydrogen, so that one can imagine it as an analog for the enolate, especially since α-diazoketones have negative charge character at the α-carbon. Inactivation of the enzyme, therefore, is believed to be the result of attempted protonation at C-4, which would generate an α-keto diazonium ion (**45**). The excellent leaving group character of the diazonium function could enable this species to react with a nearby nucleophilic residue.

B. PHOTOAFFINITY LABELING

1. *Unsaturated Ketones: Enones, Dienones, and Trienones*

The highly successful use of unsaturated ketosteroids in photoaffinity labeling of receptors was first stimulated by the work of Benisek on Δ^5-3-ketosteroid isomerases. [This work has been reviewed carefully by Benisek *et al.* (1982).] He found that the isomerase from *P. testosteroni* was inactivated specifically when irradiated at >300 nm with an unsaturated ketosteroid bound at the active site. A related isomerase from *Pseudomonas putida* proved to be very unstable to irradiation in the absence of steroid. However, by using steroidal dienones and trienones having much greater molar adsorptivities at the irradiation wavelengths (>300 nm), specific, ligand-dependent photoinactivation was obtained (Smith and Benisek, 1980).

In retrospect, it is amusing that the active site specific photoinactivation processes studied by Benisek do not appear to involve as a major component the covalent attachment of the photoreactive ligand. Rather, inactivation appears to be the result of a ligand-dependent, photostimulated reaction within the protein, which, in the *P. testosteroni* isomerase, causes conversion of aspartate-33 to an alanine by a decarboxylation, and, in *P. putida* isomerase, is the loss of a thiol group. There does appear to be a minor, active site-specific, light-induced covalent attachment of steroidal enones to the *P. testosteroni* enzyme (Hearne and Benisek, 1983), but covalent attachment to the *putida* isomerase has not been documented (Benisek *et al.*, 1982). Nevertheless, these photochemical studies of Benisek were a seminal influence on studies of androgen binding protein with Δ^6-testosterone (see below) and the subsequent studies using R5020 and R 1881 (cf. Sections III,C–E).

Extensive photolabeling studies have been carried out on androgen-binding protein (ABP), an extracellular protein produced by Sertoli cells, utilizing Δ^6-testosterone (**46**), a steroidal dienone with good affinity for this protein (Danzo *et al.*, 1980, 1982a; Taylor *et al.*, 1980a,b; Schmidt *et al.*, 1981). Molecular weight analysis by polyacrylamide-gel electrophoresis under native and denaturing conditions together with

(**46**)

cross-linking studies suggest that the native protein is a dimer composed of two subunits having slightly different molecular weights; the ratio of these subunits varies between species. Similar studies on rabbit sex steroid binding globulin (Danzo et al., 1982b) indicate that this protein is a dimer composed to two identical subunits.

A notable feature of the ABP study was that labeling efficiencies of up to 65% were obtained with prolonged irradiation; this is far higher than achievable with steroidal dienone and trienones in receptor-labeling studies. Whether this is due to the different photochemical behavior of the 4,6-dien-3-one chromophore in Δ^6-testosterone vs the 4,9-dien-3-one in R5020 or the 4,9,11-trien-3-one in methyltrienolone, or the result simply of a more favorable disposition of ABP toward photocovalent labeling, is not apparent.

The astute reader will have noted that unsaturated ketones have been utilized both as electrophilic and as photoreactive affinity labeling agents. In the latter application, where the unsaturated system is acting as an electrophilic Michael acceptor, the site of attack by the nucleophile must be unhindered, lest the rate of covalent attachment be greatly retarded. The photoreactive unsaturated ketones, on the other hand, generally have olefin termini that are mono or dialkyl substituted and thus are inert as Michael acceptors under the usual conditions of labeling. Their reactivity in the excited state involves intermediates and processes that have been discussed earlier (cf. Section II,B,2a).

2. α-Diazoketones

Three steroid-binding serum proteins, corticosteroid-binding globulin (CBG), α-fetoprotein (AFP), and thyroxine-binding prealbumin, have been labeled by steroids containing the photoreactive α-diazoketone function.

In the course of preparing some photoreactive corticosteroid derivatives to label the aldosterone receptor, Wolff et al. (1975) investigated several 21-diazopregnanes: 9α-fluoro-21-diazo-21-deoxycorticosterone, 9α-bromo-21-diazo-21-deoxycorticosterone, 21-diazo-21-deoxycorticosterone, and 21-diazoprogesterone. In competitive binding assays, these derivatives showed relatively weak affinity for the aldosterone receptor from rat kidney, but some of them bound quite well to corticosteroid-binding globulin (CBG). Using purified CBG, Marver et al. (1976) showed that 21-diazo-21-deoxy[^{3}H]corticosteroid **47** acted as a photoaffinity labeling agent for the serum protein. The attachment efficiency appeared to be quite low, but was enhanced by conducting the irradiation at $-12°C$ in a glycerol-containing buffer; presumably the

(47) (48) (49)

increased viscosity of this medium retarded the dissociation of the photoreactive species from the active site. By careful competition and fluorescence quenching studies, the labeling was shown to be irreversible and associated specifically with the steroid binding site. In addition, the buffer component Tris was shown to act as a scavenger, reducing the level of labeling of other proteins in the CBG preparation.

16-Diazoestrone (48) binds to rat AFP with an affinity somewhat greater than estradiol, and photolysis of 16-diazo[^{3}H]estrone at 300 nm causes covalent labeling of AFP with ~ 20% efficiency (Payne et al., 1980). The labeling is very selective for the steroid binding site, and the covalently labeled protein shows electrophoretic mobility on SDS–polyacrylamide gels identical to that of unmodified AFP. Through a set of careful time-course and scavenging experiments, the workers were able to establish that the covalent labeling was actually the result of two processes: About one-third was produced by a normal photoaffinity labeling reaction that was chromophore dependent and not subject to scavenging. The bulk of the labeling, however, arose from an electrophilic photoproduct generated by photolysis of 16-diazoestrone, but which reacted only slowly with AFP in a process that was subject to scavenging by mercaptoethanol. Although the nature of this electrophilic photoproduct was not elucidated, its lifetime under the conditions of the study ($t_{1/2}$ = 17 hours) would be consistent with the acylazide (49) produced by trapping of the norsteroid ketene (the result of Wolff rearrangement) by azide ion present in the buffer preparations. This suggests that mild acylating species might have utility in other steroid affinity labeling studies (cf. Section IV,B,6).

N-(Ethyl-2-diazomalonyl) derivatives of thyroxine and triiodothyronine (50) were used in a photoaffinity labeling study of thyroxine-binding prealbumin (Somack et al., 1982). Both of these derivatives have reasonably high affinity for prealbumin (although they have very low affinity for the rat liver nuclear thyroid receptor), and upon photolysis, the hormone-binding site in the serum protein is covalently labeled with very good efficiency (~ 60%). Curiously, preirradiation of the diazomalonyl derivatives, with attendant destruction of the diazocarbonyl chromophore, produces some species that could still be

(50)

induced to label the hormone-binding site of prealbumin upon continued irradiation, although with somewhat reduced efficiency. While thyroxine itself labels prealbumin covalently by irradiation in the ultraviolet (cf. Section IV,C,3), the efficiency of this labeling is much lower than that achieved by the photoproduct of diazomalonylthyroxine. Thus, the structure of this photoproduct remains a curiosity.

3. Aromatic Iodides

Aryl iodides are known to be photochemically unstable, producing aryl and iodine radicals that can undergo a variety of abstraction and coupling reactions (Wolf and Kharasch, 1965). Thus, it is not surprising that thyroxine can be used directly as a photoaffinity labeling agent for thyroxine-binding proteins. Irradiation of ^{125}I-labeled thyroxine bound to thyroxine-binding prealbumin or thyroxine-binding globulin (Somack et al., 1982) causes labeling of these proteins almost exclusively at the hormone-binding site, although with low efficiency. In addition of the compound in serum, however, cause labeling of many other proteins. The direct labeling of thyroid receptors by photolysis of thyroxine and triiodothyronine has been discussed (cf. Section III,F).

V. Conclusion

In principle, affinity labeling has always held the promise of permitting binding proteins to be covalently labeled with the selectivity inherent in the interactions of reversible ligands with the binding site. On the practical level, however, the problem has been to find suitable chemically reactive or photoactivatable derivatives of the reversibly binding ligands so that the covalent labeling selectivity could, in fact, be made manifest. While the bulk of earlier studies that utilized affinity labeling agents were directed toward homogeneous preparations of binding proteins, the extention of this methodology to more complex systems, as is the case with receptors for steroid and thyroid hormones, has proved to be a challenge. Here, the desired target is the hormone-binding site of a protein, often rarely more than partially purified and in some cases present in unpurified cell fractions or in intact cells.

While the application of the affinity labeling technique to such challenging systems is still in a relatively early stage of development, it is apparent already that the methodology is adequate to label receptors covalently with a sufficient degree of selectivity so that they can be easily detected. Hence, this novel extension of affinity labeling technology has already led to interesting comparisions of receptor physicochemical properties and subunit structure, insightful studies on receptor localization, and provocative findings of receptor dynamics within cells. Certainly, further refinement of these selective labeling techniques will continue to bring valuable new information about the action of hormones at the molecular level.

REFERENCES

Baker, B. R. (1967). "Design of Active Site-Directed Irreversible Enzyme Inhibitors." Wiley, New York.

Baker, B. R. (1970). Specific irreversible enzyme inhibitors. *Annu. Rev. Pharmacol.* **10,** 35–50.

Balasubramanian, V., and Robinson, C. H. (1981). Irreversible inactivation of mammalian Δ^5-3β-hydroxysteroid dehydrogenases by 5,10-secosteroids. Enzymatic oxidation of allenic alcohols to the corresponding allenic ketones. *Biochem. Biophys. Res. Commun.* **101,** 495–501.

Balasubramanian, V., McDermott, I. R., and Robinson, C. H. (1982). 4-Ethenylidene steroids as mechanism-based inactivators of 3β-hydroxysteroid dehydrogenases. *Steroids* **40,** 109–119.

Batzold, F. H., Covey, D. F., and Robinson, C. H. (1977). Effects of novel acetylenic and allenic steroids on the rat prostate. *Cancer Treat. Rep.* **61,** 255–257.

Bayley, H. (1983). *In* "Photogenerated Reagents in Biochemistry and Molecular Biology" (T. S. Work and R. H. Burdon, eds.). North-Holland Publ., Amsterdam.

Bayley, H., and Knowles, J. R. (1977). Photoaffinity labeling. *In* "Methods in Enzymology" (W. B. Jakoby and M. Wilchek, eds.), Vol. 46, pp. 69–114. Academic Press, New York.

Benisek, W. F., Ogez, J. R., and Smith, S. B. (1982). Design of site-specific pharmacologic reagents: Illustration of some alternative approaches by reagents directed towards steroid-hormone-specific targets. *Adv. Chem. Ser.* (198), 267–323.

Bevins, C. L., Kayser, R. H., Pollack, R. M., Ekiko, D. B., and Sadoff, S. (1980). Irreversible active site-directed inhibition of Δ^5-3-ketosteroid isomerase by steroidal 17-β-oxiranes. Evidence for two modes of binding in steroid-enzyme complexes. *Biochem. Biophys. Res. Commun.* **95,** 1131–1137.

Birnbaumer, M., Schrader, W. T., and O'Malley, B. W. (1983a). Photoaffinity labeling of chick progesterone receptor proteins: Similar hormone binding domains detected after removal of proteolytic interference. *J. Biol. Chem.* **258,** 1637–1644.

Birnbaumer, M., Schrader, W. T., and O'Malley, B. W. (1983b). Assessment of structural similarities of chick oviduct progesterone receptor subunits by partial proteolysis of photoaffinity-labeled proteins. *J. Biol. Chem.* **258,** 7331–7337.

Blohm, T. R., Metcalf, B. W., Laughlin, M. E., Sjoerdsma, A., and Schatzman, G. L. (1980). Inhibition of testosterone 5α-reductase by a proposed enzyme-activated, active site-directed inhibitor. *Biochem. Biophys. Res. Commun.* **95,** 273–280.

Bonner, J. J. (1982). An assessment of the ecdysteroid receptor of Drosophila. *Cell* **30,** 7–8.

Chang, C. H., Rowley, D. R., Lobl, T. J., and Tindall, D. J. (1982). Purification and characterization of androgen receptor from steer seminal vesicle. *Biochemistry* **21**, 4102–4109.

Chang, C. H., Rowley, D. R., and Tindall, D. J. (1983). Purification and characterization of the androgen receptor from rat ventral prostate. *Biochemistry* **22**, 6170–6175.

Cheng, S.-Y. (1983). Structural similarities in the plasma membrane 3,3',5-triiodo-L-thyronine receptors from human, rat and mouse cultured cells. Analysis by affinity labeling. *Endocrinology* **113**, 1155–1157.

Cheng, S.-Y., Cahnmann, H. J., Wilchek, M., and Ferguson, R. N. (1975). Affinity labeling of the thyroxine binding domain of human serum prealbumin with dansyl chloride. *Biochemistry* **14**, 4132–4136.

Cheng, S.-Y., Wilchek, M., Cahnmann, H. J., and Robbins, J. (1977). Affinity labeling of human serum prealbumin with *N*-bromoacetyl-L-thyroxine. *J. Biol. Chem.* **252**, 6076–6081.

Chin, C.-C., Asmar, P., and Warren, J. C. (1980). Synthesis of 2-bromoacetamidoestrone methyl ether and study of the steroid-binding site of human placental estradiol 17β-dehydrogenase. *J. Biol. Chem.* **255**, 3660–3664.

Chin, C.-C., Pineda, J., and Warren, J. C. (1982a). Spatial relationships of steroid and cofactor at the active site of human placental estradiol 17β-dehydrogenase. *J. Biol. Chem.* **257**, 2225–2229.

Chin, C.-C., Murdock, G. L., and Warren, J. C. (1982b). Identification of two histidyl residues in the active site of human placental estradiol 17β-dehydrogenase. *Biochemistry* **21**, 3322–3326.

Chowdhary, V., and Westheimer, F. H. (1979). Photoaffinity labeling of biological systems. *Annu. Rev. Biochem.* **48**, 293–325.

Cidlowski, J. A., and Richon, V. (1983). Physical characterization and purification of affinity labeled human glucocorticoid receptors. *Proc. Annu. Endoc. Soc. Meet., 65th* Abstr. No. 588, p. 227.

Cornelisse, J., and Havinga, E. (1975). Photosubstitution reactions of aromatic compounds. *Chem. Rev.* **75**, 353–388.

Covey, D. F., and Hood, W. F. (1981). Enzyme-generated intermediates derived from 4-androstene-3,6,17-trione and 1,4,6-androstatriene-3,17-dione cause a time-dependent decrease in human placental aromatase activity. *Endocrinology* **108**, 1597–1599.

Covey, D. F., and Hood, W. F. (1982a). Aromatase enzyme catalysis is involved in the potent inhibition of estrogen biosynthesis caused by 4-acetoxy- and 4-hydroxy-4-androstene-3,17-dione. *Mol. Pharmacol.* **21**, 173–180.

Covey, D. F., and Hood, W. F. (1982b). A new hypothesis based on suicide substrate inhibitor studies for the mechanism of action of aromatase. *Cancer Res. (Suppl.)* **42**, 3327s–3333s.

Covey, D. F., Hood, W. F., and Parikh, V. D. (1981). 10β-Propynyl-substituted steroids. *J. Biol. Chem.* **256**, 1076–1079.

Danzo, B. J., Taylor, C. A., Jr., and Schmidt, W. N. (1980). Binding of the photoaffinity ligand 17β-hydroxy-4,6-androstadien-3-one to rat androgen-binding protein: Comparison with the binding of 17β-hydroxy-5α-androstan-3-one. *Endocrinology* **107**, 1169–1175.

Danzo, B. J., Taylor, C. A., Jr., and Eller, B. C. (1982a). Some physicochemical characteristics of photoaffinity-labeled rabbit androgen-binding protein. *Endocrinology* **111**, 1270–1277.

Danzo, B. J., Taylor, C. A., Jr., and Eller, B. C. (1982b). Some physicochemical characteristics of photoaffinity-labeled rabbit testosterone-binding globulin. *Endocrinology* **111**, 1278–1285.

David-Inouye, Y., Somack, R., Nordeen, S. K., Apriletti, J. W., Baxter, J. D., and Eberhardt, N. L. (1982). Photoaffinity labelling of the rat liver nuclear thyroid hormone receptor with [^{125}I]triiodothyronine. *Endocrinology* **111**, 1758–1760.

Dellweg, H.-G., Hotz, A., Mugele, K., and Gehring, U. (1982). Active domains in wild-type and mutant glucocorticoid receptors. *EMBO J.* **1**, 285–289.

Dunkerton, L. V., Markland, F. S., Jr., and Li, M. P. (1982). Affinity-labelling corticoids I. Synthesis of 21-chloroprogestrone deoxycorticosterone 21-(1-imidazole) carboxylate, 21-deoxy-21-chloro dexamethasone, and dexamethasone 21-mesylate, 21-bromoacetate, and 21-iodoacetate. *Steroids* **39**, 1–6.

Dure, L. S., IV, Schrader, W. T., and O'Malley, B. W. (1980). Covalent attachment of a progestational steroid to chick oviduct progesterone receptor by photoaffinity labelling. *Nature (London)* **283**, 784–786.

Eckert, R. L., Rorke, E. A., and Katzenellenbogen, B. S. (1982). Determination of the rates of synthesis and turnover of the estrogen receptor in MCF-7 breast cancer cells using a density shift technique. *Proc. Annu. Endocr. Soc. Meet., 64th* Abst. 29, p. 87.

Eckert, R. L., Mullick, A., Rorke, E. A., and Katzenellenbogen, B. S. (1984). Estrogen receptor synthesis and turnover in MCF-7 breast cancer cells measured by a density shift technique. *Endocrinology* **114**, 629–637.

Fedan, J. S. (1983). Pharmacological and biochemical applications of photoaffinity labels. *Fed. Proc., Fed. Am. Soc. Exp. Biol.* **42**, 2825–2850.

Foster, C. M., Eisen, H. J., and Bloomfield, C. D. (1983). Covalent labeling of rat thymocyte and human lymphoid glucocorticoid receptor. *Cancer Res.* **43**, 5273–5277.

Galardy, R. E., Hall, B. E., and Jamieson, J. D. (1980). Irreversible photoactivation of a pancreatic secretagogue receptor with cholecystokinin carboxylterminal octapeptides. *J. Biol. Chem.* **255**, 2148–3155.

Gehring, U. (1979). Genetic analysis of glucocorticoid action in neoplastic lymphoid cells. *Adv. Enzyme Regul.* **17**, 343–361.

Gehring, U., and Hotz, A. (1983). Photoaffinity labeling and partial proteolysis of wild-type and variant glucocorticoid receptors. *Biochemistry* **22**, 4013–4018.

Gronemeyer, H., and Pongs, O. (1980). Localization of ecdysterone on polytene chromosomes of *Drosophila melanogaster*. *Proc. Natl. Acad. Sci. U.S.A.* **77**, 2108–2112.

Gronemeyer, H., Hameister, H., and Pongs, O. (1981). Photoinduced bonding of endogenous ecdysterone to salivary gland chromosomes of *chironomus tentans*. *Chromosoma (Berlin)* **82**, 543–559.

Hearne, M., and Benisek, W. F. (1983). Photoaffinity modification of Δ^5-3-ketosteroid isomerase by light-activatable steroid ketones covalently coupled to agarose beads. *Biochemistry* **22**, 2537–2544.

Holmes, S. D., and Smith, R. G. (1983). Identification of histidine and methionine residues in the active site of the human uterine progesterone receptor with the affinity labels 11α- and 16α-(bromoacetoxy) progesterone. *Biochemistry* **22**, 1729–1734.

Holmes, S. D., Van, N. T., Stevens, S., and Smith, R. G. (1981). Affinity labeling of the human uterine progesterone receptor with 21-, 16α- and 11α-bromoacetoxyprogesterones. *Endocrinology* **109**, 670–672.

Horiuchi, R., Johnson, M. L., Willingham, M. C., Pastan, I., and Cheng, S.-Y. (1982). Affinity labeling of the plasma membrane 3,3',5-triiodo-L-thyronine receptor in GH$_3$ Cells. *Biochemistry* **79**, 5527–5531.

Horwitz, K. B., and Alexander, P. S. (1983). In situ photolinked nuclear progesterone receptors: Subunit mass without proteolysis. *Endocrinology* **113**, 2195–2201.

Horwitz, K. B., Freidenberg, G. R., Sheridan, R. L., and Alexander, P. S. (1983). Progestins and the antiprogestin RU38 486: Effects on progesterone receptors and on proliferation of human breast cancer cells. *Proc. Annu. Endocr. Soc. Meet., 65th* Abstr. No. 581, p. 226.

Houlsey, P. R., and Pratt, W. B. (1983a). Phosphorylation of the glucocorticoid receptors by intact L cells. *Fed. Proc., Fed. Am. Soc. Exp. Biol.* **43,** 1879 (Abstr. No. 711).

Housley, P. R., and Pratt, W. B. (1983b). Direct demonstration of glucocorticoid receptor phosphorylation by intact L-cells. *J. Biol. Chem.* **258,** 4630–4635.

Ikeda, M. (1982). Identification of thiol group at the estrogen-binding site on the cytoplasmic receptor from rabbit uterus by affinity labeling. *Biochim. Biophys. Acta* **718,** 66–73.

Jakoby, W. B., and Wilchek, M., eds. (1977). Affinity labeling. "Methods in Enzymology," Vol. 46. Academic Press, New York,

Janne, O. A. (1982). Purification and photoaffinity labeling of rabbit uterine progesterone receptors. *Endocrinology* **110** *(Suppl.),* 141, Abstr. No. 248.

Jelenc, P. C., Cantor, C. R., and Simon, S. R. (1978). High yield photo-reagents for protein crosslinking and affinity labeling. *Proc. Natl. Acad. Sci. U.S.A.* **75,** 3564–3568.

Kadohama, N., Petrow, V., Lack, L., and Sandberg, A. A. (1983). Inhibitory effects of some steroidal 6-methylene derivatives on 5α-reductase activity in human and rat prostate. *J. Steroid Biochem.* **18,** 551–558.

Katzenellenbogen, J. A. (1977). Affinity labeling as a technique in determining hormone mechanisms (review). *In* "Biochemical Actions of Hormones" (G. Litwack, ed.), Vol. 4, pp. 1–84. Academic Press, New York.

Katzenellenbogen, J. A., Johnson, H. J., Jr., Carlson, K. E., and Myers, H. N. (1974). The photoreactivity of some light-sensitive estrogen derivatives. The use of an exchange assay to determine their photointeraction with the rat uterine estrogen binding protein. *Biochemistry* **13,** 2986–2994.

Katzenellenbogen, J. A., Carlson, K. E., Johnson, H. J., Jr., and Myers, H. N. (1977). Estrogen photoaffinity labels II: Reversible binding and covalent attachment of photosensitive hexestrol derivatives to the uterine estrogen receptor. *Biochemistry* **16,** 1970–1976.

Katzenellenbogen, J. A., Kilbourn, M. R., and Carlson, K. E. (1980). Photosensitive steroids as probes of estrogen receptor sites. *Ann. N.Y. Acad. Sci.* **346,** 18–32.

Katzenellenbogen, J. A., Carlson, K. E., Heiman, D. F., Robertson, D. W., Wei, L. L., and Katzenellenbogen, B. S. (1983). Efficient and highly selective covalent labeling of the estrogen receptor with [³H]tamoxifen aziridine. *J. Biol. Chem.* **258,** 3487–3495.

Katzenellenbogen, B. S., Wei, L. L., Robertson, D. W., and Katzenellenbogen, J. A. (1982). Selective cytotoxicity mediated by the estrogen receptor. *J. Cell. Biochem.* **6,** 134.

Katzenellenbogen, B. S., Miller, M. A., Eckert, R. L., and Sudo, K. (1983a). Antiestrogen pharmacology and mechanism of action. *J. Steroid Biochem.* **19,** 59–68.

Katzenellenbogen, B. S., Monsma, F. J., Jr., Miller, M. A., Norman, M. J., and Katzenellenbogen, J. A. (1983b). Characterization of the estrogen receptor and its dynamics in MCF-7 breast cancer cells using a covalently-attaching antiestrogen. *Proc. Annu. Endocr. Soc. Meet., 65th* Abstr. No. 405, p. 182.

Kayser, R. H., Bounds, P. L., Bevins, C. L., and Pollack, R. M. (1983). Affinity alkylation of bacterial Δ⁵-3-ketosteroid isomerase. *J. Biol. Chem.* **258,** 909–915.

Khan, M. S., and Rosner, W. (1977). Investigation of the binding site of human corticosteroid-binding globulin by affinity labeling. *J. Biol. Chem.* **252,** 1895–1900.

Knowles, J. R. (1972). Photogenerated reagents for biological receptor-site labeling. *Acc. Chem. Res.* **5,** 155–160.

Kunkel, G. R., Mehrabian, M., and Martinson, H. G. (1981). Contact-site cross-linking agents. *Mol. Cell. Biochem.* **34,** 3–13.

Lamb, D. J., Holmes, S. D., Smith, R. G., and Bullock, D. W. (1982). Purification of a progesterone receptor from rabbit uterus. *Biochem. Biophys. Res. Commun.* **108,** 1131–1135.

LeGaillard, F., and Dautrevaux, M. (1977). Affinity labelling of human transcortin. *Biochim. Biophys. Acta* **495,** 312–323.

Lessey, B. A., Alexander, P. S., and Horwitz, K. B. (1983). The subunit structure of human breast cancer progesterone receptors: Characterization by chromatography and photoaffinity labeling. *Endocrinology* **112,** 1267–1274.

Marcotte, P. A., and Robinson, C. H. (1982a). Synthesis and evaluation of 10β-substituted 4-estrene-3,17-diones as inhibitors of human placental microsomal aromatase. *Steroids* **39,** 325–344.

Marcotte, P. A., and Robinson, C. H. (1982b). Inhibition and inactivation of estrogen synthetase (aromatase) by fluorinated substrate analogues. *Biochemistry* **21,** 2773–2778.

Marver, D., Chiu, W.-H., Wolff, M. E., and Edelman, I. S. (1976). Photoaffinity site-specific covalent labeling of human corticosteroid-binding globulin. *Proc. Natl. Acad. Sci. U.S.A.* **73,** 4462–4466.

Metcalf, B. W., Wright, C. L. Burkhart, J. P., and Johnston, J. O. (1981). Substrate-induced inactivation of aromatase by allenic and acetylenic steroids. *J. Am. Chem. Soc.* **103,** 3221–3222.

Miller, M. A., and Katzenellenbogen, B. S. (1983a). Characterization and quantitation of antiestrogen binding sites in estrogen receptor-positive and -negative human breast cancer cell lines. *Cancer Res.* **43,** 3094–3101.

Miller, M. A., and Katzenellenbogen, B. S. (1983b). Antiestrogen binding in antiestrogen resistant variants of MCF-7 human breast cancer cells. *Proc. Annu. Endocr. Soc. Meet., 65th* Abstr. No. 159, p. 120.

Monsma, F. J., Jr., Katzenellenbogen, B. S., Miller, M. A., Ziegler, Y. S., and Katzenellenbogen, J. A. (1984). Characterization of the estrogen receptor and its dynamics in MCF-7 human breast cancer cells using a covalently-attaching antiestrogen. *Endocrinology* **115,** 143–153.

Muldoon, T. G. (1980). Molecular and functional anomalies in the mechanism of the estrogenic action of 4-mercuri-17β-estradiol. *J. Biol. Chem.* **255,** 1358–1366.

Muldoon, T. G., and Warren, J. C. (1969). Characterization of steroid-binding sites by affinity labeling. *J. Biol. Chem.* **244,** 5430–5435.

Murdock, G. L., and Warren, J. C. (1982). Isolation of histidyl peptides of the steroid-binding site of human placental estradiol 17β-dehydrogenase. *Steroids* **39,** 165–179.

Nawata, H., Bronzert, D., and Lippman, M. E. (1981). Isolation and characterization of a tamoxifen-resistant cell line derived from MCF-7 human breast cancer cells. *J. Biol. Chem.* **256,** 5016–5023.

Nikodem, V. M., Cheng, S.-Y., and Rall, J. E. (1980). Affinity labeling of rat liver thyroid hormone nuclear receptor. *Biochemistry* **77,** 7064–7068.

Nordeen, S. K., Lan, N. C., Showers, M. O., and Baxter, J. D. (1981). Photoaffinity labeling of glucocorticoid receptors. *J. Biol. Chem.* **256,** 10503–10508.

Pascual, A., Casanova, J., and Samuels, H. H. (1982). Photoaffinity labeling of thyroid hormone nuclear receptors in intact cells. *J. Biol. Chem.* **257,** 9640–9647.

Payne, D. W., Katzenellenbogen, J. A., and Carlson, K. E. (1980). Photoaffinity labeling of rat α-fetoprotein. *J. Biol. Chem.* **255**, 10359–10367.

Penning, T. M., and Covey, D. F. (1982). Inactivation of Δ⁵-3-ketosteroid isomerase(s) from beef adrenal cortex by acetylenic ketosteroids. *J. Steroid Biochem.* **16**, 691–699.

Penning, T. M., Covey, D. F., and Talalay, P. (1981). Irreversible inactivation of Δ⁵-3-ketosteroid isomerase of *Pseudomanas testosteroni* by acetylenic suicide substrates. *J. Biol. Chem.* **256**, 6842–6850.

Penning, T. M., Heller, D. N., Balasubramanian, T. M., Fenselau, C. C., and Talalay, P. (1982). Mass spectrometric studies of a modified active-site tetrapeptide from Δ⁵-3-ketosteroid isomerase of *Pseudomonas testosteroni*. *J. Biol. Chem.* **257**, 12589–12593.

Petrow, V., Wang, Y.-S., Lack, L., and Sandberg, A. (1981). Prostatic cancer. I. 6-Methylene-4-pregnen-3-ones as irreversible inhibitors of rat prostatic Δ⁴-3-ketosteroid 5α-reductase. *Steroids* **38**, 121–140.

Petrow, V., Wang, Y.-S., Lack, L., Sandberg, A., Kadohoma, N., and Kendle, K. (1983). Prostatic cancer II. Inhibitors of rat prostatic Δ⁴-3 ketosteroid 5α-reductase derived from 6-methylene-4-androsten-3-ones. *J. Steroid Biochem.* **19**, 1491–1502.

Pollack, R. M., Kayser, R. H., and Bevins, C. L. (1979). An active-site directed irreversible inhibitor of Δ⁵-3-ketosteroid isomerase. *Biochem. Biophys. Res. Commun.* **91**, 783–790.

Reiner, G. C. A., and Katzenellenbogen, B. S. (1983). A potential estradiol-based affinity label for studying estrogen receptors in human breast cancer. *Breast Cancer Res. Treat.* **3**, 304.

Reiner, G. C. A., Katzenellenbogen, B. S., Bindal, R. D., and Katzenellenbogen, J. A. (1984). Biological activity and receptor binding of a strongly interacting estrogen in human breast cancer cells. *Cancer Res.* **44**, 2302–2308.

Robaire, B., Covey, D. F., Robinson, C. H., and Ewing, L. L. (1977). Selective inhibition of rat epididymal steroid Δ⁴-5α-reductase by conjugated allenic 3-oxo-5,10-secosteroids. *J. Steroid Biochem.* **8**, 307–310.

Robertson, D. W., Wei, L. L., Hayes, J. R., Carlson, K. E., Katzenellenbogen, J. A., and Katzenellenbogen, B. S. (1981). Tamoxifen aziridines: Effective inactivators of the estrogen receptors. *Endocrinology* **109**, 1298–1300.

Roth, L. J., Diab, I. M., Watanabe, M., and Dinerstein, R. J. (1977). Autoradiography in cytopharmacology. *In* "Drug Fate and Metabolism" (E. R. Garett, and J. L. Hertz, eds.), Vol. 1, Chap. 2, pp. 27–63. Dekker, New York.

Sadler, S. E., and Maller, J. L. (1982). Identification of a steroid receptor on the surface of *Xenopus* oocytes by photoaffinity labeling. *J. Biol. Chem.* **257**, 355–361.

Schaltmann, K., and Pongs, O. (1982). Identification and characterization of the ecdysterone receptor in *Drosophila melanogaster* by photoaffinity labeling. *Proc. Natl. Acad. Sci. U.S.A.* **79**, 6–10.

Schmidt, W. N., Taylor, C. A., Jr., and Danzo, B. J. (1981). The use of a photoaffinity ligand to compare androgen-binding protein (ABP) present in rat sertoli cell culture media with ABP present in epididymal cytosol. *Endocrinology* **108**, 786–794.

Shaw, E. (1970a). Selective chemical modification of proteins. *Physiol. Rev.* **50**, 244–296.

Shaw, E. (1970b). *In* "The Enzymes" (P. D. Boyer, ed.), 3rd Ed., Vol. 1, pp. 91–146. Academic Press, New York.

Simons, S. S., Jr., and Thompson, E. B. (1981). Dexamethasone 21-mesylate: An affinity label of glucocorticoid receptors from rat hepatoma tissue culture cells. *Proc. Natl. Acad. Sci. U.S.A.* **78**, 3541–3545.

Simons, S. S., Jr., and Thompson, E. B. (1982). Affinity labeling of glucocorticoid receptors: New methods in affinity labeling. In "Biochemical Actions of Hormones" (G. Litwak, ed.), Vol. 9, pp. 221–254. Academic Press, New York.

Simons, S. S., Jr., Thompson, E. B., Merchlinsky, M. J., and Johnson, D. F. (1980a). Synthesis and biological activity of some novel, chemically reactive glucocorticoids. J. Steroid Biochem. 13, 311–322.

Simons, S. S., Jr., Pons, M., and Johnson, D. F. (1980b). α-Keto mesylate: A reactive, thiol-specific functional group. J. Org. Chem. 45, 3084–3088.

Simons, S. S., Jr., Thompson, E. B., and Johnson, D. F. (1980c). Unique long-acting antiglucocorticoid in whole and broken cell systems. Proc. Natl. Acad. Sci. U.S.A. 77, 5167–5171.

Simons, S. S., Jr., Schleenbaker, R. E., and Eisen, H. J. (1983). Activation of covalent affinity labeled glucocorticoid receptor-steroid complexes. J. Biol. Chem. 258, 2229–2238.

Singer, S. J. (1967). Covalent labeling of active sties. Adv. Protein Chem. 22, 1–54.

Smith, S. B., and Benisek, W. F. (1980). Active site-directed photoinactivation of Δ^{5}-3-ketosteroid isomerase from Pseudomonas putida dependent on 1,4,6-androstatrien-3-one-17β-ol. J. Biol. Chem. 255, 2690–2693.

Somack, R., Nordeen, S. K., and Eberhardt, N. L. (1982). Photoaffinity labeling of human thyroxine-binding prealbumin with thyroxine and N-(ethyl-2-diazomalonyl) thyroxine. Biochemistry 21, 5651–5660.

Strickler, R. C., Covey, D. F., and Tobias, B. (1980). Study of 3α, 20β-hydroxysteroid dehyrogenase with an enzyme-generated affinity alkylator: Dual enzyme activity at a single active site. Biochemistry 19, 4950–4954.

Strickler, R. C., Tobias, B., and Covey, D. F. (1981). Human placental 17β-estradiol dehydrogenase and 20α-hydroxysteroid dehydrogenase. J. Biol. Chem. 256, 316–321.

Sudo, K., Monsma, F. J., Jr., and Katzenellenbogen, B. S. (1983). Antiestrogen-binding sites distinct from the estrogen receptor: Subcellular localization, ligand specificity, and distribution in tissue of the rat. Endocrinology 112, 425–434.

Sutherland, R. L., Foo, M. S., Green, M. D., Waybourne, A. M., and Krozowski, Z. R. (1980). High affinity antiestrogen binding site distinct from the estrogen receptor. Nature (London) 288, 273–275.

Taylor, C. A., Jr., Smith, H. E., and Danzo, B. J. (1980a). Photoaffinity labeling of rat androgen binding protein. Biochemistry 77, 234–238.

Taylor, C. A., Jr., Smith, H. E., and Danzo, B. J. (1980b). Characterization of androgen binding protein in rat epididymal cytosol using a photoaffinity ligand. J. Biol. Chem. 225, 7769–7773.

Thomas, E. W. (1977). Carbohydrate binding sites. In "Methods in Enzymology," (W. B. Jakoby and M. Wilchek, eds.), Vol. 46, pp. 362–368. Academic Press, New York.

Thomas, J. L., LaRochelle, M. C., Covey, D. F., and Strickler, R. C. (1983). Inactivation of human placental 17β, 20α-hydroxysteroid dehydrogenase with enzyme-generated 16-methylene estrone. Fed. Proc., Fed. Am. Soc. Exp. Biol. 42, 643.

Tobias, B., Covey, D. F., and Strickler, R. C. (1982). Inactivation of human placental 17β-estradiol dehydrogenase and 20α-hydroxysteroid dehydrogenase with active site-directed 17β-propynyl-substituted progestin analogs. J. Biol. Chem. 257, 2783–2786.

Tometsko, A. M., and Richards, F. M. (1980). Applications of photochemistry in probing biological targets. Ann. N.Y. Acad. Sci. 346.

Turro, N. J. (1978). "Modern Molecular Photochemistry." Benjamin/Cummings, Menlo Park, California.

Turro, N. J. (1980). Structure and dynamics of important reactive intermediates involved in photobiological systems. *Ann. N.Y. Acad. Sci.* **346**, 1–17.

van der Walt, B., Nikodem, V. M., and Cahnmann, H. J. (1982). Use of un-derivatized thyroid hormones for photoaffinity labeling of binding proteins. *Proc. Natl. Acad. Sci. U.S.A.* **79**, 3508–3512.

Voigt, W., Castro, A., Covey, D. F., and Robinson, C. H. (1978). Inhibition of testosterone 5α-reductase by and antiandrogenicity of allenic 3-keto-5,10-secosteroids. *Acta Endocrinol.* **87**, 668–672.

Walsch, C. (1982). Suicide substrates: Mechanism-based enzyme inactivators. *Tetrahedron* **38**, 871–907.

Weisz, A., Buzard, R. L., Horn, D., Li, M. P., Dunkerton, L. V., and Markland, F. S., Jr. (1983). Steroid derivatives for electrophilic affinity labelling of glucocorticoid binding sites: Interaction with the glucocorticoid receptor and biological activity. *J. Steroid Biochem.* **18**, 375–382.

Westphal, H. M., Fleishmann, G., and Beato, M. (1981). Photoaffinity labeling of steroid binding proteins with unmodified ligands. *Eur. J. Biochem.* **119**, 101–106.

Wolf, W., and Kharasch, N. (1965). Photolysis of iodoaromatic compounds in C_6H_6. *J. Org. Chem.* **30**, 2493–2498.

Wolff, M. E., Feldman, D., Catsoulacos, P., Funder, J. W., Hancock, C., Amaro, Y., and Edelman, I. S. (1975). Steroidal 21-diazo ketones: Photogenerated corticosteroid receptor labels. *Biochemistry* **14**, 1750–1759.

Wrange, O., and Gustafsson, J. A. (1978). Separation of the hormone- and DNA-binding sites of the hepatic glucocorticoid receptor by means of proteolysis. *J. Biol. Chem.* **253**, 856–865.

Yamamoto, K. R., Gehring, U., Stampfer, M. R., and Sibley, C. H. (1976). Genetic approaches to steroid hormone action. *Recent Prog. Horm. Res.* **32**, 3–32.

By DOROTHY T. KRIEGER

1. Messages being communicated may have to do with cell and tissue differentiation (Grimmelikhuijzen and Schaller, 1979; Riddeford, 1980), cell proliferation (Villa-Komaroff, quoted in Kolata, 1982), or could be related to effecting responses to exogenous stimuli [i.e., food, temperature, or osmotic changes (Grimm-Jørgensen, 1980], or reproductive cues.

2. Recently, the genomic structures of the precursor molecules for Substance P (Nawa *et al.*, 1983), somatostatin (Montminy *et al.*, 1984), and VIP (Itoh *et al.*, 1983) have been reported. Each of these structures has confirmed some of the generalizations proposed to date with regard to genomic structure or precursor proteins (see pp. 18–23). In the case of Substance P, yet another peptide, kassinin (previously identified as an amphibian peptide in the tachykinin family), was found within the precursor molecule.

In the case of the vasopressin gene (see p. 23), the recent studies suggest some controversy with regard to its expression in different tissues and the nature of the vasopressin gene in normal and in Brattleboro (vasopressin-deficient) rats. Schmale and Richter (1984) have cloned the vasopressin gene from one Brattleboro animal and have demonstrated a single nucleotide deletion within the second of three axons. Such a deletion results in a frame shift, altering the amino acid sequence of neurophysin, removing the "stop" codon, and altering the sequence of what would have been the normal glycopeptide, removing its glycosylation site, which is the normal termination codon. Five of the 13 cysteine residues normally present in neurophysin are removed by the frame shift, giving rise to a precursor that may no longer be processed as is the precursor in normal animals. In this report, equal amounts of vasopressin mRNA were found in Brattleboro and normal rats, suggesting normal transcription. However, Majzoub *et al.* (1983) found dehydrated Brattleboro rats to have only 5% of the hypothalamic vasopressin mRNA of that of dehydrated rats from the parent stock of this mutation, suggesting a transcriptional defect or altered degradation. Similar to other neuropeptides, vasopressin has been detected in extra-CNS tissue (i.e., ovaries, adrenals) of normal rats. The Brattleboro rat appears to have a normal adrenal content of vasopressin-like material, as measured by radioimmunoassay, which is also biologically active (Nussey et al., 1983). Similar findings have been reported with regard to vasopressin content in ovaries of Brattleboro rats (Lim et al., 1984), suggesting that the defect in vasopressin production in the Brattleboro pituitary seems to be a tissue-specific one. It is possible that there may be a second gene for vasopressin or a closely related peptide which is expressed in the adrenal and in the ovary, or that there is tissue-specific splicing of vasopressin RNA. In support of the first possibility is the observation that there is an immunoreactive glycopeptide in adrenals but not pituitary from Brattleboro animals. Thus far, there has been no characterization of the size of vasopressin mRNA in these extra-CNS tissues.

In the case of the somatostatin gene in the rat (isolated from recombinant bacteria phage library prepared from rat liver DNA), Southern blot analysis was most consistent with the presence of a single gene encoding this peptide in this species, unlike observations in the fish, where at least two distinct somatostatin genes are present (Hobart et al., 1980; Noe and Spiess, 1983).

The precursor for VIP has been shown to contain a novel peptide of 27 amino acids, designated PHM-27, which differed by only two amino acids from PHI-27, a peptide recently isolated from porcine intestine. When the structure of h_p-GRF was reported (Guillemin et al., 1982; Rivier et al., 1982), homology to glucagon was noted. Homologies between VIP and the glucagon–secretin family had long been known (see p. 15). It is therefore not surprising that the amino-terminal region of h_p-GRF has a remarkable sequence homology to porcine PHI-27.

It has been stated (Barnstable et al., 1983) that in the field of molecular biology there are a number of important questions that have no molecular answers, while molecular biologists have arrived at answers for which they now have to discover the appropriate questions—as in the case of the strategy wherein cDNAs translated from total brain poly(A) RNA were cloned and determining which of the mRNA were exclusively synthesized in the brain. To date, more than 50 brain-specific cDNAs encoding molecules unrelated to existing peptides and of unknown function have been produced from such a study (Sutcliffe et al., 1982).

3. There is also suggestive evidence for receptor evolution. In the frog, caerulein is a strong stimulant of gastric mucosal short-circuit current, whereas mammalian gastrin is a relatively weak stimulus (Dockray, 1979). Gastrin-like peptides are absent in amphibia, whereas it has been shown that caerulein or CCK-like peptides regulate not

only gallbladder and exocrine pancreas but also acid secretion. Therefore, the divergence of gastrin and CCK in higher vertebrates allows for the independent control in such species of gastric secretion and the pancreatic and gallbladder secretion, unlike the situation in the frog. It would appear, therefore, that in the frog stomach caerulein receptors are present, while those for gastrin may be present in lesser amounts or may differ structurally from their mammalian counterparts, compatible with the absence of gastrin-like peptides in this species.

4.   Recent evidence indicates similar commitment with regard to expression in the central nervous system. When fetal rat medullary raphe neurons which contain 5HT with or without Substance P or TRH are transplanted to adult rat striatum, the grafts contain many 5HT immunoreactive cells; some Substance P- and a few TRH-immunoreactive cells are also present. Similar grafts transplanted to hippocampus or spinal cord consistently express 5HT and/or TRH. Mesencephalic raphe neurons were similarly studied, which contained similar neuropeptides and neurotransmitters. Similar findings were seen in the case of striatal transplants, whereas when mesencephalic raphe cells were transplanted into the hippocampus they exhibited predominantly 5HT-like immunoreactivity, similar to findings in spinal cord transplants (Foster et al., 1984; Schultzberg et al., 1984).

5.   Recently, a specific carboxypeptidase has been described in the adrenal chromaffin granules which appears to be selective for liberation of enkephalins from their precursor molecule (Fricker and Snyder, quoted in Kolata, 1984). In the case of nerve growth factor, the gene for which has been cloned (Ulrich et al., 1983), the γ-subunit of this factor, which is an arginine-specific protease of the serine family, was found associated with NGF and acts on the precursor molecules to remove a carboxyl-terminal fragment. The location of this fragment, however, is not at the carboxyl terminus of the mature protein; hence it may not be the major processing enzyme of the precursor molecule.

6.   In the case of peptides with diffuse CNS distribution, there may be alterations only in a localized area in disease, not reflected in assays on cerebrospinal fluid. A number of characterized "neuropeptides" are reported to be present in pituitary (immunocytochemistry, immunoassay) though evidence for synthesis has not been presented—i.e., gastrin (Rehfeld, 1978), VIP (Morel et al., 1982; Lee et al., 1984), neurotensin (Goedert et al., 1982), Substance P (de Palatis et al., 1982), renin (Naruse et al., 1981), angiotensin (Steele et al., 1982), and "brain

specific S-100 protein" (Shirasawa *et al.*, 1983), (the three latter in gonadotropins); these may also be transported to CSF. There may also be dynamic changes in peptide secretion into CSF as well as active or passive transport of a given peptide to blood and CSF, which are reflected in concentration gradients (Hyyppa and Liira, 1979).

7. These effects may also be mediated by gastrointestinal function (i.e., secretion, motility) (Bueno and Ferre, 1982). In the case of CCK, although effects have been seen with intracerebroventricular administration in sheep, which are reversed by administration of CCK antiserum (Della-Fera *et al.*, 1981), as well as with peripheral administration, a significant observation has been that total abdominal vagotomy reduced the satiating effect of peripherally administered CCK (Smith *et al.*, 1981). This has now been shown to be mediated via vagal afferent fibers (Gerard Smith, personal communication). Peripherally administered CCK-8 increases the firing rate of such fibers (Niijima, 1983). This represents yet another mechanism of neuropeptide action. It is unclear whether such fibers are responding to circulating or paracrine-secreted CCK, and what is the final effector of this pathway.

8. A major new finding has been the diverse number of neuropeptides reported to regulate pituitary hormone secretion—a far cry from the original postulate in neuroendocrinology that there were specific hypothalamic releasing hormones (see p. 3) and possibly inhibitory factors regulating the secretion of a given pituitary hormone. There is evidence of interaction of these multiple peptides to (a) facilitate pituitary hormone release, either (1) by direct actions on the pituitary, (2) related to paracrine interactions of these substances secondary to their presence in pituitary, or (3) by one peptide enhancing the effects of a second peptide by increasing receptors to the latter (Negro-Vilar, 1984); or (b) by acting directly on the CNS, leading to release of a more specific pituitary trophic factor. It is also becoming apparent, as with peptide–neurotransmitter interactions in CNS, that similar interactions occur in the pituitary (Negro-Vilar, 1984). Reports have also appeared on the regulation of given pituitary hormones by neuropeptides (Grossman, 1984; Kato *et al.*, 1984; McCann *et al.*, 1984).

9. The demonstration that a VIP-like substance is present in large granule vesicles of nonsympathetic nerve axons and terminals in the cerebral arterial wall (Lee *et al.*, 1984), and the observation that exogenously applied VIP induces dilation of cat pial arteries *in vitro* and *in vivo* (Edvinsson *et al.*, 1981; Heistad *et al.*, 1980), suggest that such a

substance serves as a transmitter for vasodilation in cerebral blood vessels. In this regard, interaction with other neurotransmitters can be considered, i.e., VIP with cholinergic mechanisms (see page 29) and serotonergic mechanisms (serotonin stimulates VIP release) (Shimatsu *et al.*, 1983).

Whether the immunoreactive EGF-like material described in forebrain and midbrain structures and pallidal areas of brain (Fallon *et al.*, 1984) serves as a mitogen in CNS development, or as a neurotransmitter, or as both, is unclear. Such material is detected in brains of 15-day-old rats, but not in those 7 to 14 days old. Staining patterns seen in animals 15 days and older are conserved throughout adulthood. EGF has a demonstrated mitogenic effect on cultured astrocytes (Simpson *et al.*, 1982). However, the peak of astrocyte proliferation is seen prior to day 15 (Skoff *et al.*, 1976).

REFERENCES TO ADDENDUM

Barnstable, C., Jessell, T., Sanes, J., Stevens, C., and Robertson, M. (1983). How molecular is neurobiology? *Nature* **306**, 14–16.

Bueno, L., and Ferre, J.-P. (1982). Central regulation of intestinal motility by somatostatin and cholecystokinin octapeptide. *Science* **216**, 1427–1429.

Della-Fera, M. A., Baile, C. A., Schneider, B. S., and Grinker, J. A. (1981). Cholecystokinin antibody injected in cerebral ventricles stimulates feeding in sheep. *Science* **212**, 687–689.

de Palatis, L. R., Fiorindo, R. P., and Ho, R. H. (1982). Substance P immunoreactivity in the anterior pituitary gland of the guinea pig. *Endocrinology* **110**, 282–284.

Dockray, G. (1979). Evolutionary relationships of gut hormones. *Fed. Proc.* **38**, 2295–2301.

Edvinsson, L., McColloch, R., and Uddman, R. (1981). Substance P: Immunohistochemical localization and effect upon cat pial arteries in vitro and in situ. *J. Physiol.* **318**, 251–258.

Fallon, J. H., Seroogy, K. B., Loughlin, S. E., Morrison, R. S., Bradshaw, R. A., Knauer, D. J., and Cunningham, D. D. (1984). Epidermal growth factor immunoreactive material in the central nervous system; Location and development. *Science* **224**, 1107–1109.

Foster, G. A., Schultzberg, M., Bjorklund, A., Gage, F., and Hokfelt, T. (1984). Immunohistochemical analysis of transmitter phenotypic expression in medullary and mesencephalic neurones transplanted to the hippocampus and spinal corts of the rat. Proceedings of the Fernstrom Symposium, "Transplantation in the Mammalian CNS," Lund, Sweden, abs. P-48.

Goedert, M., Lightman, S. L., Nagy, J. J., Marley, P., and Emson, P.C. (1982). Neurotensin in the rat anterior pituitary gland. *Nature (London)* **298**, 163–165.

Grimm-Jørgensen, Y. (1980). Effect of thyrotropin releasing hormone on ^{22}Na uptake by the pond snail *Helisoma carabaceum*. *J. Exper. Zool.* **212**, 471–473.

Grimmelikhuijzen, C. J. P., and Schaller, H. C. (1979). *Trends Biol. Sci.*, pp. 265–267.

Grossman, A. (1984). Opioid peptides and pituitary hormone secretion. *In* "7th International Congress of Endocrinology Abstracts." Elsevier, Amsterdam.

Guillemin, R., Brazeau, P., Bohlen, P., Esch, F., Ling, N., and Wehrenberg, W. B. (1982). Growth hormone-releasing factor from a human pancreatic tumor that caused acromegaly. *Science* **218**, 585–587.

Heistad, D. D., Marcus, M. L., Said, S. I., and Gross, P. M. (1980). Effect of acetocholine and vasoactive intestinal peptide on cerebral blood flow. *Am. J. Physiol.* **239**, H73-H80.

Hobart, P., Crawford, R., Shen, I., Pictet, R., and Rutter, W. (1980). Cloning and sequence analysis of cDNAs encoding two distinct somatostatin precursors found in the endocrine pancreas of anglerfish. *Nature (London)* **288**, 137–141.

Hyyppa, M. T., and Liira, J. (1979). Neuropeptide hormones in cerebrospinal fluid. Experimental and clinical aspects. *Med. Biol.* **57**, 367–373.

Itoh, N., Obata, K., Yanaihara, N., and Okamoto, H. (1983). Human preprovasoactive intestinal polypeptide contains a novel PHI-27-like peptide, PHM-27. *Nature (London)* **304**, 547–549.

Kato, Y., Shimatsu, A., Matsushita, N., Ohta, H., Tojo, K., Kabayama, Y., Inoue, T., and Imura, H. (1984). Regulation of pituitary hormone secretion by VIP and related peptides. *In* "7th International Congress of Endocrinology Abstracts." Elsevier, Amsterdam.

Kolata, G. (1982). Molecular biology of brain hormones. *Science* **215**, 1222–1224.

Kolata, G. (1984). Unique enzyme targets neuropeptide. *Science* **224**, 1417.

Lee, T. J.-F., Saito, A., and Berezin, I. (1984). Vasoactive intestinal polypeptide-like substance: The potential transmitter for cerebral vasodilation. *Science* **224**, 898–901.

Lim, A. T. W., Lolait, S. J., Barlow, J. W., Autelitano, D. J., Toh, B. H., Boublik, J., Abraham, J., Johnston, C. I., and Funder, J. W. (1984). Immunoreactive arginine–vasopressin in Brattleboro rat ovary. *Nature (London)* **310**, 61–64.

McCann, S. M., Lumpkin, M. D., Ono, N., Khorram, O., Ottlecz, A., Koenig, J., Bedran de Castro, J., Krulich, L., and Samson, W. K. (1984). Interactions of brain peptides within the hypothalamus to alter anterior pituitary hormone secretion. *In* "7th International Congress of Endocrinology Abstracts." Elsevier, Amsterdam.

Majzoub, J. A., Rich, A., van Bloom, J., and Habener, J. F. (1983). Vasopressin and oxytocin mRNA regulation in the rat assessed by hybridization with synthetic oligonucleotides. *J. Biol. Chem.* **288**, 14061–14064.

Montminy, R. M., Goodman, R. H., Horovitch, S. J., and Habener, J. F. (1984). Primary structure of the gene encoding rat prepromatostatin. *Proc. Natl. Acad. Sci. U.S.A.* **81**, 3337–3340.

Morel, G., Besson, J., Rosselin, G., and Dubois, P. M. (1982). Ultrastructural evidence for endogenous vasoactive intestinal peptide-like immunoreactivity in the pituitary gland. *Neuroendocrinology* **34**, 85–89.

Naruse, K., Celio, M. R., Takii, Y., and Inagami, T. (1981). *Proc. Endocrine Soc. Meet.*, p. 277.

Nawa, H., Hirose, T., Takashima, H., Inayama, S., and Nakanishi, S. (1983). Nucleotide sequence of cloned cDNAs for two types of bovine brain substance P precursor. *Nature (London)* **306**, 32–36.

Negro-Vilar, A. (1984). Monoamine-peptide interactions in the regulation of pituitary cell function. *In* "7th International Congress of Endocrinology Abstracts." Elsevier, Amsterdam.

Niijima, A. (1983). Glucose-sensitive afferent nerve fibers in the liver and their role in food intake and blood glucose regulation. *J. Auton. Nerv. Syst.* **9**, 207–220.

Noe, B. D., and Spiess, J. (1983). Identification, isolation and characterization of a primary cleavage product of (pre)promatostatin-II in pancreatic islets. *Proc. Endocrine Soc. Meet., San Antonio*, p. 85.

Nussey, S. S., Ang, V. T. Y., Jenkins, J. S., Chowdrey, H. S., and Bisset, G. W. (1983). Brattleboro rat adrenal contains vasopressin. *Nature (London)* **310**, 64–67.

Rehfeld, J. (1978) . Localization of gastrins to neuro- and adenohypophysis. *Nature (London)* **271**, 771–773.

Riddeford, L. M. (1980). Prothoracic ectopic hormone-secreting hormone cells in the insect brain. *Nature (London)* **285**, 615–616.

Rivier, J., Spiess, J., Thorner, M., and Vale, W. (1982). Characterization of a growth hormone-releasing factor from a human pancreatic islet tumour. *Nature (London)* **300**, 276–278.

Schmale, H., and Richter, D. (1984). Single base deletion in the vasopressin gene is the cause of diabetes insipidus in Brattleboro rats. *Nature (London)* **308**, 705–709.

Schultzberg, M., Forster, G. A., Bjorklund, A., Gage, F. H., and Hokfelt, T. (1984). Immunohistochemical studies of transplants to the rat striatum of neurones containing more than one putative transmitter. Proceedings of the Fernstrom Symposium, "Transplantation in the Mammalian CNS," Lund, Sweden, abs. P-47.

Shimatsu, A., Kato, Y., Matsushita, N., Katakami, H., Ohta, H., Yanaihara, N., and Imura, H. (1983). Serotonin stimulated vasoactive intestinal polypeptide release from rat hypothalamus in vitro. *Brain Res.* **264**, 148–151.

Shirasawa, N., Kihara, H., Yamaguchi, S., and Yoshimura, F. (1983). Pituitary folliculostellate cells immunostained with S-100 protein antiserum in postnatal, castrated and thyroidectomized rats. *Cell Tissue Res.* **231**, 235–249.

Simpson, D., Morrison, R., de Vellis, T., and Herschman, H. (1982). Epidermal growth factor binding and mitogenic activity on purified populations of cells from the central nervous system. *J. Neurosci. Res.* **8**, 453–462.

Skoff, R. P., Price, D. L., and Stocks, S. (1976). Electron microscopic autoradiographic studies of gliogenesis in rat optic nerve. II. Time of origin. *J. Comp. Neurol.* **169**, 313–334.

Smith, G. P., Jerome, C., Cushin, B. J., Eterno, R., and Simansky, K. J. (1981). Abdominal vagotomy blocks the satiety effect of cholecystokinin in the rat. *Science* **213**, 1036–1037.

Steele, M. K., Brownfield, M. S., and Ganong, W. F. (1982). Immunochemical localization of angiotensin immunoreactivity in gonadotrops and lactotrops of the rat anterior pituitary gland. *Neuroendocrinology* **35**, 155–158.

Sutcliffe, J. G., Millner, R. J., Bloom, F. E., and Lerner, R. A. (1982). Common 82-nucleotide sequence unique to brain RNA. *Proc. Natl. Acad. Sci. U.S.A.* **79**, 4942–4946.

Ulrich, A., Gray, A., Berman, C., and Dull, T. J. (1983). Human beta-nerve growth factor gene sequence highly homologous to that of mouse. *Nature (London)* **303**, 821–825.

Index

A

Acetylcholine, 2–3, 31
  effect on phosphatidylinositol turnover, 126–128
  in smooth muscle contraction, 99
Acetyl-CoA carboxylase
  biphasic response to insulin, 62, 63
  insulin sensitivity, 64–68
Actin, 98
Acylhalides, 260–261
Adenosine triphosphatase, Ca^{2+},Mg^{2+}, insulin sensitivity, 64–68
Adenovirus, 20
Adenylate cyclase
  in blowfly salivary glands, and phosphatidylinositol turnover, 144–146
  insulin sensitivity, 64–68
  uterine, effect of relaxin, 104
Adipocyte
  biphasic response to insulin, 62
  mitochondria, insulin sensitivity, 52–55
  phosphatidylinositol turnover, 119
  plasma membranes, insulin sensitivity, 52–55
  whole, insulin action in, 60
Adrenal cortex, phosphatidylinositol turnover, 138–139
Adrenal cortical carcinoma, 197
Adrenal glomerulosa cells, phosphatidylinositol turnover, 137–138
Adrenal medulla, phosphatidylinositol turnover, 135–137
β-Adrenergic agonists, in smooth muscle contraction, 99
Adrenocorticotropic hormone (ACTH), 2, 4, 13
  distribution, 28
  in memory, learning, and adaptive behavior, 32–34

precursor, 20
  in steroidogenesis, 138–139
  in temperature regulation, 38
Adrenocorticotropin-β-lipotropin, precursor, 173
Affinity labeling, 213–274
  agents, *see also* specific agent
    efficiency, 215–220
    electrophilic, 214, 220
    ligand affinity and exchange, 220
    photoactivated, 214, 216, 220
    selectivity, 215–220
  of androgen receptors, 245–247
    agents, 245–246
  application, 214
  covalent, 215–225
    advantages and limitations, 225–226
    critical factors, 215–222
    covalent attaching functions, 222–225
    electrophilic, 222–223
    photoactivated, 223–225
  of ecdysone binding proteins, 252
    efficiency, 221
    study, 226
  electrophilic, of enzymes and extracellular binding proteins, 254–262
  electrophilic vs photoactivated, applicability to intact systems, 221–222
  of enzymes, 253–266
  of estrogen receptors, 229–235
    agents, 229–231
  of extracellular binding proteins, 253–266
  of glucocorticoid receptor, 241–245
    agents, 241
  methods, 214
  photoaffinity, of enzymes and extracellular binding proteins, 263–266
  of progestin receptors, 235–241
    agents, 235–236

Affinity labeling (*continued*)
    of receptors for steroids and thyroid
        hormones, 214–215
    selectivity, 213, 214, 221
    studies, 225–253
    types, 225–229
    of thyroid hormone receptors, 247–253
        agents, 247
    of *Xenopus* oocyte preparations, 252
Albuterol, effect on erythropoietin pro-
    duction, 167
Alzheimer's disease, 40
Amino acid, excitatory or inhibitory, in
    CNS, 2, 3
Androgen binding protein, 245, 263–264
Androgen receptor
    affinity labeling, 224, 230, 245–247
    molecular weight species, 246
1,4,6-Androstatrien-3,17-dione, 261
4-Androstene-3,6,17-trione, 261
Androstenedione
    acetylenic ketone-substituted, 259
    19,19-difluoro-substituted, 260–261
    19-fluoro-substituted, 260–261
Anemia
    in chronic renal disease, 196, 203
    erythropoietin in, 165, 178, 181, 202–
        203
    sickle cell, erythropoietin in, 166
Angiotensin, 2
    in blood pressure regulation, 39
    distribution, 28
    in pain perception, 32
    in smooth muscle contraction, 99
Angiotensin II, 4
    effect on steroidogenesis, in adrenal
        glomerulosa cells, 137
Anti-insulin receptor antibody, biphasic
    response to, 62, 63
Anti-prolactin receptor antibody, 58
Aplysia
    egg-laying hormone, 19
    polypeptide hormones, multigene
        family, 19
Arachidonic acid
    effect, on erythropoietin production, 167
    physiologic source, 128–129, 152
    release, in blowfly salivary gland, 149
Aromatase, 259–260
    inactivation, 261

Aromatization, 262
Asialoerythropoietin, 171–172
    activity, effect of galactose-terminal
        glycoproteins, 171, 172
    in bone marrow culture, 173
    hydrolysis, 173
    oxidation of galactose residues, effect
        on activity *in vivo*, 171–172
Autoradiography, 228
Azides, photoaffinity attaching functions,
    225
Aziridines, electrophilic attaching func-
    tions, 223

B

Binding protein, extracellular, affinity
    labeling, 253–266
Blowfly salivary glands, phos-
    phatidylinositol turnover, 144–151
Bombesin, 4
    distribution, 27
    in feeding behavior, 37
    in pain perception, 32
    in temperature regulation, 38
Bradykinin, 4
Brain
    microdissection, 11
    synaptosomes, phosphatidylinositol
        turnover, 125–129
Brain peptides, 1–50, *see also*
        Neuropeptide
    acetylation, 24
    amidation, 24
    biosynthesis, 5, 17–23
    categories, 3, 4
    characterization, 5–8
        physicochemical, 5–6
    concentrations, 3, 4
        alterations in CNS disease, 40–41
    deacetylation, 24
    degradation, 23–26
    delineation, methods, 5–13
    detection, 5–8
    distribution, 26–29
    effects
        on adaptive behavior, 32–34
        on blood pressure, 33, 39
        on feeding, 36–37
        on learning, 32–34

on major homeostatic mechanisms, 31–40
on memory, 32–34
on pain, 31–32
on temperature regulation, 37–39
evolution and, 13–16
functions, 29–40
glycosylation, 24
immunohistochemistry, 6–8
in situ hybridization cytochemistry, 7–8
isolation, 5–8
neurophysiological studies, 8–10
new, detection, 6
processing, evolutionary changes, 15
proteolytic processing, 23–26
in psychiatric disease, 34–35
radioimmunoassay, 5–6
receptors, detection, 10
study
methods, 5–13
neuroanatomical techniques, 10–12
quantitation of cell number and density, 12
stereotaxic techniques, 11–12
therapeutic applications, 41
Bretylium tosylate, effect, on relaxin-dependent uterine cAMP increase, 104
11α-Bromoacetoxyprogesterone, 240
16α-Bromoacetoxyprogesterone, 240
21-Bromoacetoxyprogesterone, 240
N-Bromoacetyl-L-thyroxine, 255
N-Bromoacetyltriiodothyronine, 247–251

C

Caerulein, 15
Calcitonin, 4, 20
in feeding behavior, 37
precursor, 20
Calcitonin gene-related product, 6
Calcium
control of smooth muscle contraction, 98–99
in phosphatidylinositol turnover, 118–119, 121, 124, 126–127, 129–136, 138–140, 142, 144–151
in temperature regulation, 37–38
Calmodulin, effect, on smooth muscle contraction, 101

cAMP
effect on phosphatidylinositol turnover, 142
regulation, in blowfly salivary glands, 144–145
cAMP antagonist, 70
cAMP-dependent protein kinase
activation, by relaxin, 104–105
insulin sensitivity, 64–68
in smooth muscle contraction, 100–102
cAMP-independent kinase, insulin sensitivity, 64–68
cAMP-independent protein kinase, insulin sensitivity, 64–68
cAMP phosphodiesterase
effect of phospholipids, 70–71
insulin sensitivity, 64–69
Captopril, in blood pressure regulation, 39
Carnosine, 4
Catecholamine, effect on phosphatidylinositol turnover, 142, 144
Cellular communication, 1, 14
11β-Chloromethylestradiol, 231
Cholecystokinin, 2, 4
distribution, 27, 28
octapeptide
concentrations, alterations in CNS disease, 40
effect on phosphatidylinositol turnover, 128
in feeding behavior, 36–37
in pain perception, 32
processing, 15
Chorionic gonadotropin, 173
Clonidine, in blood pressure regulation, 39
Concanavalin A
biphasic response to, 62, 63
in study of ligand–receptor interaction, 57–59
Corticosteroid binding globulin, 255, 264–265
photoaffinity labeling, 224
Corticotropin-like intermediate lobe peptide (CLIP), 25
Corticotropin-releasing factor, 34
distribution, 27–29
in feeding behavior, 37
Corticotropin-releasing hormone, 2, 4

Cortisol mesylate, 241, 243–245
Cytidine monophosphate, effect, on phosphatidylinositol turnover, 127
Cytidine triphosphate, in phosphoinositide turnover, 121

D

Dansyl chloride, 261
Degenerative myoconus epilepsy, 40–41
Dexamethasone mesylate, 241, 243–245
Diacylglycerol
    from phosphatidylinositol breakdown, 118
    in phosphatidylinositol turnover, 119–122, 135, 140–141, 144–145, 149, 152
Diazirines, photoaffinity attaching functions, 224–225
N-2-Diazo-3,3,3-trifluoropropionyl-3,5,3'-triiodo-L-thyronine, 247–251
Diazocarbonyl compounds, photoaffinity attaching functions, 224–225
16-Diazoestrone, 265
α-Diazoketones, 262
    photoaffinity labeling with, 264–266
Diazonium, 262
21-Diazopregnanes, 264
Dienone, 256–257
Diet, effect on insulin metabolism, 56–57
5α-Dihydrotestosterone 17-bromoacetate, 246
Dopamine, 2, 31

E

Ecdysone
    binding protein, affinity labeling, 252
    binding sites, affinity labeling, 224
Ectopic hormone syndrome, 196
Endocrine system, evolution, 13–14
β-Endorphin, 4, 13
    acetylation, 24
    distribution, 28
    in temperature regulation, 38
Endorphins
    in feeding behavior, 36
    in memory, learning, and adaptive behavior, 32–33
    in psychiatric disease, 34–35

Met-Enkephalin, 4
Leu-Enkephalin, 4
Enkephalins, 2, 6, 26
    in blood pressure regulation, 39
    concentrations, alterations in CNS disease, 40
    distribution, 27, 28
    in memory, learning, and adaptive behavior, 32
    in pain perception, 32
    precursor, 20–22
    in psychiatric disease, 35
Enkephalinase, 26
Enone, 256–257
Enzyme-activated irreversible inhibitors, 253–254
Enzymes
    affinity labeling, 253–266
    pseudosuicide inactivation, 254
    suicide substrates, 253–254
Epidermal growth factor, 106
Epinephrine, 2, 130
    effect on phosphatidylinositol turnover, 142
Epoxides
    affinity labeling with, 255–256
    electrophilic attaching functions, 223
    steroid, 256
Erythrogenin, 174, 177
Erythroid burst-forming units, 186–187
Erythroid colony-forming units, 186–187
Erythropoiesis, 166
    control, 161–162
Erythropoietin, 161–211
    amino acid composition, 169–170
    amino acid sequence, 169–170
    apparent molecular weight, 170–171
    assay, 163–164, 181, 186–194
    bioassay vs. radioimmunoassay, 194
    biogenesis, 174
    carbohydrate composition, 169
    carbohydrate moiety, role of, 173
    cell origin, 199–202
    chemistry, 168–178
    circulating, 165
    detection, in normal human serum, 192–194
    discovery, 162
    forms, 168, 169, 177–178
    functions, 161

glycosylation, 173
heterogeneity, 169
from human urine, 178, 181–186
  hydrophobic interaction chromatography, 184–185
  lectin affinity chromatography, 186
  molecular weight, 185–186
inactivation, 181
in kidney, 175–177, 194
monoclonal antibodies, 186
precursor, 174
production
  anephric models, 194–195
  in vitro, 167–168
  and oxygen supply, 165–166
  perfusion studies, 195–196
  by renal and nonrenal tumors, 196–199, 202
  site, 194–202
protein complex, 177–178
purification, 178–186, 202
radioimmunoassay, 163, 189–192, 202
sheep plasma, 179–181
sialic acid, role of, 171–173
sources, 163, 178, 186
species differences, 163
species distribution, 162
species specificity, 162–163
standardization, 164
structure, 163
structure-function relationships, 168–178
Esters, electrophilic attaching functions, 223
Estrogen
control of relaxin receptor, 106
enones, 230
receptor
  affinity labeling, 216–217, 223, 229–235
  dynamics, 234–235
  inactivation, 216
  photoaffinity labeling, 225
  structure and function, 231–234
Estrogen synthetase, 255

F

α-Fetoprotein, 264–265
photoaffinity labeling, 224

Formylmethionylleucylphenylalanine, effects on phosphatidylinositol turnover, 122–125
Forskolin, 146

G

Gastrin, 4, 15
Gastrointestinal peptides, 3, 4
Glucagon, 2, 4, 15
Glucocorticoid
photoaffinity labeling, 223
receptor
  affinity labeling, 230, 241–245
  molecular weight species, 242, 244–245
  structure and function, 242–245
Glycogen synthase phosphatase, biphasic response to insulin, 62, 63
Glycogen synthase phosphoprotein phosphatase, insulin sensitivity, 64–68
Glycosylation, in protection from proteolysis, 173
Gonadotropin-releasing hormone, 4
Growth factor, platelet-derived, 106
Growth hormone, 4, 19, 58
Growth-hormone releasing hormone, 2, 4

H

H_4 hepatoma
insulin action in, 60–61
insulin response in, 64
Haloacetamides, affinity labeling, 254
Haloacetates, affinity labeling, 254
Halocarbonyl groups, electrophilic attaching functions, 222
Hemangioblastoma, cerebellar, 196–197
Hemoglobin
H Cape Town, 166
Kempsey, 166
Ypsilanti, 166
Hemoglobin oxygen dissociation curve, 166–167
Hepatocyte, phosphatidylinositol turnover, 119–120, 129–135, 141, 149
Hepatoma, 197
Hexestrol azide, 229–230
Histamine, effect on phosphatidylinositol turnover, 128

Hormone
  analogs, 228–229
  neurohypophyseal, 4
  polypeptide
    diversity, 18–20
    multigene families, 18–19
    splicing choices within primary transcript, 20
Huntington's disease, 40
4-Hydroxy-4-androstene-3,17-dione, 261
20α-Hydroxysteroid dehydrogenase, 256, 259
17β-Hydroxysteroid dehydrogenase, 256, 259
20β-Hydroxysteroid dehydrogenase, 240
  affinity labeling, 254–255
Δ⁵-3-Hydroxysteroid dehydrogenase, 258
Hypothalamic releasing hormones, 2, 3, 4, 26

I

Immunoglobulin, 20
Indomethacin, effect
  on erythropoietin production, 167
  on insulin mediator, 70
  on relaxin-dependent uterine cAMP increase, 104
Inositol triphosphate, 151
Insulin, 2, 4, 13, 80, 106
  action
    intracellular mediators, 51–78
    on nuclear function, 57–58
  amino acid sequences, 88–92
  binding, 95
  C-peptide, 87
  distribution, 28
  enzymes sensitive to, 64–68
  evolution, 93
  in feeding behavior, 37
  functions, 51
  genes, 85
  interaction with receptor, 51–52
  major target tissues, 51
  mediators
    from adipocyte plasma membranes, 52–55
    chemical characteristics, 68–71
    inactivation, 69

    mediators potentially related to, 58–59
    from muscle, 54–55
    number of, 61–64
    physical characteristics, 68–71
    whole cell and tissue studies, 60–61
  membrane systems sensitive to, 55–58
  processing, 88
  second messenger, 51, 52, 61
  subcellular systems responding to, 52–59
Insulin-like growth factor, 80
  amino acid sequences, 88–89
Invertebrate peptides, 3, 4, 13, 15
Iodides, aromatic, photoaffinity labeling with, 266
Iodoaromatics, photoaffinity attaching functions, 225
Ionophore A23187, effect on phosphatidylinositol turnover, 118–120, 123, 126–129, 140–141, 143, 146–147
3-Isobutyl-1-methylxanthine, in uterine contraction, 103–105
Isoproterenol, effect on uterine cAMP, 103–104

K

k_{cat} inhibitors, 254
Ketones
  acetylenic, 259
  allenic, 257–259
  unsaturated, 258–259
    electrophilic affinity labeling with, 256–257
    photoaffinity labeling, 263–266
Δ⁴-3-Ketosteroid 5α-reductase, 257, 258, 262
Δ⁵-3-Ketosteroid isomerase, 255, 257–258, 260, 263

L

β-Lipotropin, 25
Liver
  biphasic response to insulin, 62
  insulin action in, 60–61
  plasma membrane, insulin sensitivity, 55–58

Luteinizing hormone, 4, 173
Luteinizing hormone releasing hormone, 26, 30
  distribution, 28
Lymphocyte, IM-9, insulin action in, 60–61

M

Macrophage, phosphatidylinositol turnover, 122–125
Mast cell, phosphatidylinositol turnover, 119, 122–125
α-Melanocyte-stimulating hormone, 4
  deacetylation, 24, 25
  distribution, 28
  in memory, learning, and adaptive behavior, 32
  in temperature regulation, 38
Mercurials, electrophilic attaching functions, 223
4-Mercuriestradiol, 230–231, 235
6-Methylene-4-pregna-3,20-dione, 257
16-Methylene estrone, 256
Methyl trienolone, 245–246
Monoamines, 2–3
Morphine, in memory, learning, and adaptive behavior, 32
Motilin, 4
Muscle
  biphasic response to insulin, 62
  insulin action in, 60–61
Muscular dystrophy, congenital, 40–41
Myosin, 98–99
Myosin ATPase, 98–99
Myosin light chain kinase, 99–101
  in trachea, 102
  uterine, 103

N

Naloxone
  in blood pressure regulation, 39
  effects, in schizophrenia, 35
  in thermoregulation, 38
Neural pathways, demonstration, 10–11
Neurohormone, 1, 13
Neuromodulator, 30

Neurons
  cultured, patch clamp technique for, 9
  peptidergic, expression, 16–17
Neuropeptide, *see also* Brain peptides
  function, 3
  precursors, 20–23
  processing, 8
  synthesis, 8
Neuropeptide Y_y, 4
Neurophysins, 3, 4, 23
Neurotensin, 4
  distribution, 27, 28
  effect on phosphatidylinositol turnover, 128
  in pain perception, 32
  in temperature regulation, 38
Neurotransmitter, 1, 2, 3, 13
  definition, 29–30
  expression in neural tissues, ontogeny, 16–17
Neutrophil, phosphatidylinositol turnover, 122–125
Nitroanisoles, photoaffinity attaching functions, 225
Norepinephrine, 2, 30–31
  effect
    on phosphatidylinositol 4,5-bisphosphate labeling, 125
    on phosphatidylinositol turnover, 131
Nuclei, biphasic response to insulin, 62, 63

O

Opioid peptides
  in blood pressure regulation, 39
  in feeding behavior, 36–37
  in pain perception, 32
  in psychiatric disease, 34
  in temperature regulation, 38
Oxiranes, electrophilic attaching functions, 223
17β-(1-Oxo-2-propynyl)androst-4-en-3-one, 259
6-Oxoestradiol, 229, 230
  estrogen receptor affinity labeling, 217–218
Oxytocin, 2, 3, 4
  distribution, 27, 28

Oxytocin (*continued*)
in pain perception, 32
precursor, 20, 23
in smooth muscle contraction, 99

P

Pancreatic polypeptide, in pain perception, 32
Peptidase, in neural tissue, 25–26
Phentolamine, effect on relaxin-dependent uterine cAMP increase, 104
Phenylephrine, effect on phospatidylinositol turnover, 128
Pheochromocytoma, 197
Phorbol myristate, 141
Phosphatidic acid
in phosphatidylinositol turnover, 117–160
turnover, 117
Phosphatidylinositol
breakdown
in blowfly salivary glands, 118–119, 150–151
effect of serotonin, 147
in hepatocytes, 149
history, 120
synthesis, inhibition, 118
turnover
activation by hormones, 117–160
in adrenal glomerulosa cells, 137–138
in adrenal medulla, 135–137
in blowfly salivary glands, 144–150
in brain synaptosomes, 122–125
in hepatocytes, 129–135
in macrophages, 122–125
in mast cells, 122–125
in neutrophils, 122–125
in platelets, 139–144
Phosphatidylinositol 4,5-bisphosphate
in adrenal medulla, 136
degradation, 132–135
Phosphatidylinositol effect, 117–118
Phosphatidylinositol 4-phosphate, 70–71
in adrenal medulla, 136
Phosphatidylserine, 70–71
Phosphoinositide
breakdown, functions, 151–152
turnover, 117–160

Phospholipase C, 122, 148, 149
Phospholipid, in insulin action, 70–71
Phosphorylation, in control of enzyme activity, 103
Phytohemagglutinin
biphasic response to, 62, 63
in study of ligand–receptor interaction, 57–59
Pituitary peptides, 3, 4
Placenta, plasma membrane, insulin sensitivity, 56
Platelet, phosphatidylinositol turnover, 139–144
Platelet-activating factor, 143–144
in phosphatidylinositol turnover, 141–142
Polycythemia
secondary, 197
vera, 197
Polyphosphoinositides, *see also* Phosphatidylinositol; Phosphoinositide breakdown, 150
Ponasterone, 252–253
Prealbumin, 261
Pregnenolone, synthesis, 137, 139
Preprorelaxin
amino acid sequences, 86–87
forms, mRNA sequences, 84, 85
processing, 86–87
Progesterone
photoaffinity labeling, 223
receptor
molecular weight, 240
structure, 236–241
Progestin
receptor, affinity labeling, 230, 235–241
synthetic
ORG 2058, 236, 240
R 1881, 263
R5020, 235–239, 241, 242, 252, 263–264
RU 38,486, 236
Prolactin, 4, 19
mediator, 58–59
Proline endopeptidase, 26
Proopiomelanocortin, 32
posttranslational processing, 25–26
precursor, 20–22
products, 18

Propranolol, effect on relaxin-dependent uterine cAMP increase, 104
Prostaglandin, 129
effects, on uterine cAMP levels, 105
in smooth muscle contraction, 99
in temperature regulation, 38
Protease, 23
inhibitors, 23
Protein kinase C, 70, 119–120, 140, 144, 152
Pyruvate dehydrogenase
activation, by insulin, 53–55
activity, effect of lectins, 59
biphasic response to insulin, 62, 63
insulin sensitivity, 64–68

R

Receptor, *see also* specific hormone, receptor
dynamics, 227–229
function, 227–229
inactivation assays, 216–217
properties, 226–227
proteolysis, 227
structure, 226–227
Relaxin, 13, 79–115
amino acid sequences, 88–92
assay, 96
B chain, insolubility, 95
A and B chains, amino acid sequence comparison, 90–91
connecting peptide fragments, synthesis, 97
covalent structure, 82, 86–94
cDNA, cloning, 80–81
effects on uterine cAMP, 103–106
evolution, 93–94
functions, 79, 82
genes, 80–86
DNA sequences, 80–85
human, 81–82
heterogeneity, 85
history, 79–80
homology, 81–82
human, synthesis, 96–97
iodination, 106
mechanism of action, 97–106
monoclonal antibodies, 108
C-peptide, 86–88, 108

physiology
in human female, 107–108
in human male, 108
porcine, chemical synthesis, 94–96
processing, 88–93
radioimmunoassay, 107–108
receptor binding, 92–93
receptors, 106–107
regulation of uterine contractions, 97
mRNA
localization, 85–86
processing, 85
sequences, 85
source, 81
species differences, 88–93, 94
synthesis
artificial prohormone approach, 94–95
by genetically engineered micro-organisms, 95
synthetic, 94–97
targets, 79
therapeutic potential, 107, 108–109
Reserpine, effect on relaxin-dependent uterine cAMP increase, 104
Ribonucleic acid, messenger
relaxin, 85–86
transport, response to insulin, 62, 63
Ribosomal protein S6, phosphorylation, 57

S

Saralasin, in blood pressure regulation, 39
Schizophrenia, brain peptides in, 34–35
Secretin, 4, 15
Serotonin, 2, 31
distribution, 27–29
effect on phosphatidylinositol turnover, 128, 144–149
in phosphatidylinositol breakdown, 118
Sleep peptides, 4
Smooth muscle
actin and myosin, structure, 98
contraction, 98–99
hormonal regulation, 99–103
myosin light chains, 98
Somatostatin, 4, 17
concentrations, alterations in CNS disease, 40

Somatostatin (*continued*)
  distribution, 27, 28
  in pain perception, 32
  precursor, 20–22
Somatotropin, chorionic, 19
Steroid, receptor, affinity labeling, 222
Substance P, 2, 4, 17
  concentrations, alterations in CNS disease, 40
  distribution, 27–29
  effect, on phosphatidylinositol turnover, 128
  in pain perception, 32
Substance P endopeptidase, 26
Sulfonyl halides, 260–261

T

Tamoxifen aziridine, 223, 230–234
  estrogen receptor affinity labeling, 216–217
    efficiency and selectivity determination, 218–220
Δ^6-Testosterone, 263–264
Thalassemia major, 165
Thrombin, effect
  on phosphatidylinositol turnover, 142–143
  on phospholipid turnover, 139–142
Thromboxane, 129
Thyroglobulin, 173
Thyroid hormone
  binding sites, photoaffinity labeling, 224
  receptors
    affinity labeling, 247–251
    structure and function, 247–251
Thyrotropin, 4
Thyrotropin-releasing hormone, 4
  in blood pressure regulation, 39
  concentrations, alterations in CNS disease, 40
  distribution, 27, 28
  in feeding behavior, 37
  in pain perception, 32
  precursor, 22–23
  in psychiatric disease, 34
  in temperature regulation, 38
Thyroxine, 247–251, 265, 266
  photoaffinity attaching functions, 225

Thyroxine binding prealbumin, 255, 264–266
Thyroxine-binding proteins, 266
Transcortin, 241, *see also* Corticosteroid binding globulin
Tranylcypromine, effect on relaxin-dependent uterine cAMP increase, 104
Triamcinolone acetonide, 241, 242
Triiodothyronine, 247–251, 265

U

α,β-Unsaturated carbonyl compounds, electrophilic attaching functions, 223
Unsaturated carbonyl compounds, photoactivated attaching functions, 223–224

V

Vasoactive intestinal polypeptide, 2, 4, 15
  and acetylcholine, interaction, 29
  concentrations, alterations in CNS disease, 40
  distribution, 27, 28
  in pain perception, 32
Vasopressin, 2, 3, 4, 13
  arginine, 23
  distribution, 27–29
  in memory, learning, and adaptive behavior, 32–34
  in phosphatidylinositol turnover, 119, 127–134
  precursor, 20, 23
  in temperature regulation, 38

W

Wheat germ agglutinin, 59

X

Xenopus, oocytes, steroid-binding protein, affinity labeling, 252

Y

Ynones, 259–260

Date Due